Psychology of Eating

From Biology to Culture to Policy

THIRD EDITION

Emily Crews Splane, Neil E. Rowland, and Anaya Mitra

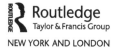

Routledge
Taylor & Francis Group

NEW YORK AND LONDON

Designed cover image: © Tara Moore/Getty Images

Third edition published 2025
by Routledge
605 Third Avenue, New York, NY 10158

and by Routledge
4 Park Square, Milton Park, Abingdon, Oxon, OX14 4RN

Routledge is an imprint of the Taylor & Francis Group, an informa business

© 2025 Emily Crews Splane, Neil E. Rowland, and Anaya Mitra

The right of Emily Crews Splane, Neil E. Rowland, and Anaya Mitra to be identified
as authors of this work has been asserted in accordance with sections 77 and 78
of the Copyright, Designs and Patents Act 1988.

First edition published by Pearson 2014
Second edition published by Routledge 2019

ISBN: 978-1-032-62138-8 (hbk)
ISBN: 978-1-032-61634-6 (pbk)
ISBN: 978-1-032-62140-1 (ebk)

DOI: 10.4324/9781032621401

Typeset in Berling
by Newgen Publishing UK

We dedicate this edition of our book to our esteemed mentor, colleague, and friend. -Emily and Anaya

Neil E. Rowland (1947–2024)

Contents

For Instructors:
Using This Book

This text is divided into 13 chapters, as described in the summary table below. Each chapter is to some extent stand-alone, so instructors may choose a different order or selection of materials. Further, although the authors have been using this as a one-semester (3-credit) elective course, covering about one chapter per week, instructors may choose to emphasize some aspects more than others, depending on their particular student population. Most chapters include "food for thought" or other offset material that could be used to initiate discussions and/or assessments. Numerous references to primary sources are cited, and these or other materials could be assigned as reading beyond the text. In addition, there are numerous online documentaries and videos that can be used as supplementary material. One of your authors (NR) has transformed this course into an entirely online format including such supplementary material. Assessment of student performance will depend substantially on the class size and format. We believe that the material encourages critical thinking and could be evaluated by essays or presentations.

Chapter	Select learning objectives	More key terms or concepts
1 Eating – You, the World, and Food	Scientific disciplines and eating; internal and external factors; discriminating real and fake facts	Motivation; hunger; satiety; body mass index; obesity; economic impact of obesity
2 Macronutrients, Micronutrients, and Metabolism	Specialist and generalist eaters; metabolism; energy input and expenditure; specific appetite	Energy density; basic structure of carbohydrate, protein, and fat; minerals and vitamins
3 You Are What You Eat: Energy Flow	Natural selection and feeding; optimal foraging and energy acquisition; portion size	Energy flow; gross energy gain; motivation and economics; meals and portion size; exercise
4 The Brain and Sensory Mechanisms of Feeding	Distinguish between monogenic and polygenic obesity; define epigenetics; role of microbiome	Basic genetics and epigenetics; genetic approaches to obesity; gut microbiota and energy balance

Chapter	Select learning objectives	More key terms or concepts
5 Brain: Outputs and Integration	Biological mechanisms of smell and taste; chemosensory gut; signals from gut to brainstem	Odorants, tastants, and receptors; brain pathways; enteric nervous system; principal gut hormones
6 Genetics, Epigenetics, and Microbiome	Brain structures and hunger; neurotransmitters; hedonic mechanisms; cortical integration	Arcuate nucleus; ventral tegmental area; leptin; orbitofrontal cortex; fMRI; hunger and satiety systems
7 Basic Learning Processes and Eating Behavior	Associative learning mechanisms in eating; food preferences and aversions; conditioned satiety	Food learning and postingestive consequences; contextual cues; learning what and how much
8 The Development of Eating Behaviors	Effect of pre- and early postnatal factors; regulation of energy balance; external influences	Suckling; independent eating; caloric regulation; parenting style; media/marketing and children
9 Social Influences on Eating	Traditional role of cuisine; direct and indirect influences on eating; role of food provider	Cultural rules; examples of cuisine; perception and attitudes to food; commensal food consumption
10 Mood and Food, Cravings and Addiction	Connection between mood and eating; stress; biological and psychological aspects of craving	Serotonin; chocolate; food addiction – description and neurobiology; opioids; reward pathway
11 Eating Disorders and Treatment	Definitions and symptoms of anorexia, bulimia nervosa, and binge-eating disorder, believed causes, and treatments	Eating disorders classification; risk factors; biopsychosocial approach; treatments; animal models
12 Personal Weight Loss Strategies in Obesity	Weight management by diet and exercise; intermittent fasting and diets; therapies against obesity	Benefits of exercise; fad diets; chrononutrition; fitness and mobile apps; weight loss medications; bariatric surgery
13 Institutional Approaches to Healthful Eating	Interventions; overpopulation and sustainability; technological innovation; food waste	Industry and government roles; environmental impact of food production; genetic modification

Preface

People are obsessed with food. If you do not have enough food, which was almost always the case for our distant ancestors, your thoughts and actions are directed toward obtaining food. Even in today's world, in which we have plenty of "mouth ready" food available, people spend large amounts of time thinking about food or rituals in which food plays a prominent role. Huge for-profit industries have been built on these human proclivities, ranging from advertising and marketing, to production and competitive retailing of an increasing array of tasty foods, to weight management or loss and medical treatment of obesity-related diseases.

Have you ever stopped to ask why humans are so attracted to food, or whether that trait is unique to humans? This book attempts to pose these questions and to explore answers. We firmly believe that psychological science is the only academic discipline that is capable of spanning and integrating the vast range of subdisciplines that are relevant to the topic. In this text, we focus on "normal" eating: How did it evolve, how does it develop and become manifest in modern society, and what functions does it fulfill? We also address contemporary problems associated with eating. We have a chapter devoted to diagnosable eating disorders, including anorexia and bulimia nervosa; however, from a perspective of sheer numbers and adverse economic impact, eating too much and becoming obese is a much bigger problem. Thus, much of the book is focused on explanations of, and possible solutions to, what is often called an obesity epidemic.

The first edition (2014) of this book arose out of an undergraduate special topics course, "Psychology of Eating," that we first taught over 20 years ago. Our impetus then, and today, is to present an integrative or capstone course for undergraduates who simply want to learn more about their own eating or those who may be contemplating a career in one of the for-profit industries mentioned earlier or in an associated medical, regulatory, or nonprofit activity. With 70% of the adult population in the USA, and many other countries, and 25% of children now classified as overweight or obese, this field will provide considerable employment opportunities for the foreseeable future! Our book may also serve as background material from which to launch directed discussions or writing at a more advanced (e.g., graduate) level. Most of the chapters include citations to primary or additional resources.

Most human behaviors have both biological and sociocultural determinants. Eating is an excellent example of this interaction of biology and culture and, in addition, revolves around commodities (i.e. foods) that have their own defined physical and chemical properties. In other words, you cannot understand eating without knowing something about nutrition, energy, genes, chemical sensing, and brain structures. This book contains essential information about each of these, although it would have been easy to fill a whole book with just these topics. Instead, we have tried to present them at a level that will be accessible to typical psychology majors. Even if your main interest is in the sociocultural topics, learning elements of the biological foundations will enrich your understanding. Conversely, we do not believe that exclusive focus on biology enables you to appreciate the complexity of human thought that dominates people's actions about what, when, and how much to eat.

The third edition has been slightly rearranged from the second, in part based on our own usage of the material. Thus, most of the biological material is in the first part, followed by the sociocultural material and, finally, the broader impact. Newer weight-loss medications have been added to this edition as well as information about food allergies. However, insofar as possible, each chapter has been written to stand alone so that the material can be sequenced in different ways to suit different approaches. In the expanded last chapters of the book, we consider the global impact of obesity, its causes, and ways to mitigate the inherent unsustainability of the present trajectory. At its core, is it possible to cool the flames of the love affair that humans have with food?

We want to thank the editors and staff at Taylor & Francis for encouraging this third edition and for their help throughout the production process.

CHAPTER 1

Eating – You, the World, and Food

After reading this chapter, you will be able to

- Understand the relevance of diverse scientific disciplines to the psychology of eating.
- Understand the derivation of body mass index and its relation to health and obesity.
- Recognize the personal and society-wide economic burdens that are associated with problematic eating, including overweight or obesity and anorexia nervosa.
- Recognize that both internal and environmental factors contribute to eating behavior.
- Understand the internal sensations that produce eating or absence of eating.
- Discriminate reliable, factual sources of information from "fake facts."

We all engage in eating behavior, sometimes with pleasure or regret, but often just because it's mealtime. At its core, eating is a transaction, or rather several classes of transaction. The first transaction is between you, your body and its physiology, and the consumable item(s) in front of you. The second type of transaction is interpersonal, the bonds formed between you and the people with whom you are eating. For our hunter-gatherer ancestors, these were perhaps the main transactions, in part because the quality, safety, or security of the food could not be assured. A third type of transaction is recent in origin, but now dominant, and that is the business aspect. In most countries today, food production, processing, and marketing are business propositions, and food preparation is often performed by unknown agent(s) such as retail sellers and restaurant personnel.

Commercialization of eating has brought with it a relentless tsunami of marketing and advertising about food products and a plethora of advice or information on what we should or should not eat, why we should eat a certain amount or way, and with what objective. As a result, eating has changed from a relatively simple act of sharing what the hunters or gatherers brought home on any given day, a world for which our pre-historic physiology was adapted, to a more complex situation in which eating is a series of decisions made among competing media messages about food and/or the purpose

DOI: 10.4324/9781032621401-1

or goals of that eating episode. Many of the food messages invoke underlying scientific (including medical) concepts, yet the public has an imperfect understanding of those concepts and, as a result, is unable to evaluate information objectively and is susceptible to believing false claims or fake facts.

This introductory chapter has three principal aims. The first aim is to advocate that psychological science provides the integrative approach necessary to understand these complex transactional aspects of eating behavior. The second aim is to introduce some of the key terms or concepts related to eating and one of its consequences, body weight. The third aim is to start to discuss some guidelines or tools by which real facts might be discriminated from the fake facts that permeate mass media about eating.

PSYCHOLOGY: THE INTEGRATIVE SCIENCE

"You are what you eat" is a phrase that contains elements of truth and yet conceals a more fundamental question of why you eat, with follow-up questions of what, where, when, and how much. If you think about eating as a scientific problem, it quickly becomes apparent that many disciplines are involved, including psychology, neuroscience, biology, nutrition, economics, and more. A well-rounded approach to eating behavior must include each of these elements. Psychological science is an integrative discipline that is uniquely well positioned to bridge the streams of scientific thought that are relevant to eating and its problems (Figure 1.1). This text does not assume or require a substantial background in any specific discipline, but it does assume or imply a scientific approach.

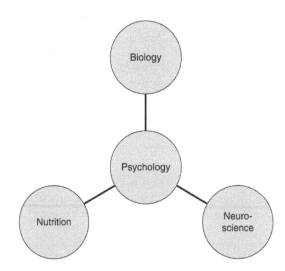

FIGURE 1.1 Psychology occupies an interdisciplinary integrative role with regard to feeding behavior

Several books or monographs bear the title or subtitle "Psychology of Eating," including those by Capaldi (1996), Logue (2015), Ogden (2010), and our first edition

(Rowland & Splane, 2014), but we believe this text is the most integrative of the relevant science disciplines. Many other texts or monographs deal with the limited topic of eating disorders such as anorexia nervosa or bulimia nervosa. While these are serious and potentially fatal disorders, their incidence is an order of magnitude less than that of the conditions of overweight or obesity. These latter conditions, which together occur in almost 40% of adults worldwide and 70% in the U.S., are seriously detrimental to health (Dahlgren et al., 2018; Flegal et al., 2012; NDC Risk Factor Collaboration, 2016; Ogden et al., 2014).

From a historical or evolutionary perspective, it can be argued that the primary purpose of eating is (or was) to maintain an organism at a high level of physical strength in order to survive the rigors of life. This argument applies to both animals and humans and predicts, minimally, that eating should, over time, yield nutrients sufficient in quantity and quality to avoid weakness due to malnutrition and to support reproduction of the species. Societal advances in many domains – civilization in a broad sense – have greatly improved access to and quality of food. One result of that has been a much longer life expectancy, and this has introduced a new purpose, namely the connection(s) between food, health, and longevity.

You are probably familiar with the term "unhealthy food" or its converse, healthy food. It is used in many messages, including media of all types, about food. But what does it mean? From a public health perspective, this concept might describe whether a food is contaminated with pathogens or poisons. Instead, common usage is a future projection that long-term consumption of that food carries a statistically higher probability of poorer health and/or a shorter lifespan. That probabilistic inference also assumes abnormal or excessive consumption of the food. That is, "unhealthy food" is not an intrinsic property of the food: It is the behavioral interaction with that food that is unhealthy. It's a case of what psychologists call external attribution: Blame an unwanted outcome on outside or environmental factors. When you next read, hear, or are even tempted to use the adjectives "unhealthy" or "healthy" in relation to food, stop and think about the assumptions behind those terms! Several chapters in this book will address factors that influence this critical interaction between person and food.

MEASURING UNDERWEIGHT, OVERWEIGHT, AND OBESITY

Earlier, we used the terms overweight and obese, and many of us have vaguely formed preconceptions about what they mean. In fact, they have a very precise scientific meaning that is based on pragmatic and simple biometric measurements of weight and height. Such measures are commonly made by medical or paramedical professionals, but can be made with reasonable accuracy by most people. Body mass index (BMI), a derivative metric, is body weight in kilograms divided by the square of height in meters (see Box 1.1 and Table 1.1). There are many published and online BMI calculators to make this easy. Ranges of BMI are widely used to categorize health and health outcomes. In particular:

- BMI less than 18.5 = underweight.
- BMI 18.6–24.9 = normal or healthy.
- BMI 25–29.9 = overweight (also known as pre-obese).
- BMI over 30 = obese (class I = 30–34.9, class II = 35–39.9, etc.).

TABLE 1.1 Body mass index

WEIGHT	4'8"	4'9"	4'10"	4'11"	5'0"	5'1"	5'2"	5'3"	5'4"	5'5"	5'6"	5'7"	5'8"	5'9"	5'10"	5'11"	6'0"	6'1"	6'2"	6'3"	6'4"	6'5"
lbs (kg)	142cm	147	150	152	155	157	160	163	165	168	170	173	175	178	180	183	185	188	191	193	196	
260 (117.9)	58	56	54	53	51	49	48	46	45	43	42	41	40	38	37	36	35	34	33	32	32	31
255 (115.7)	57	55	53	51	50	48	47	45	44	42	41	40	39	38	37	36	35	34	33	32	31	30
250 (113.4)	56	54	52	50	49	47	46	44	43	42	40	39	38	37	36	35	34	33	32	31	30	30
245 (111.1)	55	53	51	49	48	46	45	43	42	41	40	38	37	36	35	34	33	32	31	31	30	29
240 (108.9)	54	52	50	48	47	45	44	43	41	40	39	38	36	35	34	33	33	32	31	30	29	28
235 (106.6)	53	51	49	47	46	44	43	42	40	39	38	37	36	35	34	33	32	31	30	29	29	28
230 (104.3)	52	50	48	46	45	43	42	41	39	38	37	36	35	34	33	32	31	30	30	29	28	27
225 (102.1)	50	49	47	45	44	43	41	40	39	37	36	35	34	33	32	31	31	30	29	28	27	27
220 (99.8)	49	48	46	44	43	42	40	39	38	37	36	34	33	32	32	31	30	29	28	27	27	26
215 (97.5)	48	47	45	43	42	41	39	38	37	36	35	34	33	32	31	30	29	28	28	27	26	25
210 (95.3)	47	45	44	42	41	40	38	37	36	35	34	33	32	31	30	29	28	28	27	26	26	25
205 (93.0)	46	44	43	41	40	39	37	36	35	34	33	32	31	30	29	29	28	27	26	26	25	24
200 (90.7)	45	43	42	40	39	38	37	35	34	33	32	31	30	30	29	28	27	26	26	25	24	24
195 (88.5)	44	42	41	39	38	37	36	35	33	32	31	31	30	29	28	27	26	26	25	24	24	23
190 (86.2)	43	41	40	38	37	36	35	34	33	32	31	30	29	28	27	26	26	25	24	24	23	23
185 (33.9)	41	40	39	37	36	35	34	33	32	31	30	29	28	27	27	26	25	24	24	23	23	22
180 (81.6)	40	39	38	36	35	34	33	32	31	30	29	28	27	27	26	25	24	24	23	22	22	21
175 (79.4)	39	38	37	35	34	33	32	31	30	29	28	27	26	25	24	24	23	22	22	21	21	20
170 (77.1)	38	37	36	34	33	32	31	30	29	28	27	27	26	25	24	24	23	22	22	21	21	20
165 (74.8)	37	36	34	33	32	31	30	29	28	27	27	26	25	24	24	23	22	22	21	21	20	20
160 (72.6)	36	35	33	32	31	30	29	28	27	27	26	25	24	24	23	22	22	21	21	20	19	19
155 (70.3)	35	34	32	31	30	29	28	27	27	26	25	24	24	23	22	22	21	20	20	19	19	18
150 (68.0)	34	32	31	30	29	28	27	27	26	25	24	23	23	22	22	21	20	20	19	19	18	18
145 (65.8)	33	31	30	29	28	27	27	26	25	24	23	23	22	21	21	20	20	19	19	18	18	17
140 (63.5)	31	30	29	28	27	26	26	25	24	23	23	22	21	21	20	20	19	18	18	17	17	17
135 (61.2)	30	29	28	27	26	26	25	24	23	22	22	21	21	20	19	19	18	18	17	17	16	16
130 (59.0)	29	28	27	26	25	25	24	23	22	22	21	20	20	19	19	18	18	17	17	16	16	15
125 (56.7)	28	27	26	25	24	24	23	22	22	21	20	20	19	18	18	17	17	16	16	15	15	15
120 (54.4)	27	26	25	24	23	23	22	21	21	20	19	19	18	18	17	17	16	16	15	15	15	14
115 (52.2)	26	25	24	23	22	22	21	20	20	19	19	18	17	17	16	16	16	15	15	14	14	14
110 (49.9)	25	24	23	22	21	21	20	19	19	18	18	17	17	16	16	15	15	15	14	14	13	13
105 (47.6)	24	23	22	21	21	20	19	19	18	17	17	16	16	16	15	15	14	14	13	13	13	12
100 (45.4)	22	22	21	20	20	19	18	18	17	17	16	16	15	15	14	14	14	13	13	12	12	12
95 (43.1)	21	21	20	19	19	18	17	17	16	16	15	15	14	14	13	13	13	12	12	12	12	11
90 (40.8)	20	19	19	18	18	17	16	16	15	15	15	14	14	13	13	13	12	12	12	11	11	11
85 (38.6)	19	18	18	17	17	16	16	15	15	14	14	13	13	13	12	12	12	11	11	11	10	10
80 (36.3)	18	17	17	16	16	15	15	14	14	13	13	13	12	12	11	11	11	11	10	10	10	9

Note: Obese >30; overweight 25–30; normal 18.5–25; underweight <18.5.

Source: Body-mass-index-chart.gif

After adolescence, an individual's height does not change appreciably; thus, change in the BMI of an adult most often reflects changes in body composition such as fat content. There is strong epidemiological evidence that elevated body fat content is associated with diseases such as hypertension, diabetes, osteoarthritis, and cancer (Wagner & Brath, 2012). High BMI often correlates with high body fat content, although there are notable exceptions or limitations. For example, athletes in strength sports typically have elevated muscle mass, and hence high BMI, but this does not reflect excessive fat. Further, BMI does not take into account potential gender, ethnic, or body frame differences. Excess fat in the central or abdominal region (more common in males) imparts increased risk of developing cardiovascular disease, whereas the same extra fat in the hips (more common in females) does not carry the same risk (Arsenault et al., 2012). A simple estimate of distribution of body fat is waist circumference and/or the ratio of waist to hip circumferences.

BOX 1.1 HOW DID BMI BECOME A STANDARD?

In 1943, the Metropolitan Life Insurance Company published actuarial tables of ideal weight for height for the purposes of calculating health risk and insurance premiums. American physiologist Ancel Keys argued vigorously about the inadequacies of these tables and proposed instead the use of BMI (Keys et al., 1972). This index was not new at that time, but was devised in the mid-19th century by Belgian mathematician Adolphe Quetelet in his use of anthropometric statistics to define "l'homme moyen" – the average man. Quetelet's index, now called BMI, is weight (strictly, mass) divided by height squared. Mass refers to substance, whereas weight depends on gravitational force, but, since most of us live at 1 g, the terms are commonly used interchangeably in the field of health or nutrition. The universal measurement system of science is CGS (centimeter–gram–second), and BMI is expressed in CGS units for weight and height (viz., kg/m^2). Use of other units (e.g., pounds and inches) requires a multiplicative constant to convert to CGS-based BMI values and is incorporated into most electronic BMI calculators.

BOX 1.2 DO THE MATH

Imagine a 5'2" female starting college at 120 lbs. Over the next year she gains the mythical "freshman 15 (pounds)." Use an online calculator to compute BMI at the start and end of her first year. The next year, she gains an additional "sophomore 15." What is the new BMI at the end of the second year? How do these BMIs map to weight categories? Her friend is a 6'2" male weighing 160 lbs at the start of his freshman year, and he has the same gain of 15 lbs each year. What are his BMI numbers and categories? (Answers are at the end of this chapter.)

Using BMI as the index, overweight and obesity are a global problem. The World Health Organization (WHO) has compiled longitudinal data on BMI from over 19 million adults in 200 countries (www.who.int/gho/ncd/risk_factors/overweight/en/NDC; NCD Risk Factor Collaboration 2016). Figure 1.2 shows one summary result from that report: The average BMI, shown as an average for men and women, rose from 21.9 to 24.3 kg/m^2 between the years 1975 and 2014. This represents an increase of almost 3% per decade. Also shown in Figure 1.2 are BMI means for the U.S. dating from 1965, as published by the Centers for Disease Control (www.cdc.gov/obesity/data/prevalence-maps.html), summarized by Zimmerman (2011) and extrapolated by us from the WHO

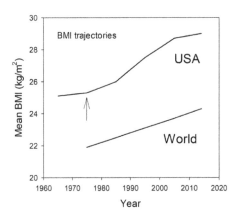

FIGURE 1.2 Mean body mass index (BMI) across time for the U.S. and for the world. Data are based on the WHO-NCD report (2016). The arrow shows the approximate onset of faster increase in the U.S. (data from Zimmerman, 2011)

data. Perhaps not surprisingly, the WHO and CDC data show that Americans have a higher average BMI than the rest of the world, but the rate of increase since 1975 has been similar in most world regions, and, from the U.S. data, there was a marked acceleration in this rate during the late 1970s (Box 1.3).

BOX 1.3 MARKETING OR ADVERTISING?

Given the upward inflection in rate of change in BMI in the late 1970s, Zimmerman (2011) considered what underlying factors might have changed at about that time. In an affluent country such as the U.S., food availability was not a plausible answer, neither was a major change in dietary constituents or in physiological makeup of the population. He concluded instead that there was a coincident dramatic rise in food marketing, including:

1 **Product innovation**: For example, the number of items available in supermarkets rose from ~8,000 in 1975 to 40,000 by 2000 because of expanding variations of a product (e.g., cereal).
2 **Price**: For example, supersizing for little added cost or bundling as in meal packages.
3 **Place**: Availability in more places, such as vending machines and convenience outlets.
4 **Promotion**: For example, product placement, sponsorship, and endorsements.

Industry expenditures on marketing have grown much faster than expenditures on direct advertising over this time frame, testament to effectiveness at the cash register – and at the waistline. As we said, "unhealthy food" is not about the food per se but the interaction between food and the consumer: We might consider adding marketing as a third factor.

The data presented so far are averages for approximately equal numbers of men and women in each cohort. However, the datasets reveal gender, regional, and socioeconomic differences. In the case of gender, women have higher incidence of overweight and/or obesity (BMI over 25) than men in some countries, but that difference is reversed in many European countries. In affluent countries with higher mean BMI, individuals in the lower socioeconomic categories have higher BMI than those in higher categories. This relation is reversed in less affluent countries, perhaps because the poor simply cannot obtain sufficient food and thus tend to be underweight. Regional heterogeneity for the U.S. is revealed in data published by the Centers for Disease Control and Prevention (CDC; www.cdc.gov/obesity/data/prevalence-maps.html), with the highest prevalence of obesity in Alabama, Arkansas, Louisiana, Mississippi, and West Virginia. Further, the prevalence of obesity (BMI ≥ 30) was twice as high (35%) in middle-aged adults compared with late teens (17%), reflecting the developmental trajectory of the problem.

QUESTIONS TO ASK YOURSELF

These considerations give rise to several questions, including:

- Is overweight or obesity abnormal if it occurs in more than 50% of the population?
- Can't we just raise the BMI criterion for obesity as the population gets heavier?
- Is obesity bad for you?
- If obesity is caused by eating too much, how do we know what is too much?
- Why doesn't our biology stop us?

Talking Point 1.1

Discuss some or all of these five questions with your peers. Did you come up with any clear answers or agreement, or not?

Many of these questions are the topics that we will discuss and challenge you to think about throughout the pages of this book. The fact remains that obesity causes distress for many individuals and detracts from physical health. Since obesity itself is now considered a disease, it may be more accurate to say someone "has obesity" rather than "is obese." Treatment of obesity takes an enormous fraction of the health care budget, regardless of whether the funds are public or private. In the U.S., some 20% of the annual health care budget is estimated to go toward the treatment of obesity-related diseases (Cawley & Meyerhoefer, 2012), and the projected loss of workplace productivity alone will approach $500 billion per year by 2030 (Wang et al., 2011). Less affluent countries are not and will not be able to allocate substantial portions of their budget to health care in general or obesity in particular, and, especially in those regions, obese individuals will experience reduced quality of life or life expectancy. The foregoing focus on obesity is not intended to marginalize the very serious problems of anorexia and bulimia nervosa, because these also have extremely serious personal, societal, and economic impact.

In Chapter 2, we will consider in detail the energy-related aspects of eating and their implications for development of abnormal BMI. But, at a gross level, it is understandable that overweight is caused by eating more than the body needs (i.e., energy expenditure), and underweight is caused by eating less than energy expenditure. Body mass index or changes in it ultimately are founded in eating behavior, but eating behavior is surprisingly hard to measure reliably over a long period. That brings us back to a previous question: What is the goal of eating in this 21st century?

WHAT IS THE GOAL OF EATING?

Often, people eat because they feel hungry. Hunger is a subjective sensation – it can only be measured by self-report. A common way of measuring hunger is using a visual analog linear scale, one end of which might be labeled "not hungry" and the other end "very hungry." These scales have been validated as predicting subsequent food intake (e.g., Parker et al., 2004), although other types of questionnaire have been used. The most easily understood occasion for hunger is one that develops following an extended period without eating, or eating very little. You may have experienced a period of food deprivation or been on a diet. If you're like most people, your thoughts and actions become progressively more dominated by food. If you are hungry right now, you might start sketching food in your notebook or looking up restaurants on your electronic device! Also, you are more likely to engage in behaviors that bring you in contact with food – visiting the vending machine/cafeteria or ordering food to be delivered to you. And maybe you become less picky about what you will eat – perhaps potato will do just fine instead of parfait. Without much conscious effort, all of these feelings, thoughts, and behaviors lead us to food.

The concept of hunger has solved the problem of mechanism, right? No, and, if it had, then this would be an extremely short book! Instead, it has reframed the question to: What is it that makes us hungry? And there's a second question: If food is available all the time, do we eat only when we are hungry, or are there times we eat when we are not hungry? The latter is an important question because, if there are times that we eat when we are not hungry, or even that we start eating at different levels of hunger on different occasions (i.e., there is a different threshold), then there will not be a strong one-to-one or quantitative correspondence between hunger and behavior. Think again about the time when you were without food for an extended period of time. Did your sensation of hunger get more and more intense as time went by, or did it come and go in waves? In general, people rate their hunger as increasing with time since food and decreasing after eating (Barkeling et al., 2007). Many theories of feeding now talk about satiety or fullness rather than hunger. Satiety is usually defined as the absence of hunger.

All animals eat, and the study of the feeding behavior of animals can give us important insights into human behavior. Further, for animals that have similar feeding habits to our own (i.e., mammalian omnivores, such as rats), there is every reason to believe that some of the physiological and brain mechanisms underlying feeding are similar to our own. Although many aspects of feeding and the brain can be directly studied in humans, and many examples will be given in this book, there are some scientific procedures and measures that we cannot perform in humans, and we instead turn to suitable animal models to address the questions. Most such research uses rats or mice, and we will occasionally refer to such studies. All animal research is highly regulated and reviewed by both institutional and national professional entities with regard to rigorously humane treatment and scientific necessity. Likewise, all research with humans is regulated by institutional review boards and includes not only aspects of safety but also confidentiality of records.

BIOMEDICAL OR ENVIRONMENTAL APPROACHES?

Overeating and obesity are significant 21st-century problems for individuals and society, as are other eating disorders such as anorexia nervosa. How do we best address and aspire to solve these problems that are, as we noted earlier, essential problems of interaction or transaction between individuals, their food, and the food environment?

The biomedical approach advocates that these problems are best solved by direct manipulation or treatment of an individual, either because something internal is broken or malfunctioning, or because the treatment will change the way in which the individual interacts with food. One example of this is the popular concept of taking drugs to suppress appetite, which will be treated further in Chapter 12. The mode of action of such drugs in relation to overweight or obesity is to change some aspect of the physiology or brain such that food is more filling and/or less attractive. These drugs are meant to change the body's internal signals related to food; evaluating this approach requires a background in the physiology and brain mechanisms of feeding.

The environmental approach considers that nothing is fundamentally broken within the majority of overweight individuals, but rather it is the environment – broadly defined – that is causing the problems. Indeed, the obesity epidemic has been fueled by increases in the energy content and amount of food available, its advertising and marketing, and a generally low level of physical activity, factors that together form a so-called obesogenic environment. Are there effective ways in which this obesogenic environment can be "treated" and, if so, by whom? This is a difficult issue because the food environment is heavily influenced by economic forces that constrain behaviors of business entities ranging from production to retail, behaviors that are partially shaped by consumer demand but also are designed in turn to influence consumer demand. One approach that has frequently been tried in relation to individuals combating an obesogenic environment is that of diets and diet programs. These are, effectively, devices to achieve cognitive restraint – for example, by restricting times of eating or by consuming smaller amounts of a smaller range of foods. Diets, dieting, and restraint are discussed later in this text.

Talking Point 1.2

In relation to human health, make one list of desirable and another list of undesirable types of changes in the food-related environment that have occurred during the past few decades. Then, compare your lists with those of your classmates. Do some changes occur on both lists? What could you personally and/or as a society do to eliminate the undesirables?

FAKE FACTS – HOW DO I KNOW WHAT I READ IS THE TRUTH?

Let's end this chapter with our third stated objective. Increasingly, we live in a world replete with information and immediate access. A major emergent problem is how to recognize truth or credible sources. The fact is that most media, whether primarily written, spoken, or pictorial, are vying for the attention of would-be consumers. Science is a system for acquiring, storing, and communicating replicable facts and observations. Much of that communication occurs via scientific journals (some are now exclusively online, and most are available online through your library and/or through public access sites such as PubMed). Most of these journals require that authors submit their manuscript for criticism or review by experts in the field (i.e., *peer review*) and follow up with an adequate response to those comments in a revision prior to publication. Journals that require peer review thus confer a certain standard of scientific credibility. This generally works well, but there are rare instances in which the system breaks down, including improper data analysis or even data falsification. Because of this, several funding agencies and journals have instituted more comprehensive standards of data reporting, analysis, and transparency.

Strong scientific hypotheses are best tested using narrow or specific experimental designs, but that approach runs the risk that those results might not generalize to other situations. Thus, replication of a scientific finding or conclusion by other, different groups of investigators, potentially using somewhat different methods or designs, is the hallmark of an established fact. Review articles that summarize several different published studies on a topic, including meta-analyses which effectively assess the "consensus finding" on a question from all of the relevant published studies, are very useful resources for real facts.

If you step away from peer-reviewed articles, the search for the truth is more of a crapshoot. There are any number of for-profit organizations that disseminate free-access "infomercials" that may contain elements of truth but ultimately are trying to sell you something – such as a healthy food or a guaranteed diet, neither of which are objectively demonstrable for a particular consumer. Many academic and non-academic organizations promulgate popular press releases, and these likewise should be avoided as a sole source: They do serve a useful function by drawing attention to a topic, but the journalists who write these articles are evaluated by the popularity, not by the accuracy, of their work. Bottom line, if you are reading or viewing a piece that seems too good to be true, it is! In this book, we are trying to stick to established or well-agreed-upon facts. Whenever we advance our opinion or a speculation, we will try to identify it as such.

ANSWER TO THE "DO THE MATH" BMI CALCULATION

Initially, the female has a BMI of about 22, normal weight category. One and two years later, her BMIs are 25 and 28, respectively; she has become substantially overweight.

Initially, the male has a BMI of about 21, normal weight category. One and two years later, despite the same weight gain in pounds, his BMIs are 22.5 and 24, respectively, still in the normal range. The principal reason for the smaller change in BMI in the male for the same weight gain is his greater height (74″ vs 62″, a 19% difference).

GLOSSARY

Anorexia nervosa	An eating disorder in which a person drops to a dangerously low body mass index, often with distorted body image, in which they refuse to eat sufficient quantities of food to sustain themselves.
Body mass index (BMI)	Body weight (in kg) divided by height (in m) squared: Thus, the unit is kg/m^2. This is the most commonly used clinical measure to define underweight (<18.5), normal body weight (18.5–24.9), overweight (25–29.9), obese class I (30–34.9), obese class II (35–39.9), obese class III (>40).
Bulimia nervosa	An eating disorder characterized by cycles of out-of-control eating (bingeing) followed by restrictive compensatory behaviors including self-induced vomiting.
Fullness	A subjective sensation relating one's current state to the (comfortable) fullest that one could imagine after eating a large meal.
Hunger	Internal (unpleasant) sensation that diverts our thoughts and actions to acquiring and eating food; one cause of hunger is a prolonged period since last eating.
Hunter-gatherer	Refers to a human or lifestyle in which all or most food is obtained by foraging – hunting for wild animals and gathering naturally occurring plants, fruits, and so on. Only a few such societies are still in existence, but our distant ancestors all pursued this nomadic lifestyle.
Meta-analysis	A review paper or article that compiles and summarizes data from many or all of the published papers on a given topic and presents the prevailing averages and conclusion(s).
Obese	Term formally defined by body mass index >30 kg/m^2.
Obesogenic	Term used for an environment (or specific food) that promotes the development of obesity.
Overweight	Term formally defined by body mass index between 25 and 30.

Peer review	In the field of scientific publication, peer review means that an author's manuscript is sent (by the editor) to one or more experts in that field for their comments, critiques, and assessment of whether the manuscript is suitable for publication in that journal. If relevant, the editor then will require that reviewers' critiques be incorporated into a revised manuscript.
Satiety	The absence of hunger. It is closely related to the sensation of fullness.

REFERENCES

Arsenault, B.J., Beaumont, E.P., Despres, J.P., & Larose, E. (2012). Mapping body fat distribution: A key step toward the identification of the vulnerable patient? *Annals of Medicine, 44*, 758–772.

Barkeling, B., King, N.A., Naslund, E., & Blundell, J.E. (2007). Characterization of obese individuals who claim no relationship between their eating pattern and sensations of hunger or fullness. *International Journal of Obesity, 31*, 435–439.

Capaldi, E.D. (1996). *Why we eat what we eat: The psychology of eating.* Washington, DC: American Psychological Association.

Cawley, J., & Meyerhoefer, C. (2012). The medical care costs of obesity: An instrumental variables approach. *Journal of Health Economics, 31*, 219–230.

Dahlgren, C.L., Wisting, L., & Ro, O. (2018). Feeding and eating disorders in the DSM-5 era: A systematic review of prevalence rates in non-clinical male and female samples. *Journal of Eating Disorders, 5*, 56. doi:10.1186/s40337-017-0186-7

Flegal, K.M., Carroll, M.D., Kit, B.K., & Ogden, C.L. (2012). Prevalence of obesity and trends in the distribution of body mass index among US adults, 1999–2010. *Journal of the American Medical Association, 307* (5), 491–497.

Keys, A., Karvonen, N., Kimura, N., & Taylor, H.L. (1972). Indices of relative weight and obesity. *Journal of Chronic Diseases, 25*, 329–343. [Reprinted in *International Journal of Epidemiology*, 2014].

Logue, A.W. (2015). *The psychology of eating and drinking*, 4th ed. New York: Brunner-Routledge.

NCD Risk Factor Collaboration. (2016). Trends in adult body-mass index in 200 countries from 1975 to 2014: A pooled analysis of 1698 population-based measurement surveys with 19.2 million participants. *Lancet, 387*, 1377–1396.

Ogden, C.L., Carroll, M.D., Kit, B.K., & Flegal, J.M. (2014). Prevalence of childhood and adult obesity in the United States, 2011–12. *JAMA, 311*, 806–814.

Ogden, J. (2010). *The psychology of eating: From healthy to disordered behavior*, 2nd ed. Malden, MA: Wiley-Blackwell.

Parker, B.A., Sturm, K., MacIntosh, C.G., Feinle, C., Horowitz, M., & Chapman, I.M. (2004). Relation between food intake and visual analogue scale ratings of appetite and other sensations in healthy older and young subjects. *European Journal of Clinical Nutrition, 58*, 212–218.

Rowland, N., & Splane, E.C. (2014). *Psychology of Eating.* Harlow, UK: Pearson Education.

Wagner, K.-H., & Brath, H. (2012). A global view on the development of noncommunicable diseases. *Preventative Medicine, 54* (suppl.), S38–S41.

Wang, Y.C., McPherson, K., Marsh, T., Gortmaker, S.L., & Brown, M. (2011). Health and economic burden of the projected obesity trends in the USA and the UK. *Lancet, 378*, 815–825.

Zimmerman, F.J. (2011). Using marketing muscle to sell fat: The rise of obesity in the modern economy. *Annual Review of Public Health, 32*, 285–306.

CHAPTER 2

Macronutrients, Micronutrients, and Metabolism

After reading this chapter, you will be able to:

- Understand the concepts of bioenergetics, metabolism, energy input, and expenditure.
- Recognize the three macronutrients, carbohydrates, proteins, and fats.
- Understand the needs for and functions of minerals and vitamins, and specific appetites.

ENERGY, BIOENERGETICS, AND METABOLISM

Bioenergetics is defined as the study of the transformation of energy in living organisms. The term energy is used in its definition in physics: The property of matter that endows a capacity to perform work. Metabolism is defined as the chemical processes that occur within a living organism to maintain life. Thus, energy, bioenergetics, and metabolism are all essential components of the so-called fire of life. Quite literally, organisms exploit chemical energy present in food and transform it into energy as molecules that are suitable to sustain operation of their component cells, including those that directly allow behavior such as heart, muscles, and brain. Different organs within our body require or use energy in different amounts, and the total energy use per unit of time by an organism is called its metabolic rate. Metabolic rate has two principal components for consideration:

- **Basal metabolic rate or BMR**: Rate of energy use when at rest or asleep. Processes involved include maintaining body temperature, breathing, and blood circulation.
- **Activity-related metabolism**: Additional energy (e.g., muscular, heart, breathing) used as a result of an ongoing physical activity. The more intense the activity, the greater this component.

Both these types of metabolic rate are related to body size. The relationship of metabolic rate to body mass across adults of many species differing in size (e.g., mice, dogs, humans) is not linear but is closer to a power function of $(\text{body mass})^{2/3}$. For most people, BMR

DOI: 10.4324/9781032621401-2

accounts for 60–70% of metabolism. BMR is an inescapable or involuntary cost of living. In contrast, the amount of activity-related metabolism has some elective or voluntary component.

Metabolism is expressed in energy units. One common unit is the kilocalorie (kcal): 1 kcal = 1,000 calories, where one (small) calorie is the amount of energy needed to heat 1 g of water by 1°C. Kcal is used extensively by food scientists, but the SI (international system of units) instead uses joules and kilojoules (kJ). A joule is 4.184-fold smaller than a calorie: As an approximation, you can use multipliers of 4 (kJ to kcal) or ¼ (kcal to kJ) to interconvert these units. For example, if you heat a 250 g cup of water from room temperature to boiling (a rise of about 80°C), you would need 80 × 250 calories = 20,000 calories = 20 kcal, or approximately 80 kJ (actually 84). This is the amount of energy that could be derived by complete combustion of one level teaspoon (5 g) of sugar in a lab calorimeter. Biological metabolic processes are not as efficient as a calorimeter; the energy actually derived from a particular food is known as its metabolizable energy.

Almost all the energy produced from food by animals comes via aerobic metabolism, meaning that air, and specifically oxygen, is required. Metabolism is a complex physiological science, and what follows is a very simplified presentation of some essentials (see, for example, Wilson [2015] for more detailed discussion).

The universal chemical or molecule used to drive cellular processes is adenosine triphosphate (ATP). ATP is a high energy state molecule (adenosine with three attached phosphate groups in a chain) that acts as an energy source or donor (Figure 2.1). These phosphate groups can be removed sequentially by enzymatic reaction(s) to yield lower energy forms – adenosine diphosphate and adenosine monophosphate. The phosphate groups are transferred to recipient molecules which then are transformed into an active form to execute their specific biological function. The used or dephosphorylated ATP then can be regenerated by an enzyme (ATP synthase) that is powered by a proton gradient or pump called the chemiosmotic potential which is set up in the citric acid cycle (Figure 2.2). This latter is a cycle of chemical transformations fueled by aerobic metabolism of nutrient-derived fuels. These reactions occur in mitochondria, which are specialized organelles inside each cell. The most metabolically active cells usually have more mitochondria than less active cells.

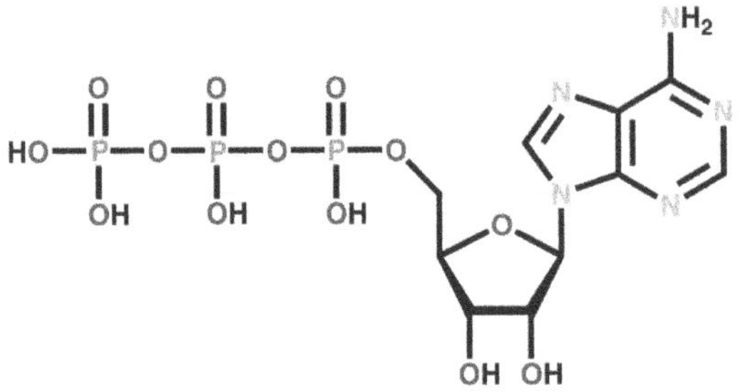

FIGURE 2.1 Structure of ATP

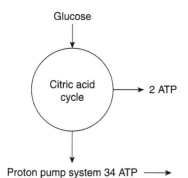

Glucose

Citric acid cycle

→ 2 ATP

Proton pump system 34 ATP ⟶

FIGURE 2.2 Simplified schematic of aerobic metabolism showing a common fuel, glucose, entering the citric acid cycle (several chemical steps are not shown) and subsequent generation of ATP. The theoretical maximum yield is 36 molecules of ATP from 1 molecule of glucose, although the actual yield is usually only ~30

Macronutrients are energy-yielding molecules used in the citric acid cycle to generate ATP. There are three classes of macronutrient:

- Carbohydrates (net metabolizable energy approximately 4 kcal or 17 kJ per gram).
- Proteins (net metabolizable energy approximately 4 kcal or 17 kJ per gram).
- Fats, also called lipids (net metabolizable energy approximately 9 kcal or 38 kJ per gram).

The energy density of a food is its energy yield per unit weight of food (e.g., kJ per gram) and depends on the relative amounts of the three macronutrients present in that food. As a rule, foods with the highest energy density are high in fat content. Conversely, foods with the lowest energy density, such as vegetables, have high amounts of water, which yields no energy, or other non-metabolizable constituents such as dietary fiber. We will now consider each of these macronutrient classes in more detail.

Talking Point 2.1

Most foods have nutrition labels, but have you ever looked at these closely? Collect some labels from foods in your kitchen and compare and discuss these with your classmates. Are there any macronutrient contents or energy densities that you found surprising? Did any foods contain more than 40% fat? Were some labeled "low fat," and, if so, how low is low?

BOX 2.1 DO THE MATH

1   Suppose your body expends 2,700 kcal per day – just a bit higher than the average person. If this energy were derived entirely from stored fat, how many grams of fat would you need to use per day?

2   If an individual weighs 200 lbs and has 30% body fat (probably in the overweight category), how many kilograms of fat does he or she carry (use the approximation

that 2 lbs = 1 kg). If that person stopped eating completely, but daily energy expenditure remained the same, how long would it take for their fat stores to be completely depleted?

3   Suppose instead the person goes on a diet and consumes only half as much per day (i.e., 1,350 kcal). How long would their stored fat now last until depleted? If he or she set a more reasonable goal of losing half of their stored fat (i.e., to 15% of body weight), how long would it take to achieve this on the same strict diet? (Answers are at the end of this chapter.)

In chemical structure, the simplest naturally occurring carbohydrates are monosaccharides such as glucose (also known as dextrose), fructose (abundant in fruits), and galactose (in milk). They consist of a core ring of one oxygen atom and four or five carbon atoms (Figure 2.3). Monosaccharides usually have a sweet taste and are commonly known as sugars or simple sugars. Once eaten, these are absorbed rapidly from the digestive system and lead to a rapid increase in the concentration of that sugar in our blood stream (a "sugar rush"). These blood-borne sugars then are either used immediately for energy in the processes mentioned in the previous section or stored (see below).

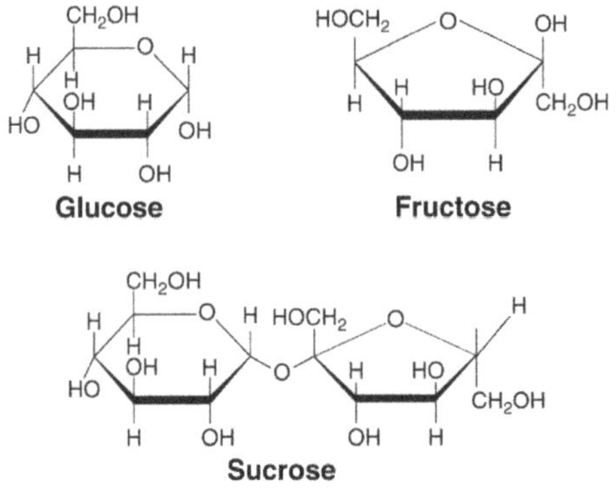

FIGURE 2.3 Structures of monosaccharides glucose and fructose, and the disaccharide sucrose that is formed by joining these two components

The size of the spike (more technically, the integrated area under the curve of blood glucose versus time) in blood sugar per standard or unit weight of a food eaten is known as its glycemic index (Figure 2.4). By convention, the glycemic index of pure glucose is set at 100. High-carbohydrate foods such as rice or potatoes have glycemic indices of 70 or more, while beans and fruits are typically 55 or lower (Foster-Powell et al., 2002), meaning that the spike in blood glucose is substantially smaller. Foods with a high glycemic index exacerbate diabetes, and so patients with this metabolic disease are often advised to eat foods with a relatively low glycemic index. The glycemic load of a food takes into account the actual weight of carbohydrate per serving and may be a more practical number to track in relation to a particular dietary regimen (Figure 2.4).

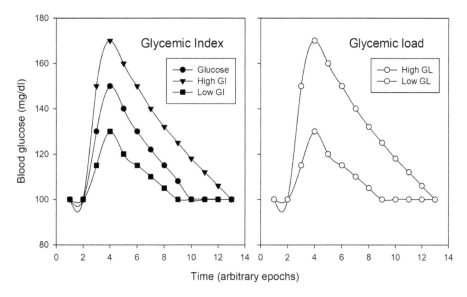

FIGURE 2.4 Diagram illustrating glycemic index (GI; left panel) and glycemic load (GL; right panel). GI: Changes in blood glucose level over time after consumption (starting at time 2 and for a short duration thereafter) of the same mass of glucose, a high GI food, or a low GI food. GL: Changes in blood glucose level over time after consumption of large or small portions of the same food

The next class of sugars is disaccharides, so named because they have two core monosaccharide rings joined by an oxygen bridge (Figure 2.3). The most common include:

- Sucrose (common or cane sugar) = glucose joined to fructose.
- Maltose (malt sugar) = glucose joined to glucose.
- Lactose (milk sugar) = glucose joined to galactose.

When these disaccharides are eaten, they first are broken apart by digestive enzymes in the gut into their component monosaccharides, which are then absorbed into the blood stream. The globally common condition of lactose intolerance, symptoms of which include diarrhea and bloating, occurs because the enzyme that breaks lactose apart is not present after infancy. Since mother's milk is the natural food of all infants, early-life loss of this enzyme would have been selected against evolutionarily. Most adults with lactose intolerance can consume milk products if the lactose is broken down by prior fermentation, such as in production of yogurt or kefir.

Complex carbohydrates, also known as starches or polysaccharides, consist of many molecules of monosaccharides joined together to form polymers. In plants, amylose (a head-to-tail or linear polymer) and amylopectin (a branching polymer) are common classes of starch, and, when these plants are eaten as a food source, they are broken down in the gut into the component monosaccharides before absorption. In part because this process takes time to get to completion, the glycemic index of complex carbohydrates is lower than for glucose. High fructose corn syrup (HFCS) has, for economic reasons, largely replaced sucrose as a sweetener in food processing. It is produced industrially from starch in corn first by the starch being broken down into glucose, and then some of that glucose being converted to fructose by an enzymatic process. HFCS 55, which is the nomenclature for 55% of the glucose so converted, has sweetness comparable to sucrose. HFCS is a mixture of monosaccharides and has a high glycemic index.

Talking Point 2.2

Using a table of glycemic index and load (available on many websites), estimate the average glycemic load of all the food you eat in a typical day. What is the range of these estimates in your class? How would you change your diet to reduce the load by 10%? How does glycemic load compare with the glycemic index of these items? Why are people diagnosed with diabetes recommended a low glycemic diet?

Cellulose is a structural component of plants and, like amylose, is a glucose polymer. Because the bridging oxygen atoms are in a different position in the molecule than for amylose, humans have a limited physiologic ability to break it down into glucose. For this reason, cellulose passes through the human gastrointestinal tract in more or less undigested form (see also the section on microbiome in Chapter 6) and is known as dietary fiber. This fiber, along with water, produces distention of the gut and may feel filling or satiating. It should be added that some animal species, notably herbivores, are able to break down cellulose from the vegetation that they eat into glucose.

In animals and humans, circulating glucose that is not used immediately for ATP production is converted into a storage form called glycogen. Glycogen is present in cells as globular or ball-like structures with a core molecule (glycogenin) and both branched and straight chains of up to about ten glucose molecules radiating out. During periods of fasting, glucose molecules can be cleaved from these glycogen balls to provide a source of glucose when none is being absorbed from the gut. Formation of glycogen from glucose dissipates some energy, and so the net energy that can be derived from glycogen for metabolism is a little less than the dietary energy consumed. Some mechanisms of storage and mobilization are discussed later.

PROTEINS

Proteins are made from structural units called amino acids that are joined head-to-tail to form chains of various lengths. Structural proteins are often several hundred amino acids long, whereas many short chain proteins (e.g., <50) are mobile signaling molecules called peptides.

Twenty amino acids occur naturally (Table 2.1); each of these amino acids differs in shape, size, and physicochemical properties. (Amino acids exist in two mirror image forms, l- and d-, but for our purposes only the l-forms occur naturally and are of biological use.) The overall properties and function of a specific protein are determined by the specific sequence of amino acids. Some amino acids are hydrophilic (water-loving), and proteins with a high fraction of these are themselves soluble in water or neutral salt solution. Examples found in common foods include albumins (e.g., in milk and eggs) and globulins (e.g., in vegetables and nuts). Other amino acids are hydrophobic (repel water), and proteins with a high fraction of these are insoluble in water (e.g., casein in curdled milk).

TABLE 2.1 Dietary essential and non-essential amino acids	
Essential	Non-essential
Arginine	Alanine
Histidine	Asparagine
Isoleucine	Aspartate
Leucine	Cysteine
Lysine	Glutamate
Methionine	Glutamine
Phenylalanine	Glycine
Threonine	Proline
Tryptophan	Serine
Valine	Tyrosine

In the gut, food-derived proteins are broken down into their constituent amino acids, which are then absorbed and are rebuilt into specific proteins or peptides, including structural proteins, enzymes, and signal molecules, or they are used for energy production. Some amino acids can be made in the body, but others cannot and must be diet-derived: These are called essential amino acids (see Table 2.1). An imbalanced protein is one that is low or deficient in one or more of the essential amino acids. Eating only an imbalanced protein will not provide sufficient amounts of one or more of the essential amino acids and will lead to an inability to synthesize all or sufficient of the proteins essential for body function. Most proteins from animal sources are balanced or high quality, whereas many plant proteins are not. Vegans and vegetarians must carefully mix their protein sources to obtain an overall balance.

Protein-to-calorie ratio is also often used as an indication of adequacy of protein intake in relation to total energy consumed. Pre-adult animals, including humans, have the greatest need for proteins (to grow new structure). A protein-to-calorie ratio below about 10% is associated with growth hindrance; that is, even if adequate calories are consumed, malnutrition occurs if there is insufficient protein.

FATS (LIPIDS)

Fats are esters, a chemical combination of one molecule of glycerol and three molecules of fatty acids (Figure 2.5). Chemically, fatty acids are relatively long carbon-based chains. The links between adjacent carbon atoms in these chains can be single chemical bonds (saturated) or double bonds (unsaturated). Saturated fats are lipids in which all of the side chain bonds are saturated: These give the overall molecule a long profile and tend to be solid at room temperature (e.g., lard and other animal-derived fats). Unsaturated fats are lipids in which all three fatty acids contain some double bonds that give the overall molecule a ball-like profile and tend to be liquid at room temperature (e.g., olive oil and most other plant-derived fats). There are graded degrees of unsaturation, depending on the number of unsaturated bonds. Monounsaturated fats (MUFA) have one double bond per chain, whereas polyunsaturated fats (PUFA) have two or more. Partial hydrogenation is a food production process in which some of the unsaturated bonds of an oil are saturated, such as producing margarine from oil.

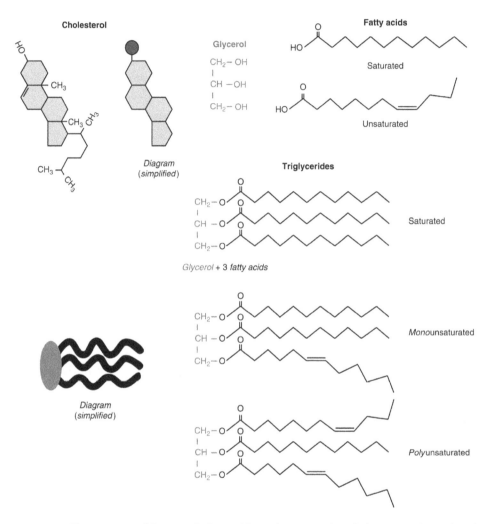

FIGURE 2.5 The structure of fatty acids formed from three ester bonds between glycerol and fatty acids. The different classes of fatty acids discussed in the text are indicated. Also shown is cholesterol which, although not a fatty acid, is a cardiovascular health risk

It has been claimed that eating relatively high amounts of saturated fats is detrimental to health, in particular cardiovascular health, because they may increase the levels of cholesterol in the blood. By contrast, unsaturated fats are sometimes called heart healthy, and many restaurants no longer fry food using saturated fats. However, the evidence for this distinction is not always clear-cut (e.g., Siri-Tarino et al., 2010), and a stronger argument can be made for deleterious effects of high-fat diets of any kind (Harcombe, 2018).

Some fatty acids can be made or rearranged by chemical reactions in our body; those that cannot be so formed are called essential fatty acids, meaning that they must be derived from our diet. Essential fatty acids include PUFAs known as n-3 or omega-3 and n-6 or omega-6. Oily fish such as salmon, herring, and sardines have a particularly high content of n-3 PUFA.

Triglycerides have to be broken down into free fatty acids in the gut by enzymes called lipases. Free fatty acids can be used directly for energy production or can be stored in adipose tissue. Humans have multiple different adipose tissue depots, and these on average contain 87% triglycerides by weight and very little water (fats repel water). This latter observation is why adipose tissue, at ~9 kcal/g, is the densest form of energy storage.

Most foods are mixtures of all three macronutrient classes. The energy density of a food depends not only on its relative content of fat compared with protein and carbohydrate, but also on the amount of non-energetic constituents such as water or fiber that it contains. Table 2.2 shows the typical relative sizes of major energy stores in an average-weight human. It is clear that plasma carries only a tiny fraction, that adipose tissue triglycerides contain at least 80% of the total, that glycogen (in muscle and liver) is about 2%, and that metabolizable protein is a substantial but ideally little-used source.

TABLE 2.2 Typical distribution of energy sources in a 70-kg human

Class	Source	Energy content (kJ)
Carbohydrates	Plasma glucose	350
	Liver glycogen	2,000
	Muscle glycogen	6,000
Metabolizable protein	Muscle, skin, gut	85,000
Lipids	Plasma triglyceride + fatty acids	150
	Adipose tissue triglyceride	450,000

Talking Point 2.3

Make a list of the sources of fat that you eat in a typical day – including in fried food, meat, baked products, and so on. Using food labels or a web source, break this down as best as you can into saturated and unsaturated categories. Discuss how you could reduce saturated fat intake.

MICRONUTRIENTS

In addition to energy-yielding macronutrients, a relatively large number of non-energetic dietary components are essential constituents for the structure and function of our bodies. The principal categories of these are salts and vitamins. Water is a non-caloric necessity but, compared with food, it has a separate set of regulatory systems. In addition to the water in beverages that we drink, foods contain variable amounts of water; it could thus be argued that we also eat water. We will not pursue aspects of fluid balance or thirst in this text (see Rowland [2022] for a comprehensive treatment).

Salts

Chemically, salts are molecules that contain positively charged cations of a metallic element such as sodium and negatively charged anions such as chloride. Most foods contain a mixture of salts, some in larger amounts than others, and those salts derive from the soil or other substrate in which plants grow. Animals contain specific salts, but those are accumulated from the plants and animal products that they eat. Given a balanced diet, it is likely that our salt requirements are met, but salt deficiencies can occur in eating disorders (see Chapter 10) and in absorption problems such as after bowel surgery.

The most abundant ion in our body is calcium (~1,000 g for an adult), followed by phosphate (~750 g). Our bones are made primarily of calcium phosphate, and deficiency of calcium leads to bone loss and diseases such as osteoporosis. Calcium is also vital in a great many intracellular processes, including release of hormones and neurotransmitters. Other ions that are abundant in our bodies include sodium, potassium, and chloride, which are the principal constituents of the fluid inside and surrounding most of the cells in our body. Other diet-derived salts that are present in much smaller amounts in the body include chromium, cobalt, copper, fluoride, iodide, iron, magnesium, manganese, molybdenum, selenium, sulfide, and zinc.

Insufficiency or deficiency of one or more of these ions interferes with a spectrum of physiological processes for which these ions are essential components or catalysts, but most usually deficiency of any of them is associated with a common symptom of tiredness or lethargy. One of the most prevalent of these deficiencies is iron. Iron is an essential component of hemoglobin, the oxygen-carrying molecule in red blood cells, and insufficient iron is associated with anemia and resulting low oxygen-carrying capacity. Excessive loss of blood, including during menstruation or with repeated blood donation, can result in anemia and may be resolved by taking iron or mineral supplements.

These various salts or minerals generally are present in food in trace amounts; their weak taste is usually masked by the food itself. Sodium chloride (table salt) occupies a special niche. Table salt is added to many of our foods, either at the commercial production stage or during cooking or eating, the latter being because many of us like or prefer a salty taste. Indeed, we have taste mechanisms that are narrowly tuned to the taste of sodium ions. This will be expanded upon in later chapters, particularly Chapter 4. For now, it is sufficient to note that sodium is unique among the salts insofar as humans and many animals exhibit a taste-driven specific appetite for sodium, or salts of sodium, when they are deficient in sodium. This is commonly known as salt appetite. Sodium is lost continuously in urine and sweat, and many salt or electrolyte-containing drinks are available especially for athletes and people who work in hot environments.

Talking Point 2.4

You have heard that high levels of dietary salt (sodium chloride) are undesirable, especially for people with high blood pressure or certain other physiological conditions. The daily amount of salt that is recommended for an adult is about 2 g. Examine food labels to estimate how much salt you consume daily (be sure to include any salt you sprinkle on your food). Also, most prepared food, such as pizza, is loaded with salt, so be sure to count that too!

Vitamins

Vitamins are defined as chemicals that are essential in small amounts for life but are not made in the body. They are found in many natural foods and are involved in a large number of physiological processes in the body. As is the case for minerals, a balanced diet will normally provide adequate amounts of the various vitamins, but deficiency in one or more vitamins is associated with often diffuse symptoms that include (again) tiredness. Vitamins can be placed in one of two categories (Table 2.3). Water soluble vitamins cannot be stored in appreciable amounts in the body and require continuous replenishment from diet. Fat soluble vitamins require dietary fat for absorption but are stored to some extent in fat depots. Prophylactic vitamin supplements are particularly recommended for children and the elderly, as well as in certain chronic surgical or other medical conditions.

TABLE 2.3 Classes of vitamins or vitamin families

Fat soluble vitamins (One member of each family shown)	*Water soluble vitamins* (Together, B vitamins are also known as the B-complex)
A (retinol)	B1 (thiamin)
D (cholecalciferol)	B2 (riboflavin)
E (α-tocopherol)	B3 (niacin)
K (phylloquinone)	B5 (pantothenic acid)
	B6 (pyridoxine)
	B7 (biotin)
	B9 (folate)
	B12 (cobalamin)
	C (ascorbic acid)

SPECIALIST AND GENERALIST EATERS

In the first chapter, we noted that our hominid ancestors were hunter-gatherers: They ate whatever was available and are classified as omnivores. Here are some basic classes of eaters found in the animal kingdom, with the implication that the foods are consumed in their natural forms, without preparation.

- Omnivore – an animal eating or having the capability of eating most food types or classes.
- Carnivore – an animal eating exclusively or predominantly meat.
- Piscivore – a carnivorous animal eating primarily fish.
- Insectivore – a carnivorous animal (or plant!) that eats primarily insects.
- Herbivore – an animal eating exclusively or predominantly green plant material.
- Frugivore – herbivore or omnivore preferentially eating fruits.
- Granivore – animal that eats predominantly seeds.

People who exclude animal source foods (ASF) from their diet – namely, vegans, fruitarians, and vegetarians – generally consume less energy, with a lower proportion from fat, and more fiber, potassium, and vitamin C, than do ASF-eaters. Likewise, people who exclude ASF often have a lower BMI and positive long-range health outcomes associated with lower BMI. These types of diet restrictions are personal choices, driven by ethics, religious, or health concerns. They differ from food likes or dislikes of an individual that arise from taste, flavor, and experience eating that food. These latter will be discussed in subsequent chapters in this book. The aspect that ties all of these various food classes together is that they are composed (in varying proportions) of macronutrients that supply our bodies with the energy to function. It is this aspect to which we now turn our focus. All of these types of eaters are dependent on local flora and fauna to provide their food. Because the availability of one or more types of foods often varies with season of the year (Table 2.4), some degree of dietary flexibility is essential. Further, because single foods rarely contain all the essential macro- or micronutrients, some degree of dietary variation was necessary for our ancestors to achieve adequate growth and performance.

TABLE 2.4 Irregular or unpredictable nature of food sources for terrestrial mammals

Classification	Example	Strategic solution	Comment
Seasonal availability of specific item(s)	Fruits, berries, nuts	Find alternative foods during out-of-season	Food storage is viable for non-perishables
General seasonal decline of food	Harsh winters or arid summers	Migration, hibernation, prior fat accumulation	For coastal dwellers, fish may be available
Intermittency of food availability	Encounters with prey species	Improve probability by learning prey patterns	Intermittent fasting diets (Chapter 11) similar

In the modern food world, the goal has shifted from basic survival to performance, health, and longevity. Most of us have adequate food supplies, choices, and access to knowledge about nutrition, yet often choose to restrict the food types we eat, as in these examples:

- Vegan – a person or diet that excludes all meat and animal products.
- Fruitarian – allowing only plant matter that can be gathered without harming the plant.
- Vegetarian – a person or diet that excludes all meat and some other animal products.
- Lacto-ovo vegetarian – a person or diet that excludes meat but includes milk and eggs.
- Pollo-pescatarian – a person or diet that includes chicken and fish, but not red meat.

Talking Point 2.5

According to www.foodallergy.org/resources/facts-and-statistics, some 10% of American adults and children have a food allergy, and 200,000 require emergency medical treatment each year. Teenagers and young adults are the most likely to have serious or fatal food-related anaphylaxis. The most persistent allergies into adulthood are to peanuts and tree nuts and to fish or shellfish. For people with such allergies, the best strategy is to avoid eating these foods, but these are also impacting people without allergies: for example, schools prohibit nut snacks, and airlines do not serve peanuts.

Survey your class, friends, or family and assess how many people report food allergies and to what specific food or foods. Discuss with your class how you think these allergies come about and to what extent it is justified to apply food restrictions to the >90% who do not have an allergy. If you have a food allergy, share the experience with your class.

Let's review and apply your knowledge. Take some time to answer these chapter questions:

- What are the main types of dietary self-restriction found in today's society?
- What are the subdivisions of carbohydrates? What are some sources of these?
- Describe the subdivisions of fats and what makes them different. Which are the most healthful, and which can be detrimental to health?
- What is essential about essential amino acids and fatty acids? How could you most easily ensure that your diet contains adequate amounts of these?
- What are the three main ways that energy expenditure occurs? Can these be influenced by factors under our control? Explain. What accounts for the majority of energy output?

ANSWERS TO THE "DO THE MATH" ENERGY CALCULATIONS

1   Three hundred grams of fat per day yield $300 \times 9 = 2,700$ kcal.
2   The individual carries 30% of 200 lbs = 60 lbs, or approximately 30 kg of fat. At 300 g per day, this would last 100 days.
3   On a 50% diet, it would last twice as long – 200 days. To lose half the fat (to 15%) on the 50% diet would take half that time – 100 days. Reasonable weight loss on a strict diet takes months to achieve. Commercial dietary claims of massive weight loss in a short time are fake facts.

GLOSSARY

Activity-related metabolism	The energy expenditure above basal that can be attributed to physical activity.
Adipose tissue	Tissue aggregates or depots that are made of cells that store large amounts of triglycerides.
Aerobic metabolism	Biochemical cycles that use oxygen in transformation of food-derived fuels into cellular energy.
Amino acids	Series of 20 naturally occurring molecules containing an organic acid ($^-$COOH) and an amine ($^-$NH2) group.
Animal source food (ASF)	A food derived from animals, including meat, eggs, and milk products.
Basal metabolic rate	The rate at which energy is expended when a person is at physical rest.
Cellulose	A fiber made up of glucose molecules, but joined in such a way that they cannot be broken down and used for energy by humans and many other animals. It is one of the most common dietary fibers.
Chemiosmotic potential	A chain of reactions inside cells that involves transferring protons (H^+) between molecules (or electrons in the other direction) that eventually generate most of the ATP in cells.
Citric acid cycle	A cyclic chain of chemical reactions that transforms metabolic fuels into energy.
Complex carbohydrate	Also known as starch. A metabolizable molecule composed of many glucose molecules joined in either linear (amylose) or branched (amylopectin) chains. To be nutritionally useful, these chains must be broken down to glucose by enzymes in the digestive tract.
Dietary fiber	Refers to large molecules derived from plants that are not broken down by human and some other animal digestive systems, and so no energy can be derived. These molecules pass essentially unchanged through our digestive tract and constitute bulk or "roughage."
Disaccharide	A carbohydrate formed by chemical union of two monosaccharide rings. Examples include sucrose (glucose + fructose) and lactose (glucose + galactose).

Energy balance	The difference, over a suitable time frame, between energy input as food and energy expenditure as metabolic rate.
Energy density	The metabolizable energy of a food. A given foodstuff is usually a mixture of the three macronutrients, plus non-nutritive constituents such as water. Foods with high water or fiber content have low energy density. Foods with high fat content have high energy density.
Enzyme	A complex protein that catalyzes or facilitates the conversion of one or more different molecules into a product (or products) in an enzymatic reaction. Enzymes are usually highly specific, catalyzing only one specific reaction.
Essential amino acid	Any one of 10 (of the 20) naturally occurring amino acids that cannot be made in the body. These have to be obtained by eating food containing adequate amounts.
Essential fatty acid	A fatty acid that is required (in small amounts) but cannot be synthesized in the body: It must be derived from specific food(s).
Fatty acid	A carbon-based chain ending with an organic acid ($^-$COOH) group that is a component of dietary fat. It is usually esterified with glycerol to form triacylglycerol molecules.
Glycemic index	The increase above basal in blood glucose level, integrated across time until it returns to baseline, following consumption of a unit weight of a food. By convention, pure glucose has an index of 100, and other foods are compared with this standard.
Glycemic load	A similar concept to glycemic index, but in relation to a specific food item, accounting for the actual amount of carbohydrate in that item.
High fructose corn syrup (HFCS)	Inexpensive and widely used sweetener in manufactured foods. Corn starch is broken down into glucose, and then some of the glucose is enzymatically converted into fructose (which makes it sweeter).
Imbalanced protein	A protein that is deficient in one or more essential amino acids.
Iron	An element (Fe) that is essential to several biological reactions in our body. For example, iron is part of the hemoglobin complex that carries oxygen in our bloodstream.

Kilocalorie	A common unit in which to express energy intake. It may be referred to as calories (as in your diet), but this is technically incorrect because one calorie is one-thousandth of a kilocalorie and is defined as the amount of energy required to raise the temperature of 1 g of water by 1°C.
Kilojoule	The international unit for expressing energy intake, used in most places outside the U.S.A. It is approximately 4.2 times smaller than a kilocalorie.
Macronutrient	An energy-yielding food component of carbohydrate, protein, or fat classes.
Metabolic rate	The rate at which energy is expended over a suitable period of time. It includes basal metabolic rate, energy cost of physical activity, and that used to generate excess heat (thermogenesis).
Metabolism	Complex series of chemical reactions inside the body that transform nutrients into the heat and energy necessary to sustain life.
Metabolizable energy	The actual energy yield derived from unit mass (most usually 1 g) of a macronutrient. The metabolizable energies of carbohydrates, proteins, and fats are approximately 4, 4, and 9 kilocalories per gram (kcal/g) or 17, 17, and 38 kilojoules per gram (kJ/g), respectively.
Mitochondria	Energy-generating organelles inside cells.
Monosaccharide	Also known as simple sugar; a carbohydrate in which each molecule consists of a single basic ring of four to five carbon atoms and one oxygen atom. Examples include glucose, fructose, and galactose.
Omnivore	An animal that usually eats or is able to digest foods from a wide variety of sources.
Protein	A protein is typically a chain of several hundred amino acids joined chemically. The order in which the amino acids are joined is specified by our genes, and different sequences give rise to different proteins that have various functions in our bodies, such as structural proteins or enzymes that catalyze specific chemical reactions.

Saturated fats	Triglyceride molecules in which the three fatty acid chains contain only saturated (single) bonds in the carbon backbone.
Specific appetite for sodium	Taste-guided behavior seeking sodium salts in the environment.
Starches	Generic name for glucose polymers, most usually in plants, that can be broken down for usable energy.
Thermogenic	Chemical or physiological reaction or series of reactions that generate heat.
Triglyceride	An ester of glycerol and fatty acids. Fatty acids can be saturated or unsaturated, and the latter occur either as monounsaturates (MUFA) or polyunsaturates (PUFA, notably some fish oils).
Unsaturated fats	Triglyceride molecules in which one or more of the three fatty acid chains contain unsaturated (double) bonds in the carbon backbone.
Vitamins	Compounds that occur in trace amounts in various foods and are essential for optimal metabolic and other life processes.

REFERENCES

Foster-Powell, K., Holt, S. H. A., & Brand-Miller, J. C. (2002). International table of glycemic index and glycemic load values: 2002. *American Journal of Clinical Nutrition, 76,* 5–56. doi:10.1093/ajcn/76.1.5

Harcombe, Z. (2018). US dietary guidelines: Is saturated fat a nutrient of concern? *British Journal of Sports Medicine.* doi:10.1136/bjsports-2018-099420

Rowland, N. E. (2022). *Thirst and body fluid regulation: From nephron to neuron.* Cambridge: Cambridge University Press (274 pp). doi:10.1017/9781108878166

Siri-Tarino, P. W., Sun, Q., Hu, F. B., & Krauss, R. M. (2010). Meta-analysis of prospective cohort studies evaluating the association of saturated fat with cardiovascular disease. *American Journal of Clinical Nutrition, 91,* 535–546. doi:10.3945/ajcn.2009.27725

Wilson, D. F. (2015). Programming and regulation of metabolic homeostasis. *American Journal of Physiology, Endocrinology and Metabolism, 308,* E506-17. doi:10.1152/ajpendo.00544.2014

CHAPTER 3

You Are What You Eat

Energy Flow

> **After reading this chapter, you will be able to**
> - Understand the process of natural selection as it applies to feeding behavior.
> - Understand the concept of energy and its flow through organisms.
> - Apply the concept of optimal foraging to the economics of energy acquisition.
> - Interpret the relation of portion size in the modern world to these concepts.

In Chapter 2, we described the constituents of food and how these are stored in the body. It could be argued that the sole purpose of eating, at least in an evolutionary sense, is to grow or maintain those energy reserves. For many species and especially omnivores, food is not a constant or continuously available commodity. Indeed, in many instances, food acquisition must be opportunistic or dependent upon the proximity or availability of food item(s). We start this chapter with an evolutionary context.

HOMINID EVOLUTION

The theory of evolution attributed to Charles Darwin proposed that species evolve by a very slow process called natural selection. This means that a species will change, over a long time span, if that change allows the individuals or group to exploit or compete for resources better than their ancestors or competitors. These individuals are said to have higher biological fitness because they live to produce more offspring inheriting the fitness traits encoded in their genes. Most scientists are swayed by overwhelming evidence that humans and all living entities past and present are products of natural selection. At the behavioral level, choices and decision making are crucial cognitive manifestations of natural selection, enhancing survival and fitness in a particular environment.

Fossil records show that the earliest hominids appeared about 4.5 million years ago; they were hunter-gatherers – food acquisition was central to their survival. In the next 4–5 million years of hominids' existence, prior to the emergence about 200,000 years ago of modern humans (*Homo sapiens*), species of *Australopithecus* and *Homo* evolved only to suffer extinction. A common theme of hominid evolution is the progressive alteration of body shape or size, including stature becoming more erect, altered jaw and tooth structure (adapting to different foods), and the development of a bigger brain. This large

DOI: 10.4324/9781032621401-3

brain has allowed communication and cooperation for food resources, culture, agriculture, and technology.

The human brain has some 100 billion specialized cells called neurons. Big brains come at a significant cost because neurons are relative energy gluttons (Table 3.1). If we compare ourselves with nonhuman primates of similar body size (chimpanzees), brain size is twofold to threefold higher in humans. At birth, the human brain weighs about 500 g, or 15% of typical newborn body mass, and that brain may account for up to 85% of the total energy budget or metabolic rate. By age 2, the brain has grown to near adult size (modifications of brain connectivity continue at least into late adolescence), whereas the body is still only about 20% of adult size. This large and disproportionate early development of the brain in humans poses uniquely large demands on energy intake by human infants. This is manifest prenatally as rapid fetal development through the assimilation of nutrients circulating in the mother's bloodstream. Postnatally, these demands are met by innate behaviors and digestive systems that are optimal for obtaining and absorbing nutrients from milk, traditionally provided by the mother. In Chapter 8, we discuss the ontogeny of feeding in infants and children. Maternal milk is an animal source food (ASF), high in fat and energy density, that provides all of the necessary nutrients for growth until the infant is able to be weaned to fully independent feeding.

TABLE 3.1 Approximate sizes and energy use of brains in hominids			
	Brain weight (g)	Brain weight as % body weight	Brain metabolic cost (% of MR)
Adult chimpanzee	500	1	10*
Human newborn	500	15	85*
Adult human	1400	2	20

* Assuming a metabolic rate per unit brain weight similar to adult humans.

ENERGY FLOW

Almost all animal and plant life on this planet exists in a thin and fragile shell, extending from a little below sea level to about 5 km above, and essentially the only source of new energy for life in that shell is electromagnetic radiation from the sun. Plants harness the energy from that radiation and transform it into chemical energy that is stored in molecules and later released as energy (notably, ATP) to drive cellular reactions and interactions (see Chapter 2). Animals harness that chemical energy as food, either derived directly from eating plants or indirectly by eating other animals and ASFs.

To understand eating, you must understand energy flow through an organism. This can be illustrated in oversimplified form by analogy to a bank account. This has one source of input, currency, be that in cash or electronic format, and is analogous to food we eat. Some deposits may be bigger than others and they may occur at irregular intervals, but they have a common currency in which they can be expressed (e.g., dollars). A bank account also has outputs in the form of withdrawals, some of which might occur on a regular basis (e.g., rent), and some of which are occasional (e.g., buying a birthday present). These outputs are expressed in the same currency as the inputs. If, over a given time period, the inputs exceed the outputs, then the balance in the bank account increases. On the other hand, if outputs exceed inputs, then the balance in the account decreases. Returning to a living organism, when its "energy account" is depleted below a critical level, it cannot function and will die of starvation. Thus, in order to live and do the things for which our bodies have evolved, we must have an adequate source of food and the physiological mechanisms to both store and mobilize the energy in that food. Unlike each dollar in the bank account, all calories are not quite equal. That is because, as noted in Chapter 2, living organisms are less efficient at extracting energy from food than a chemical calorimeter burning it. This efficiency varies with the type or complexity of the food and endogenous factors such as genes or current stores. We use food more efficiently when we are energy depleted, as in starvation or chronic dieting.

Metabolic rate is a continuous albeit fluctuating energy requirement, yet food intake is not continuous and most usually occurs in episodes. Thus, the system(s) that regulate energy flow must be able to accommodate this temporal mismatch and do so by creating internal food buffers – mostly as stored fat and, to a lesser extent, as glycogen. We often refer to feeding episodes as meals, but this concept is not as simple as it may appear. You probably have your own concept of what constitutes a meal: Perhaps it has to do with how much food is consumed, the time of day, or the social milieu within which the eating occurs. Those are all person-centered, modern factors. But let's go back to our own (and animals') evolutionary past for a broader perspective.

The food habits of many animals were and remain source-to-mouth, in part because small food items often cannot be transported and/or stored conveniently. Absent transportation, the pattern of eating such a food is determined by the frequency with which it is encountered and the amounts at each discrete encounter. Episodes of eating may be punctuated by rest or sleep periods, and these could be used to define boundaries. Most animals show a daily or circadian rhythm to their eating: They are often either nocturnal or diurnal feeders, with the remainder of the 24-hour cycle spent in a rest or sleep state.

Thus, for opportunistic or other reasons, the actual loading of food energy through the mouth is relatively brief and episodic contrasted with the continuous needs for energy for use in metabolism and physical activity. Once food has been swallowed to the stomach it is digested, in a process that involves enzymatic breakdown and passage (via peristalsis) along the intestine until the usable energy is absorbed across the wall of the intestine into the bloodstream. This process of digestion is not instantaneous, but it is most rapid soon after eating and slows in an approximately exponential manner until compete after 2–3 hours, depending mainly on the size of the meal or snack. Thus, while digestion somewhat smooths the energy input across time, it is still very much fluctuating and/or intermittent.

Talking Point 3.1

In an average day, how long do you spend in the act of eating (don't include thinking about, waiting for, or driving to food)? Survey your class or friends for their answers. You might find that the outcome is surprisingly small and is only a tiny fraction of 24 hours. How is that eating distributed in time? Many people eat in two to four large episodes per day, which we call meals (e.g., breakfast, lunch, dinner), and several small episodes, which we call snacks. Again, survey your class or friends for their responses.

Some animals, and in particular humans, have developed strategies to carry and hoard larger food items in a secure location. These individuals are called central place foragers, and there is either a complete or partial temporal disconnect between acquisition and consumption of food. Humans are highly accomplished central place foragers. With embellishments including social food sharing and, more recently, central production of food in agriculture, we have developed into occasional eaters. Because hunters and gatherers leave the central location during the day, feeding episodes both before and after the daily activities were most likely to conform to what we now consider a meal (e.g., breakfast and dinner). Even within the modern context of plentiful food for meals, humans have a wide variation in their proclivity to snack or otherwise exhibit so-called chaotic eating (Schüz et al., 2017; Zimmerman et al., 2018).

Talking Point 3.2

Dieticians and other people who give advice about eating often talk about "listening to your body signals" in relation to hunger and satiety. Based on the text, including the concept of opportunism, discuss whether you think there has been evolutionary pressure to develop satiety mechanisms that have **strong** control over behavior and especially termination of eating. If, instead, such controls are relatively weak, do you think strategies to "enhance satiety" are a useful approach to reducing overall food intake through dieting? (See also Chapter 12.)

PERIODICITY OF FOOD INTAKE

The foregoing questions about how much time eating occupies is part of a larger organizing principle of timing or periodicity. There are three broad classes of rhythms:

- Ultradian, or less than a typical day (24 hours). One application to feeding is the timing between meals or large eating episodes. In most cultures, humans eat three meals spaced by about 6 hours and then have a 12-hour period without meals.
- Circadian, or daily. Under normal circumstances, these are locked or entrained to the light–dark cycle, although other entrainers can be effective, including access to food restricted to the same time every day.
- Infradian, or more than 24 hours. Seasonal changes in type or abundance of food are among factors that can drive these rhythms, although they are not prominent in modern humans and will not be mentioned further.

As mentioned before, the intermittent feeding implied by the above periodicities requires the ability to store energy in internal stores and to mobilize it for immediate energy use. In the ultradian case, a meal is eaten, and then eating stops, which corresponds to what we call satiation or satiety. The absence of food intake in the following between-meals interval defines satiety. Satiety is thought to be strongest at the end of and soon after a meal, when the absorption of nutrients from the gut is maximum, and storage of excess energy occurs. As time since the last meal increases, so the rate of absorption slows, and satiety is less potent. Eventually, satiety wanes so that it no longer is effective, fuel mobilization predominates, and a state of hunger occurs. Hunger then motivates food seeking and eating, so restarting the meal-to-meal cycle.

Superimposed on this ultradian cycle is a circadian cycle, which sets a context for storage or mobilization at different phases of the day–night cycle. Our human ancestors ate during the day, although modern humans have a number of available strategies, including artificial illumination, that allow more flexibility in feeding times. Human newborns demand food about every two hours, day and night – much to the dismay of the parents – but the circadian component develops over the next few months, and infants then sleep all night.

These various rhythms are executed or enabled by oscillations in a large number of hormones and transmitters (see Chapter 5). And it should be emphasized that these underlie probabilities of eating and are not absolute determinants. Next, we will briefly describe the autonomic nervous system, which is particularly involved in the storage and mobilization aspects of internal body stores.

AUTONOMIC NERVOUS SYSTEM

Some aspects of feeding, and especially food acquisition and the episodic act of eating, are conscious activities. For solid food, humans engage chewing (masticatory) muscles, and the force and frequency of chewing will depend on the physical characteristics of the food item such as size, hardness, and the size of each bite. Bite size is often limited by food processing or preparation such as cooking or packaging and/or the implements used to handle that food (e.g., fork, chopsticks). These were probably less important considerations in our distant ancestors. Normally, adequate chewing of food into smaller parts is followed by reflexive swallowing, although, as noted elsewhere, there must be ejection mechanisms, such as for inedible husks or undesirable taste. Many of these complex acts involve the tongue and rapid feedback of somatosensory information such as texture and mouth position into motor reflexes. These details are beyond the scope of this text, but it is relevant to note that chew then swallow episodes typically occur in contiguous clusters called **feeding bouts**.

Most of the aspects of passage of food through the gut and its absorption, energy storage, and release occur automatically. One component of swallowing is peristalsis, starting in the esophagus, to propel each food bolus (mouthful after chewing) into the stomach. This is achieved by progressive unidirectional constriction of muscles to produce a wavelike progression. Additionally, peristalsis is a critical component of moving food through the gastrointestinal tract as it is digested, and region-specific radial and longitudinal muscles achieve appropriate vigor of propulsion. These smooth muscle movements along the gut are reflexive – there is little or no voluntary control.

Another involuntary aspect of digestion, and later storage or mobilization of the energy in that food, is via the **autonomic nervous system**. This part of the peripheral nervous system sends executive signals from the brain to all internal organs, such as heart, liver, blood vessels, and adipose tissue (fat). The autonomic nervous system has two, usually opposing, divisions. The **sympathetic** division uses norepinephrine (NE) as its primary transmitter and dominates during activities such as hunting or gathering food. The **parasympathetic** division uses acetylcholine (ACh) as its primary transmitter and dominates during relaxed times such as digesting a meal. Almost all organs receive both sympathetic and parasympathetic inputs – an analogy is both gas pedal and brake. The optimal function of these systems requires sensory information from the peripheral organs. As will be described in Chapter 4, most of these organs contain specific receptors which transform or transduce a relevant variable into action potential(s) that go to the brain. Of specific relevance to eating, sensory receptors for energy-related molecules, including glucoreceptors for glucose, are found in many organs, including the liver and parts of the brain.

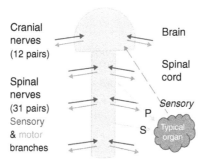

FIGURE 3.1 Schematic of the human peripheral nervous system. Spinal nerves are arranged as 31 sensory and motor pairs along the cord. The brain has 12 cranial nerves (although not all are paired; detail omitted for simplicity). Most peripheral organs receive sympathetic (S) and parasympathetic (P) innervation, and some of them send sensory signals to the brain

Food for Thought

We asked earlier how long you spend eating. The answer was probably less than 1 hour, but let's be generous and equate this to 4% of each 24-hour period. This means that the remaining 96% is not spent consuming. Thus, all of our daily energy is "loaded" during 4% of the time. The remainder is spent in early and late post-meal phases. In the early phase, food is being absorbed in excess of current needs, and the excess is stored, primarily as glycogen and fat. This storage process is orchestrated mainly by the autonomic nervous system (parasympathetic division), which controls the secretion of hormones and other internal actions to optimize the disposition of the incoming energy. In the late phase, food absorption is very low and less than current metabolic requirements, and so an appropriate amount of stored energy has to be retrieved (mobilized). This too is primarily orchestrated by the autonomic nervous system, but now the sympathetic division. We will not include further details, but you should know the general concept because various parts of this text mention sympathetic or parasympathetic effects on energy flow. An important point is that autonomic outflow is controlled by many regions of the brain, including the hypothalamus and brainstem.

OPTIMAL FORAGING

The last part of this chapter addresses aspects of food acquisition. Optimal foraging theories propose that individuals of a given species adopt the best possible set of behaviors in a given environment, including the balance between meal-eating and grazing strategies discussed above. Although energy balance is at the core of foraging theory and will be the focus of our discussion, another consideration is that foraging is not risk-free. Injury or loss of life during foraging is an energy-gathering cost that affects the inclusive fitness of a population or species.

From a perspective of energy balance, foraging behavior is associated with increased physical activity and a resultant higher metabolic rate. Thus, some fraction of the energy yield of food has to be repaid as the cost of obtaining that food, as in this equation:

Gross energy gain = metabolizable energy in food − energy used in foraging

Both basal metabolic rate and the cost of exertion are roughly proportional to body mass. Thus, a lean or light individual will have more gross energy gain from a particular quantity of food than a fatter or heavier individual. Weight loss is an effective way of reducing obligatory energy expenditure. When food is scarce or expensive and foraging costs high, being heavy is an energetic disadvantage. Conversely, if food is abundant and foraging costs are low, being heavy is not a disadvantage in the short term, and excess intake will be stored in the body as fat. From this theoretical perspective, obesity is the inevitable product of an obesogenic environment in which plentiful food is frequently available at low cost. Before considering some aspects of obesogenic environments, we next discuss exercise-related energy output.

ENERGY OUTPUT: EXERCISE

Every anti-obesity intervention, including diet, drugs, or surgery, comes along with the qualifier "and exercise." Reduction of intake is necessary but is more effective in a context of increased energy expenditure. Every aspect of modern life is replete with devices, such as automobiles and elevators, that decrease personal energy expenditure. Thus, compared with our ancestors, whose energy expenditure was in natural foraging, we often have to manufacture exercise.

The energy cost of exercise increases with body weight and with the intensity and duration of the activity. To compensate for differences in body weight, energy output is most often expressed in metabolic equivalent of task (MET) units, where 1 MET is defined as 1 kcal/kg body weight/hour. Thus, for a 70-kg (154-lb) person, 1 MET equals 70 kcal/hour, while, for someone twice the weight (140 kg; 308 lbs), 1 MET equals 140 kcal/hour. Basal metabolic rate (BMR) is only slightly less than 1 MET, and so, to a good approximation, the MET value of an activity reflects the fold-increase above BMR. Table 3.2 shows the approximate MET values associated with a number of activities. Since BMR is about 24 METs per day, to increase that by only 10% would require at least 1 hour of brisk walking.

TABLE 3.2 MET values associated with various physical activities	
Physical activity	*MET range*
Sleeping, watching television	0.9–1.0
Typical desk work, light housework, slow walking	1.5–2.5
Brisk walking, heavy housework, golf (walking)	3.0–5.0
Fast walking/jogging (5 mph), exercise bicycle/flat cycling, casual sports	5.5–7.5
High intensity or uphill exercise, heavy manual labor	8–11
Trained athlete at maximum exertion	>20

BOX 3.1 DO THE MATH

1 Suppose your BMR is 1 MET and you spend an entire 24-hour period doing absolutely nothing: What is your total energy expenditure in MET-hours? (1 MET-hour = 1 kcal/kg). Next day, you decide to get up and go for a brisk walk (at 4 METs) for 1 hour and collapse back on the couch for the other 23 hours. What is your energy expenditure? (In this and the examples below, the MET value of activity includes the basal rate of 1 MET.)

2 Another day, you increase the duration of your brisk walk to 2 hours: What is your expenditure? And another day you get up off the couch for just 1 hour and run at 7 mph at 8 METs: What is your expenditure now?

3 Then you get a job: Routine office work (8 hours at 2 METs) and commuting by public transportation (1 hour at 2 METs), with the remaining 15 hours at home doing nothing; again, what is your expenditure? Next, you still have your job, but on the way home you stop at the gym for a 1-hour moderate-to-vigorous workout at 8 METs: What is your expenditure?

4 Last, you weigh about 150 lbs and, for simplicity, assume that 1 MET = 75 kcal/hour. Your gym has a "juice bar" and they sell a 300-kcal, 20-ounce smoothie (this is a fairly typical size) that you just can't resist. For how much **extra time** would you have to do your gym workout to offset the calories in the smoothie? (Answers at the end of the chapter.)

Many people simply don't have or don't allocate sufficient time for moderate exercise and/or are unwilling or unable to perform high-intensity exercise in order to make a very large increase in their daily energy expenditure. And, even if an individual exercises at a level that for most people is quite intense, one average snack or beverage can completely undo the energy benefit. Exercise is a good idea because it has other benefits besides calorie burning, but it is not a good idea to think that exercise alone can solve obesity. Small movements over a long period of time can have cumulative beneficial effects, which is why there is interest in promoting workplace strategies such as stand-up desks, exercise ball chairs, or simply stretching or standing from time to time. Standing up and either walking or stepping in place only during the advertisements while watching TV almost doubled energy expenditure during an entire viewing period (Steeves et al., 2012).

Talking Point 3.3

Many people agree that exercise would be a good idea, but seem to be unable or unwilling to put that belief into action. Why is this so difficult? How many resolutions to walk or jog regularly are broken? How many pieces of home exercise equipment lie unused? How many gym memberships are allowed to lapse? Can you find any data on these, or cite personal experience?

MOTIVATION AND THE ECONOMICS OF FOOD

Given these limitations to stimulating energy output, we return to the input side of the equation. We left off with optimal foraging theory which, in part, regards the individual as ready to take optimal advantage of a food resource whenever it appears. We describe this type of person or animal as an **opportunistic eater**. In an environment in which food is scarce, being highly opportunistic is essential to survival. In an environment in which food is plentiful and easily available, being an opportunistic eater promotes greatly increased consumption.

Optimal foraging theory places a measurable cost, usually in energy units, on acquisition of food. However, for most of the urbanized and industrialized modern human world, food has become a commodity, and very little physical effort is expended in obtaining it. Instead, the effort takes the form of a token – money (and, implicitly, time acquiring that token) – that is exchanged for the commodity in an economic transaction.

One branch of economics is the study of consumer demand for a commodity as its cost or unit price changes. The relationship is called a demand function (Figure 3.2). One index that is commonly used is elasticity and is founded on the concept that a fixed amount of resource (e.g., money, energy) is available for that resource. For example, a 20% increase in price would decrease demand by 20%; if the actual decrease in demand were less than 20%, then the demand would be relatively inelastic, whereas, if the decrease in demand were more than 20%, the demand would be relatively elastic.

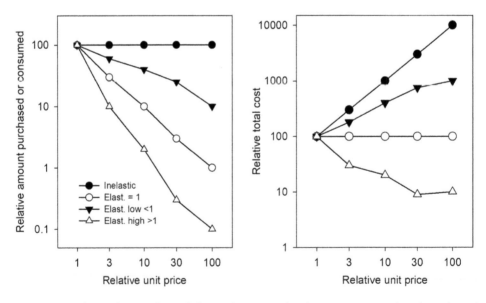

FIGURE 3.2 Left panel: Hypothetical demand curves – the change in amount (number of units) purchased or consumed as a function of unit price. (Note that both axes are logarithmic.) Shown are function for elasticity = 1, low (<1) and high (>1) elasticities, and for the case of complete price insensitivity (inelastic). The right panel shows the relative change in total cost that would result from these demand curves

A meta-analysis of demand elasticity for food derived from over 160 diverse studies published between 1938 and 2007 (Andreyeva et al., 2010) found that the mean price elasticity was less than 1.0 (i.e., all goods had relatively inelastic demand curves), with the lowest elasticity for staples such as eggs. However, purchase and consumption are not necessarily identical. Purchased food may be used in at least three ways: Food consumed to meet immediate energy needs, excess food that is consumed and stored as adipose tissue, or food stored in a cache such as a pantry.

Are the same general principles of food demand found in modern humans? In a virtual snack purchase study reported by Epstein et al. (2018), subjects were asked how many 30-g portions of a preferred snack they would buy at each of a range of prices, ranging from free to prohibitively expensive. The snacks were in either a low energy density category (e.g., fruits, vegetables) or high energy density (e.g., cookies, chips). For simplicity, we have averaged these two categories, because the results were only modestly different. Despite the very large differences between the conditions and prices of the human and mouse studies, there is impressive agreement between the results. In both species, demand is relatively inelastic (i.e., a tenfold increase in price produced only a twofold decrease in demand within these price ranges).

Most real-life studies in humans, such as potential taxation on sugar-containing drinks, have examined price increases of only a few percent, and, while there are short-term declines in demand for that item (presumably an alternative is purchased), the long-term effectiveness of such a strategy may not be as great because consumers become used to the higher price.

Talking Point 3.4

The typical price for a 30-g serving of chips or cookies from vending machines is about $2. Suppose you typically eat such a snack every day but, unannounced, the vendor increases the price by 25% to $2.50. Will you be 25% less likely to purchase your snack, or will you simply accept the fact that this is the new price? By how much would the price need to increase in order to change your behavior? What implications do these results have for dietary moderation in humans if barriers such as restriction or taxation were to be considered? These animal experiments used a single food, but humans live in a more varied food world. What do you think would be the effect if only certain foods were so taxed?

Talking Point 3.5

Whether eating in a restaurant or purchasing food at a supermarket, actual payment is usually a single event, more like an appetitive cost. In many restaurants, payment is after eating, but you know and accept that cost before you order the food. In contrast, most vending machines are effectively pay as you eat. Do you think that these two modes of payment would have different effects on human meal size or frequency, as they did in the rodent studies? Why or why not?

That brings us to the question of what determines meal or portion size in modern humans? Table 3.3 shows the typical portion sizes and energy yield of Western-style foods now and 20 years ago. In most cases, the portion size and energy intake have doubled, which has led to an overall recalibration of what is considered a normal portion or, consonantly, portion distortion. For example, a muffin today is still made of more or less the same ingredients as 20 years ago, but it's more than twice the mass and energy. Even our beverages have changed – as shown in Table 3.3 – with a more than threefold increase in mean size and associated energy load of soda served or (not shown) in drinks such as coffee which have increased dramatically in energy content as more energy-dense additives such as cream are used.

TABLE 3.3 Average U.S. portion size today and 20 years ago				
	20 years ago		Today	
Food item	Portion	Kcal (kJ)	Portion	Kcal (kJ)
Bagel	3″ (8-cm) diam.	140 (588)	6″ (15-cm) diam.	350 (1,470)
Cheeseburger	1	333 (1,400)	1	590 (2,480)
Spaghetti & meatballs	1 cup sauce + 3 small meatballs	500 (2,100)	2 cups sauce + 3 large meatballs	1,020 (5,040)
Soda	6.5 oz. (192 ml)	82 (344)	20 oz. (591 ml)	250 (1,050)
Fruit muffin	1.5 oz. (42 g)	210 (882)	5 oz. (140 g)	500 (2,100)

Source: www.nhlbi.nih.gov/health/educational/wecan/eat-right/distortion.htm

You might be surprised to know that the typical diameter of dinner plates has increased during the past 25 years from 10″ to 12″, representing a 44% increase in area. In almost every example in Table 3.3, the dispensed portion size is not under the control of the consumer – it is determined by the food industry. The food industry is responding to actual or perceived consumer demand, including how to maintain that demand or market in the future. The cost of manufacturing or producing food today is typically only a small fraction of its retail price. Much of the retail cost is fixed as personnel costs, building rent, and insurance and is not related to food mass or energy yield. It costs very little more to the provider to serve a large compared with a small portion. Thus, increased portion size is an inexpensive way for a business to attract customers. Industry advocates often consider that a large dispensed portion size gives customers a choice – that is, they may choose to eat only part of the portion. In practice, however, people are very poor at exercising this choice: Instead, they subscribe to the "clean plate club" and tend to eat everything that is served, so that an increase in served portion size does increase consumption.

Several studies have reported that the amount of an item self-served and/or consumed is influenced by the size of the bowl, container, or implement used (Wansink & Kim, 2005). However, not all studies have found this effect when varying container or serving size. Rolls et al. (2007) examined the amount of macaroni and cheese lunch consumed as a function of plate size. One critical difference between these two sets of studies is that the former occurred in social eating situations, while the latter was conducted in individual cubicles. Rolls et al. suggest that the individual eating condition in their studies might be the critical difference from the social eating situations used by Wansink and colleagues.

The rate of eating also influences the amount consumed. This was first described by Dr. Horace Fletcher who, in the 19th century, advocated that food should be chewed exactly 32 times(!) before being swallowed. In an empirical test of the effectiveness of this strategy of fletcherism in young women, Andrade and colleagues (2008) presented a test lunch with directions to eat either quickly or slowly. Subjects were tested under both conditions, on different days, and in random order. The lunch was a large (600 g) portion of seasoned ditalini pasta (small unit size) and water, and subjects could eat as much as they liked. In the fast-eating condition, subjects were given a large spoon and told to consume their meal as rapidly as possible with no pauses between bites; their average meal duration was 8.6 min. In the slow-eating condition, subjects were given a small spoon and were told to take small bites and chew each mouthful 20–30 times; their average meal duration was 29.2 min. However, despite this three-to-fourfold longer eating time, intake was only 11% less in the slow compared with the fast condition, giving only limited endorsement of fletcherism. Other studies have suggested that chewing, rather than simply slowing the rate at which food reaches the stomach, seems to be critical. An evolutionary trend in hominids has been a decrease in the size of molar teeth, indicating a shift in diet from raw plant material that required extensive chewing to animal source food (ASF) and/or cooked food that requires less chewing (Rowley-Conwy, 2001; Walker, 1981).

Talking Point 3.6

Do you ever make a conscious effort to eat slowly? Many modern or pre-prepared foods require little or no chewing, and most of our food comes in bite (mouthful) sizes or is easily made into a convenient bite size using a knife and fork – rather than with our molars! Which food that you eat routinely do you chew the most, and which the least? How does that correlate with portion size and/or calories per serving?

QUESTIONS TO ASK YOURSELF

Let's review and apply your knowledge. Take some time to answer these chapter questions.

- Explain optimal foraging theory. What factors influence energy expenditure in foraging?
- Describe food economics using the terms unit price and access cost.
- Discuss the impacts of increased portions and serving containers over the last 20 years on energy intake.
- What is fletcherism? What is its involvement in food economics?

ANSWERS TO "DO THE MATH" MET CALCULATION

1 4 hours at 1 MET is 24 METs or 24 kcal/kg body weight. The brisk walk adds 3 for a total of 27 (the 4 METs of walking is only 3 METs above the 1 MET basal that would have occurred anyway).

2 The 2 hour walk adds 2 × 3 METs above baseline = 30. The 1 hour run is 1 × 7 above baseline = 31.

3 Total of 9 hours at 2 METs (= 18) and 15 hours at 1 MET (= 15) for total of 33. The gym stop adds 8 METs but subtracts 1 hour of home sedentary time (= 14): 18 + 8 + 14 = 40.

4 You would have to burn off 300/75 = 4 METs which, if your workout was a run at 8 METs, would take half an hour. Walking at 4 METs would take one hour.

GLOSSARY

Access cost	Sometimes also called procurement or foraging cost: The cost, in relevant currency, of gaining access to a commodity (e.g., time spent traveling to a restaurant).
Commodity	A good that can be purchased or exchanged for tokens or other goods. Organized food collection and distribution (agriculture, business) has turned food into a commodity.
Consummatory cost	The cost (in suitable units of measurement) of eating a unit such as a mouthful of food once the food is nearby. Example: Price at a food vending machine.
Demand function	The relationship between consumption or demand for a commodity and its price, most usually unit price.
Elasticity	A mathematical description of the curvature of the demand curve. If demand does not change with price, the demand is inelastic. If one commodity is more vital (say, for survival) than another, you would expect a higher elasticity for the less essential commodity.
Energy	In physics, energy is a force or entity that is necessary for performing mechanical work. In biology, the same concept of energy is embodied in specific molecules that drive biological reactions (including mechanical movement such as walking) essential for life.

Evolution	The change in inherited (genetic) traits or characteristics across generations in a species. When, over a long period, such changes have become large, a new species is definable.
Fletcherism	Extensive chewing of each mouthful of food, with the goal of slowing eating rate.
Gene	Segment of the genome that encodes a single heritable trait – the smallest functional unit.
Metabolic equivalent of task (MET)	A MET is defined as 1 kcal/kg body weight/ hour. For a given person or body size, MET units provide a useful way of expressing intensity of activities.
Natural selection	First proposed by Charles Darwin, the heritable mechanism by which new species can evolve by competition or biological fitness, usually with more surviving offspring.
Obesogenic environment	An environment in which calorically dense foods are available at low cost, thus promoting excess intake and, ultimately, obesity.
Opportunistic eater	Term we use to imply that an optimal strategy for feeding in an uncertain food environment is to take advantage of each and every feeding opportunity that comes along.
Optimal foraging theory	A general theory that individuals will adopt the best possible set of food acquisition behaviors in a given environment to maximize net energy gain.
Unit price	The cost (in relevant currency, e.g., energy, money, time) to acquire a unit of a commodity once it has been reached. Most usually applied to situations in which each unit is the same (e.g., a pellet of food or a slice of pizza), but could also be applied to a derived quality such as kcal.

REFERENCES

Andrade, A. M., Greene, G. W., & Melanson, K. J. (2008). Eating slowly led to decreases in energy intake within meals in healthy women. *Journal of the American Dietetic Association*, *108*, 1186–1191.

Andreyeva, T., Long, M. W., & Brownell, K. D. (2010). The impact of food prices on consumption: A systematic review of research on the price elasticity of demand for food. *American Journal of Public Health*, *100*, 216–222.

Epstein, L. H., Stein, J. S., Paluch, R. A., MacKillop, J., & Bickel, W. K. (2018). Binary components of food reinforcement: Amplitude and persistence. *Appetite*, *120*, 67–74.

Rolls, B. J., Roe, L. S., Halverson, K. H., & Meengs, J. S. (2007). Using a smaller plate did not reduce energy intake at meals. *Appetite, 49*, 652–660.

Rowley-Conwy, P. (2001). Time, change and the archaeology of hunter-gatherers: How original is the "Original Affluent Society"? In C. Panter-Brick, R. H. Layton, & P. Rowley-Conwy (eds.), *Hunter-gatherers: An interdisciplinary perspective* (pp. 39–72). New York: Cambridge University Press.

Schüz, B., Revell, S., Hills, A. P., Schüz, N., & Ferguson, S. G. (2017). Higher BMI is associated with stronger effects of social cues on everyday snacking behaviour. *Appetite, 114*, 1–5.

Steeves, J. A., Thompson, D. L., & Bassett, D. R. (2012). Energy cost of stepping in place while watching television commercials. *Medical Science and Sports Exercise, 44*, 330–335.

Walker, A. (1981). Diet and teeth: Dietary hypotheses and human evolution. *Philosophical Transactions of the Royal Society of London, Series B, 292*, 7–64.

Wansink, B., & Kim, J. (2005). Bad popcorn in big buckets: Portion size can influence intake as much as taste. *Journal of Nutrition Education and Behavior, 37*, 242–245.

Zimmerman, A. R., Johnson, L., & Brunstrom, J. M. (2018). Assessing "chaotic eating" using self-report and the UK National Diet and Nutrition Survey: No association between BMI and variability in meal or snack timings. *Physiology and Behavior, 192*, 64–71.

CHAPTER 4

The Brain and Sensory Mechanisms of Feeding

After reading this chapter, you will be able to

- Describe the main subdivisions of a vertebrate (including human) nervous system.
- Describe the principal parts of neurons and their input–output functions.
- Understand the concept of neurotransmitters and chemical phenotype.
- Describe the principal mechanisms and pathways of olfaction (smell).
- Describe the principal mechanisms and pathways of gustation (taste).
- Understand the concept of enteroendocrine signaling by the gut.

BASIC ORGANIZATION OF THE BRAIN

Over millions of years, brains have evolved from simple distributed networks of neurons to the complex centralized structures that we find in today's vertebrates. The nervous system of vertebrates consists of central and peripheral components. The central nervous system comprises a spinal cord, which is a long, thin bundle of neural tissue enclosed in a protective bony vertebral column, and a brain, which is a prominent enlargement at one end of the cord. The overall and relative sizes of the brain and spinal cord vary considerably from species to species. Species with large bodies tend to have larger brains, disproportionately so in humans and some cetaceans.

The peripheral nervous system brings sensory signals to the brain and sends out executive signals to our various skeletal muscles and internal organs (see Figure 4.1). The signals used by the central and peripheral nervous systems are electrical, primarily action potentials in specialized cells called neurons. While there are many sizes and shapes of neurons, they are characterized by an extensive information gathering zone (dendrites and cell body), a single and sometimes very long conduction zone called the axon, and an output zone of terminals which form contacts with other neuron(s) via small gaps called synapses. Action potentials allow rapid point-to-point communication over relatively large distances within the nervous system. Most synapses use chemicals called neurotransmitters to send signals (i.e., information) from their output zone. Neurons are

DOI: 10.4324/9781032621401-4

often classified by the subset of transmitter(s) that they use: For example, glutamatergic neurons use glutamate as their primary transmitter, and their phenotype is known as glutamatergic. In fact, many neurons use two or more co-transmitters.

In addition to neural connections, brains have very rich blood supplies – the human brain weighs about 2% of body weight and yet uses 20% of the blood pumped by the heart. Signaling molecules – hormones – are released by various endocrine glands into the bloodstream. These have the potential to provide chemical signals to the brain provided receptors for those hormone(s) are located at strategic locations in the brain, and the hormones have access to those receptors. The brain normally protects itself from such a barrage of chemicals via a blood–brain barrier, and the strategic locations mentioned above usually have a reduced barrier.

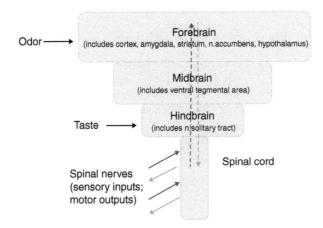

FIGURE 4.1 Diagram of spinal cord progressively enlarging to form hindbrain, midbrain, and forebrain divisions. All of these divisions are extensively and reciprocally connected. A few of the prominent structures within each division are shown. Note that odor (via olfactory tract) and taste (via cranial nerves 7, 9, and 10) signals enter different divisions of the brain

The brain itself can be described as several regions. One simple, gross classification proceeds rostrally (forward) from the spinal cord – the hindbrain, midbrain, and forebrain, as shown diagrammatically in Figure 4.1. All vertebrates share the same basic pattern, although the relative sizes differ between species. In adult humans, the brain weighs about 1,350 g. The outermost layers of the brain form the cerebral cortex, which has a highly convoluted or folded structure and is among the largest of all species'. The brain of newborn infants is about one-third this weight, with less cortical development. By comparison, rats and mice are often used as laboratory models of eating and yet have brains weighing about 2.0 and 0.2 g (i.e., ~1,000-fold smaller than humans), respectively, with only small and non-convoluted cerebral cortices.

The brain is an information processing device and, like a computer, has inputs and outputs. Most of the inputs come from specialized receptors in and all over the body that convert a particular stimulus – for example, chemicals in the case of taste and smell – into the main currency of action potentials within the nervous system. These inputs arise mainly from nerves, which are bundles of axons, going into the spinal cord, brainstem, or higher levels of the brain. All levels of the brain are involved in complex behaviors such as eating; the information processing becomes more specific and/or integrated as signals pass from hindbrain to forebrain. The rest of this chapter examines the three principal sources of sensory signals related to food and eating: olfaction (smell), gustation (taste), and enteric (gut content).

OLFACTION

One of the important sensory inputs in relation to feeding is the sense of smell, or olfaction. There are two food-relevant components. Orthonasal olfaction is basically sniffing the ambient environment and using this information to either approach or avoid the odor source, which often is not yet in view, depending on its quality. You have probably been attracted to the smell of fresh bread in the bakery around the corner, or a home dinner being prepared in the kitchen. We are naturally repelled by the smell of potentially harmful substances, including rotten food. In contrast, retronasal olfaction occurs when we are eating or chewing food, the act of which releases volatile chemicals in the mouth that diffuse via the retronasal passage from the back of the oral cavity into the nasal cavity. When you have a cold, this passage is partly blocked, and this accounts for why foods are not as attractive; altered sense of smell is also a common symptom of both acute and long COVID-19 infection (Xydakis et al., 2021). Apart from the different routes by which odorants reach the nasal cavity, the sensory surface called the olfactory epithelium is accessed by both types.

An odorant is an air-borne or volatile molecule. The intensity of an odor depends on the numbers or concentration of molecules in the air reaching the nasal cavity. For example, how do you know you are getting closer to that bakery? This occurs by chemotaxis, moving from regions of low to high concentration of desirable odorants. Most odors, such as fresh bread and many foods, are composed of many and sometimes hundreds of constituent odorants. In the simplest hypothetical combination, two odorants (A and B) might be present in two different relative amounts. High A with low B would probably smell quite different than low A with high B. With many constituents, then, the possible number of combinations becomes very large.

ODORANTS AND RECEPTORS

How do our nose and brain make sense of the input to identify one of thousands of smells that we can name? The chemical analysis of odorant molecules is performed by some 400 chemically distinct detectors called olfactory receptors. These are embedded in a thin surface membrane called the olfactory epithelium which lines part of the roof of the nasal cavity. In humans, it measures about 3 cm × 3 cm and has several thousand receptors embedded in and projecting just below the epithelium for optimal contact with odorant molecules. These receptors are on the dendrites of olfactory sensory neurons, and the axons of these neurons terminate in glomeruli in the olfactory bulb. Each glomerulus (the singular of glomeruli) receives input from several receptor neurons that are scattered across the epithelium, but, remarkably, all these neurons express the same receptor type (see Figure 4.2).

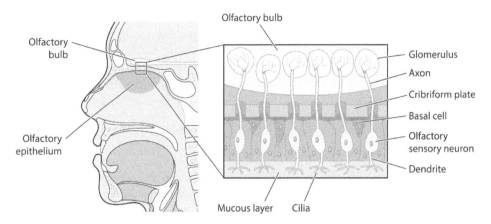

FIGURE 4.2 Diagram of the human olfactory system, including the olfactory epithelium, olfactory sensory neurons, glomeruli, and olfactory bulb

Olfactory receptors all belong to a superfamily called G-protein coupled receptors (GPCRs). GPCRs are chains of at least 300 amino acids that thread through the cell membrane seven times, forming three domains or loops outside the cell; these form a more or less unique three-dimensional pocket or "nest" for binding their matching ligands. Different GPCRs have different amino acid sequences in these loops that yield different-shaped pockets. Some of these receptors seem to have a high threshold for activation and respond to a relatively narrow range of odorant shapes, while others seem to have a low threshold for activation but respond to a broad range of odorant shapes (Yu et al., 2015). Thus, the moment-by-moment activity of each glomerulus reflects the degree of activation of its corresponding GPCR, integrated across the epithelium. Glomeruli are relay stations: They collect incoming signals from olfactory nerves and transmit them to the dendrites of mitral cells that are located in the main olfactory bulb. Axons of mitral cells then send action potentials to the brain via the olfactory tract.

OLFACTORY PROJECTIONS TO THE BRAIN

The brain areas that receive the action potentials arriving in thousands of axons from the mitral cells have to decode these signals. Each unique profile or pattern of incoming signals codes a particular odorant quality, distinct from another, according to what is known as a combinatorial code. The intensity of the odorant is coded in part by the frequency of the action potentials (i.e., number of action potentials in unit time): Many action potentials mean a high intensity, and vice versa. One key feature of this system is that, if a completely new odorant is encountered, the brain will recognize or decode it as new by virtue of a novel pattern of incoming action potentials.

Axons of the mitral cells form the olfactory tracts. These run caudally and enter the front of the brain, including parts of the telencephalon such as the cortex and amygdala. The amygdala is involved in emotional processing, and olfaction may, in a direct way, be able to influence mood or affect. Indeed, some odors can elicit feelings of either extreme pleasure or disgust. Various parts of the frontal cortex, including the insular and orbitofrontal divisions, are where odor memory, complex odor discrimination, and flavor are computed.

Odor memory is typically very good: You may not smell an odor for years but, when re-exposed, you recall the object or occasion of the prior exposure. Can you recall smells from your early childhood, such as your grandmother's kitchen? Newborn infants with minimal prior olfactory experience and an undeveloped frontal cortex can make odor discriminations, such as distinguishing their mother from other women (Cernoch & Porter, 1985). However, by age 80 most humans have impaired olfactory discrimination (a form of what is called hyposmia) and this decline is accelerated in Alzheimer's disease (Mesholam et al., 1998). Concussions from frontal head trauma – many related to sports – may be associated with either temporary or permanent anosmia – the complete loss of olfaction (Van Toller, 1999; Varney et al., 2001). In the case of permanent anosmia, axons of the olfactory receptor neurons are severed where they pass through a perforated bone, the cribriform plate, due to movement of the brain relative to the skull during trauma. Anosmic people report that food tastes bland, and they have a range of other psychological symptoms including personal isolation and emotional blunting (Van Toller, 1999).

BOX 4.1 DO YOU SMELL WHAT I SMELL – OR WHAT YOUR DOG SMELLS?

Scientists often make a distinction between macrosmatic species such as dogs, which have a well-developed sense of smell that is vital to their existence, and microsmatic species such as humans, for whom olfaction is not generally as important as other senses such as vision. Humans often use dogs to detect very low concentrations of odorants, such as hunting dogs that can detect the scent of prey or a buried object such as a truffle, and police and rescue dogs that can find concealed people, drugs, or bombs. What is the basis of this difference in sensitivity or acuity? There are probably several contributing factors. First, although the size of the olfactory bulb and number of olfactory receptor neurons are not always greatly different, the relative size may be; thus, a dog's olfactory bulb is a larger fraction of its total brain size than a human's is (Quignon et al., 2012). Second, the number of different GPCRs encoded in the genome is typically a little higher in macrosmatic compared with microsmatic species, but the difference in the fraction of those genes that encode functional receptors is greater (e.g., 80% in dogs versus 30% in humans), the balance being nonfunctional or pseudogenes (Rouquier & Giorgi, 2007). Third, the patterns of sniffing, the structure of the nasal cavity, and the flow patterns of air through it differ greatly between dogs and humans (Craven et al., 2010). In addition, macrosmatic species have a well-developed vomeronasal organ, which functions a lot like a second, parallel olfactory system.

Talking Point 4.1

Have you ever experienced loss of smell, or do you know someone who is anosmic? Were there symptoms other than loss of smell, such as those listed earlier? Can you be sure that the anosmia is causing these other symptoms, or instead that anosmia is one of several independent results from the trauma? What happens to your sense of smell when you have a cold? What difficulties with everyday life might anosmic people encounter?

GUSTATION

Taste and smell are closely interrelated; when we talk about different tastes (strawberry, lemon, etc.), we often mean odors in combination with taste. This combination is called flavor and will be discussed later. Pure taste is important for detection and recognition of the many food components that have little or no odor, such as salt. Unlike olfaction, for which there are hundreds of receptors, the number of receptor types involved in taste is far fewer, and they are organized into discrete classes of sensation. Only some of the taste receptors belong to the GPCR superfamily; others are ion channels (Table 4.1).

TABLE 4.1 Six basic taste qualities, receptor types, and typical tastant or ligand

Taste quality	Receptor(s)	Typical tastants
Salty	ENaC (ion channel, type I cell)	Sodium chloride
Sweet	T1R2 + T1R3 (GPCR dimer, type II cell)	Sugars, artificial sweeteners
Bitter	T2R (GPCR, many variants; type II cell)	Quinine, caffeine
Umami	T1R1 + T1R3 (GPCR dimer, type II cell)	Monosodium glutamate
Sour	Otop 1 (ion channel, type III cell)	Citric acid, vinegar
Fat	CD36 and GPR120	Linoleic acid

The five primary taste classes are sweet, salty, sour, bitter, and umami (Roper & Chaudhari, 2017). The recent addition of a possible sixth taste, fat, has considerable support, but research is ongoing (Jaime-Lara et al., 2023). A lipase (enzyme) released in the oral cavity seems to be required to break down triglycerides (fats) into glycerol free fatty acids, and the free fatty acids are what are detected by the relevant taste receptors.

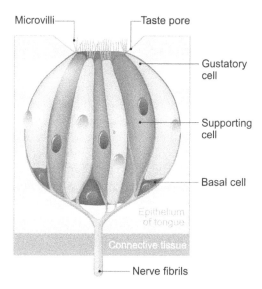

Microvilli

Taste pore

Gustatory cell

Supporting cell

Basal cell

Epithelium of tongue

Connective tissue

Nerve fibrils

FIGURE 4.3 Diagram of a taste receptor on the tongue. The bud itself is made of cells containing the taste receptors and other supporting cell types, as well as afferent nerve fibers

BOX 4.2 TASTE BUD TURNOVER

Some sensory cells, such as photoreceptors in your eyes and hair cells in your ears, are with you for life. That is, they have little or no capacity to be renewed if they are fatally damaged. Taste cells are almost at the other end of this spectrum – they typically have a life of only a few weeks after which they are replaced. The lower part of a taste bud is enriched in genes associated with cell cycle and stem cells (Hevezi et al., 2009), suggesting that new taste cells are made there, then migrate toward the tip of the bud, but eventually die. However, the part of the taste neurons (dendrites) that contacts the taste bud is not renewed. Thus, taste nerves are continually being paired with new cells; nonetheless, our sense of taste does not suddenly change.

TASTE PATHWAYS AND THE BRAIN

Different populations of taste buds release transmitter(s) when stimulated, and these are received by the adjacent dendrites or sensory neurons. The axons of these sensory neurons then coalesce to form sensory nerves. Anterior regions of the tongue are served by the facial nerve (the seventh cranial nerve, or CN7), whereas posterior regions are served by the glossopharyngeal nerve (CN9). Also, a branch of the vagus nerve (CN10) innervates the throat regions. Other mouth sensations, including information about texture and temperature, are additionally relayed via the trigeminal nerve (CN5). Completely unlike the olfactory tracts that enter the front of the brain, these taste-relaying nerves enter the hindbrain. CN7 and 9 synapse in the front or rostral part of the nucleus of the solitary tract (NST). CN10 synapses in the rear or caudal part of the NST (see enteric nervous system, below).

Most of the afferent taste fibers, as well as cells in the NST, are broadly tuned, meaning that they are activated by more than one prototypical tastant. Many cells in the NST respond to temperature or touch rather than, or in addition to, taste, and, at least in rats, the timing of firing in the NST is modified by ongoing licking behavior (Roussin et al., 2012). Cells within the NST that respond to taste stimulation of the tongue appear to be broadly tuned: They respond to more than one class of tastant. Thus, recognition of particular tastes involves recognition of patterns of responding across a large population of NST cells. As in many sensory systems, the taste pathways, including NST, respond better to a change of stimulus than to a sustained stimulus.

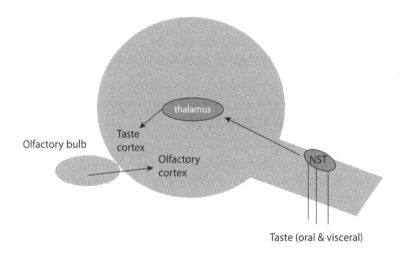

FIGURE 4.4 Schematic of brain pathways for taste and smell. Olfactory information enters the front of the brain, and taste information enters through the brainstem

CHEMICAL SENSING AND THE ENTERIC NERVOUS SYSTEM

Once you swallow something, does it become part of your body? Is your skin the largest sensory surface in your body? You may be surprised to learn that the answer to both these questions is no. It is not until nutrients are absorbed through the walls of the intestine into the bloodstream that they become an integral part of the consumer. The gastrointestinal (GI) tract can thus be thought of as a food tube with the mouth its top end (Figure 4.5). The role of this food tube is to process the foods that we eat into energy-yielding molecules that can be absorbed across the walls of the tube and to discard the unwanted material, ultimately as feces.

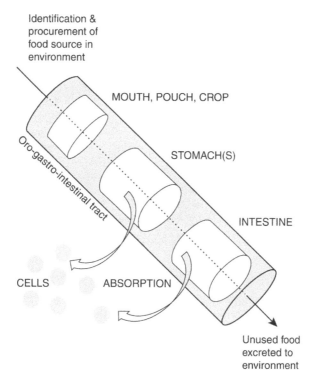

Identification &
procurement of
food source in
environment

MOUTH, POUCH, CROP

Oro-gastro-intestinal tract

STOMACH(S)

INTESTINE

CELLS   ABSORPTION

Unused food
excreted to
environment

FIGURE 4.5 The gastrointestinal tract depicted as a food tube. Nutrients are extracted, to serve as energy for the cells of the body, at various points along the tract

When food is consumed, it first passes through the mouth with its complement of chemical receptors, then passes to the stomach where it is partly broken down. From there, it passes to the small, or upper, intestine where further processing and absorption of nutrients occur and finally to the large, or lower, intestine where the process of absorption is completed. The food tube in humans is about 6 m (20′) long and is highly folded to fit into the abdomen. Further, the inner surface of the intestine is highly convoluted, with trenches and ridges such that the absorptive surface area is an astonishing 250 m², the size of a (doubles) tennis court.

The walls of the food tube are made up of several cell types and have both sympathetic and parasympathetic innervation to form an enteric nervous system. Additionally, a subset of cells that secrete hormones are located throughout the gastrointestinal tract and collectively form the enteroendocrine system, which is the largest hormone-secreting organ in the body. One of the surprising features of these cells is that they die and are replaced every few days. Research on precursor or progenitor cells that mature or differentiate into replacement enteroendocrine cells suggests a new organization or nomenclature (Table 4.2; Engelstoft et al., 2013).

TABLE 4.2 Partial list of gut endocrine cells and their function

Cell type and location	Hormone(s) produced	Principal function(s)
Gastroendocrine (stomach)	Ghrelin	Stimulates hunger in the brain
	Gastrin	Causes gastric acid secretion
Enteroendocrine (throughout GI tract)	Serotonin	Gut motility; fasting metabolism
	Somatostatin	Inhibits hormone secretion
Enteroendocrine (regional specificity)	Peptide YY (PYY) Cholecystokinin (CCK) Glucagon-like peptide (GLP-1)	All induce satiation or satiety; slow gastric emptying; promote insulin secretion (incretin action)

A subset of cells, called gastroendocrine cells, are found in the lining of the stomach, and each secretes only one hormone: Table 4.2 shows that one type secretes ghrelin. One action of ghrelin takes place in the brain to stimulate hunger. Other gastroendocrine cells secrete gastrin, the primary function of which is to release gastric acid in the stomach, which in turn aids in breaking down food.

Enteroendocrine cells arise from two principal progenitors. The first type produces cells that are found scattered throughout the intestine and secrete just one or two hormones, some of which are shown in Table 4.2. One such hormone, serotonin, stimulates gastric motility (which propels food through the food tube) and, in fasting, it has metabolic effects on liver and adipose tissue. Serotonin is also a neurotransmitter in the brain: You can read about the distinction between hormones and transmitters in Box 4.3. The second category of enteroendocrine cells, found at different locations along the intestine, each typically express gene(s) for and secrete multiple peptides, four of which are listed. The predominant hormone for any given cell is determined by the location in the gut where the progenitor cell arose, but these hormones all share a common set of functions. They are released by the presence of food-associated molecules in the gut (i.e., during and after eating) and produce inhibition of food intake: They are satiation or satiety hormones; see Box 4.3). They also slow gastric emptying and stimulate secretion of insulin from the pancreas. Within a few minutes of onset of feeding, food-associated molecules or derived signals have also been shown to increase or prolong an ongoing feeding bout (Sclafani, 2013).

BOX 4.3 SIGNAL MOLECULES: NEUROTRANSMITTERS, MODULATORS, AND HORMONES

You've heard the expression that the left hand doesn't know what the right hand is doing, but, in a more general sense, the body – and in particular the brain – has to continuously monitor what the rest of the organism (or another nearby organism) is doing. The simplest form of cell-to-cell signaling is via signal molecules that are secreted or released by one cell and are recognized by specific receptors for those molecules on the surface of or inside the recipient or target cell(s). Animals need to have systems for transfer of these signals across potentially long distances. The bloodstream is one such system, with signals known as hormones released at one location and reaching every part of the body (although only places with relevant receptors will receive that signal). In the brain, neurons transmit chemical signals in two ways, either by specific release across very narrow gaps called synapses or over somewhat longer distances by releasing the substance from a non-synaptic region. The substance then diffuses between neurons until recognized by receptor(s), but its concentration declines as distance from the source increases. Thus, synaptic transmission is essentially point-to-point or private communication, whereas modulators and hormones are more broadcast mechanisms. Further, within classical synaptic transmission, there are both fast (ionotropic – fractions of a second) and slower (metabotropic – seconds to minutes) mechanisms; most hormones and modulators also are in this slower class. In relation to feeding, there are clearly some contextual conditions such as hunger or satiety for which it is not important to have fast communication, and these could be influenced by hormones, but actions such as picking up and eating a food do require precise and rapid sequences of movements.

Because they respond (i.e., secrete hormones) in response to food-related stimuli, these enteroendocrine cells must also have receptor(s) to recognize food. Many of the sensory mechanisms that accomplish this do so via receptors that are similar or identical to those in taste buds, except that we are not consciously aware of enteric sensing (Mayer, 2011). The signals to the brain are of two main types: Action potentials in sensory afferents of the vagus nerve and specific hormones that are released into the bloodstream (and thence to the brain) as a result of specific enteroendocrine cell stimulation. For completeness, we note there are also receptors in the food tube for stimuli such as toxins and physical stretching, and this information goes to the brain via spinal afferent neurons. Primary vagal afferents first synapse in the brain in the rostral NST. The linear organization of the NST from gut (back) to mouth (front) reinforces the idea that the sensory surface of the gut is best viewed as a continuation of the mouth.

Peptide hormones such as those secreted by enteroendocrine cells normally cannot access the brain because of a structural feature called the blood–brain barrier. However, a few tiny regions have a reduced blood–brain barrier and do allow peptides to diffuse from blood to brain tissue. The two such regions of relevance to feeding are the area postrema and the arcuate nucleus. The area postrema is situated between the left and right sides of the NST and, together with a motor (movement) output region, makes up what is known as the dorsal vagal complex. The dorsal vagal complex thus receives both blood-borne and neural signals about the physical and chemical status of the gastrointestinal tract and the food therein (Young, 2012).

Insulin and Leptin

Before leaving the subject of peripheral hormones and signaling, we must introduce two other hormones. Insulin is a peptide hormone released from β-cells in the pancreas when blood glucose levels rise, such as during and after a meal, to reduce food intake in hungry animals. It is thus believed to induce satiation and/or satiety in addition to numerous peripheral effects such as facilitating glucose storage in various tissues. Walls of the β-cells contain glucose sensors (actually glucose transporters that move glucose across the cell membrane). Other chemical triggers for insulin release include cholecystokinin (CCK) and glucagon-like peptide (GLP-1) released from enteroendocrine cells. There is also a so-called cephalic phase of insulin release: It takes several minutes after the beginning of a meal for food to start being absorbed, and yet insulin secretion starts almost immediately or even in anticipation of food. Sensations of taste and smell trigger a neural signal to the pancreas, whence the term cephalic – involving the brain. A functional role of such cephalic reflexes may be to prepare the body for the arrival of food. The rapid time-course of insulin release is compatible with a role in satiation, and, consistent with this view, injecting small amounts of insulin into rats' brains decreases food intake via receptors in the brain. Another hormone released from the pancreas, glucagon, has almost opposite effects, but will not be discussed in this text, in part because its effects on behavior are less dramatic.

Leptin is a peptide hormone and is released from adipose tissue, generally in proportion to fat mass. It also reduces food intake in animals and is believed to be a satiety agent. While there are modest fluctuations in leptin levels during and between meals, it is more likely that it is an average or sustained level of leptin that serves to set a contextual function. Leptin is one of many molecules now known to be released from adipose tissue, and some of the others may be involved in feeding, but the case for leptin is the most compelling at this time.

In the next chapter, we will describe how the brain uses these and other food-related signals, and in which brain regions, to organize complex food-related behaviors.

QUESTIONS TO ASK YOURSELF

Let's review and apply your knowledge. Take time to answer these chapter questions:

- What is the basic outline of a mammalian nervous system?
- How do we "smell" different odors in our environment? Why is smell important?
- What are the six primary tastes? How are these encoded (receptors, etc.)?
- Summarize the neuroanatomy of taste. Make a sketch of the pathway for taste information, from receptors in the tongue to the hindbrain.
- What are the main functions of the enteroendocrine system? Name three peptides released from this system that inhibit food intake.

GLOSSARY

Afferent	Refers to a pathway that transmits input signal(s) toward the region of interest.
Anosmia	Inability to smell; hyposmia is impaired smell. These often occur in the elderly, or after concussive brain trauma.

Arcuate nucleus	Small nucleus at the base of the hypothalamus in the brain, situated on each side of the ventral part of the third ventricle. Has a weak blood–brain barrier, and so circulating small molecules such as peptides can gain access to this nucleus and activate (or inhibit) the neurons.
Area postrema	Small midline nucleus in the brainstem, located on the floor of the fourth cerebral ventricle. Has a "weak" blood–brain barrier, and so circulating small molecules such as peptides can gain access to this nucleus and activate (or inhibit) the neurons.
Behavioral satiety sequence	A sequence of behaviors that normally occurs immediately after the end of a natural meal; in rodents, this normally starts with grooming and ends with sleeping or resting.
Central nervous system	The major organ, located at the top of the spinal cord, in which sensory inputs are decoded and perceived and appropriate actions are organized. Also called the brain, this weighs about 1,350 g in humans.
Chemotaxis	Behavior that is moving along a concentration gradient of a chemical, such as an odorant. Moving up the gradient toward higher concentrations means approaching the source of the odorant.
Cholecystokinin (CCK)	A hormone released from cells in the upper part of the digestive tract in response to stimulation by food. Some of this released CCK contacts receptors on sensory nerve endings in the gut, and these generate neural signals to the brain (NST).
Combinatorial code	An encoding scheme whereby one type of receptor is activated by more than one odorant molecule type, and any one odorant activates more than one receptor type. The code to identify the odorant thus depends on a specific pattern and relative intensity of stimulation across receptors.
Convoluted or convolution	Refers to a surface made from an essentially two-dimensional sheet but folded like a fan to form ridges and trenches, thereby greatly increasing the surface area within a small three-dimensional space.
Endocrine gland	A gland that, when stimulated (usually by a chemical trigger), releases one or more specialized hormones into the blood circulation.

Enteric nervous system	A comprehensive network of neurons that are involved in the various sensory and motor functions of the gastrointestinal tract. It is also popularly known as the "gut brain," although, for the most part, we are not consciously aware of its functions.
Enteroendocrine cells	Specialized cells in the wall of the gastrointestinal tract that secrete hormones in response to stimulation by specific nutrients.
Fatty acids	Cleaved or hydrolyzed from triglycerides, fatty acids may function as the tastants for fat.
Flavor	A property ascribed to a food resulting from the combination of its taste and smell qualities.
Frontal cortex	The front lobe of the brain, particularly large in humans, that is involved in many high-level behaviors such as decision making and receiving distinct olfactory and gustatory inputs to several subdivisions. Flavor most likely is integrated at this level of the brain.
Gastroendocrine cells	Specialized cells in the wall of the stomach that secrete hormones in response to nutrient status. For example, ghrelin is released during fasting.
Gastrointestinal (GI) tract	Also called the food tube; it is the tube that connects the mouth to the anus. If straightened out, it would be about 20′ long. Because the walls are highly ridged or convoluted, the actual surface area is up to 100 times that of your external skin! The role of the GI tract is to detect and selectively absorb desired nutrients to fuel cells of the body.
Ghrelin	A 28-amino-acid peptide, produced by specific cells in the wall of the stomach. Ghrelin has to be chemically modified (acetylated) to yield an active form that acts in brain and other tissues via growth hormone secretagogue receptors (GHS-R). An appetite stimulant, it is considered a hunger hormone.
Glomerulus (plural glomeruli)	A spherical structure located in the olfactory bulb of the brain where synapses form between the terminals of olfactory receptor neurons and the dendrites of mitral (and other) cells that project to the brain. Each glomerulus is "odor coded": It receives input from many receptor neurons, but all of these express the same specific receptor type.

Glucagon	A peptide hormone secreted by α-cells of the pancreas, usually during fasting, that functions to raise blood glucose levels by breaking down stored glycogen into glucose.
G-protein coupled receptor (GPCR)	A superfamily of receptors, including ~400 olfaction-specific instances in the human olfactory system, that, upon binding a ligand (e.g., odorant for olfaction) at the outer surface of a cell, initiate a cascade of G-protein-mediated events inside the cell.
Heterodimer	A chemical moiety formed by association of two different moieties that together have a different or expanded function than either has alone.
Hormone	A specific chemical, usually released into the bloodstream from an endocrine gland, that activates target cells in strategic locations of the body by interacting with a corresponding receptor.
Incretins	A group of metabolic hormones that enhance production of insulin by the pancreas and thereby act to decrease blood glucose levels.
Insulin	A peptide hormone secreted by β-cells of the pancreas, usually during and after eating, that serves to promote storage of absorbed nutrients as glycogen and triglycerides.
Leptin	Peptide hormone released from adipose tissue cells into the bloodstream. To an approximation, it serves as an integrated marker of fat content in the body.
Ligand	The ligand for a receptor is a molecule, like a hormone or transmitter, that binds to specific site(s) on that receptor and causes a temporary biological change, such as receptor activation or blockade.
Nucleus of the solitary tract (NST)	A long, skinny nucleus of cells (one on each side of the brain) found in the brainstem. It is the first region in the brain contacted by incoming neural signals from the gut and from the tongue. Synonymous with the nucleus of the tractus solitarius (NTS), derived from the Latin nomenclature.
Neurons	Specialized cells found in peripheral and central nervous systems that collect, integrate, and transmit electrical signals via axons over relatively long distances.

Odorant	Molecules emitted from a source, dispersed in a carrier medium, and detected by receptors.
Olfactory bulb	Front or rostral part of the brain that contains glomeruli and mitral cells whose output axons form the olfactory tracts and project rearward or caudally to various brain regions.
Olfactory epithelium	One of four basic types of tissues found in animals. Epithelial tissues are composed of densely packed cells and line most structures in the body. The olfactory epithelium refers to the corresponding tissue (approximately 9 cm² in humans) in the roof of the nasal cavity.
Olfactory receptors	Protein molecules on olfactory receptor neurons. Their three-dimensional shape forms a binding site or pocket for odorant molecules that have a corresponding shape. As a result of this binding, the receptor initiates a cascade of chemical events inside the receptor neuron.
Olfactory receptor neuron	Specialized neuron (bipolar) class whose dendrites express the olfactory receptors and whose axon projects to and synapses in a glomerulus in the olfactory bulb. Each neuron expresses only one type of olfactory receptor and projects to only one glomerulus.
Orthonasal olfaction	Occurs when volatile molecules are inhaled (sniffed) into the front of the nasal cavity.
Retronasal olfaction	Occurs when volatile molecules are released in our mouth as we chew food, and these enter the nasal cavity via a channel from the roof of the mouth.
Tastant	A molecule that, by virtue of its shape and other characteristics, stimulates taste receptor(s) on the tongue and gives rise to a sensation of taste.
Taste buds	Onion-shaped structures composed of many cells, including taste receptor cells, that are embedded in the tongue and shaped to allow tastant molecules access to the taste receptors. There are three main taste cell types (I, II, and III), with type II carrying the GCPR-linked taste receptors.
Umami	From the Japanese for "pleasant savory taste"; it is a basic taste category, received or transduced by a specific class of taste receptors. The prototypical tastant is the common food additive monosodium glutamate (MSG).

Vagus nerve (CN10)	A mixed nerve (both sensory afferents to the brain and efferent motor fibers from the brain) that innervates a large number of organs in the chest and abdomen.

REFERENCES

Cernoch, J. M., & Porter, R. H. (1985). Recognition of maternal axillary odors by infants. *Child Development, 56*, 1593–1598.

Craven, B. A., Paterson, E. G., & Settles, G. S. (2010). The fluid dynamics of canine olfaction: Unique nasal airflow patterns as an explanation of macrosomia. *Journal of the Royal Society Interface, 7*, 933–943.

Engelstoft, M. S., Egerod, K. L., Lund, M. L., & Schwartz, T. W. (2013). Enteroendocrine cell types revisited. *Current Opinion in Pharmacology, 13*, 912–921.

Hevezi, P., Moyer, B. D., Lu, M., et al. (2009). Genome-wide analysis of gene expression in primate taste buds reveals links to diverse processes. *PLoS ONE, 4*, e6395.

Jaime-Lara, R. B., Brooks, B. E., Vizioli, C., et.al. (2023). A systematic review of the biological mediators of fat taste and smell. *Physiological Review, 103*, 855–918.

Mayer, E. A. (2011). Gut feelings: The emerging biology of gut–brain communication. *Nature Reviews Neuroscience, 12*, 453–466.

Mesholam, R. I., Moberg, P. J., Mahr, R. N., & Doty, R. L. (1998). Olfaction in neurodegenerative disease: A meta-analysis of olfactory functioning in Alzheimer's and Parkinson's diseases. *Archives of Neurology, 55*, 84–90.

Quignon, P., Rimbault, M., Robin, S., & Galibert, F. (2012). Genetics of canine olfaction and receptor diversity. *Mammalian Genome, 23*, 132–143.

Roper, S. D., & Chaudhari, N. (2017). Taste buds: Cells, signals and synapses. *Nature Reviews Neuroscience, 18*, 485–497.

Rouquier, S., & Giorgi, D. (2007). Olfactory receptor gene repertoires in mammals. *Mutation Research, 616*, 95–102.

Roussin, A. T., D'Agostino, A. E., Fooden, A. M., Victor, J. D., & DiLorenzo, P. M. (2012). Taste coding in the nucleus of the solitary tract of the awake, freely licking rat. *Journal of Neuroscience, 32*, 10494–10506.

Sclafani, A. (2013). Gut–brain nutrient signaling: Appetition vs satiation. *Appetite, 71*, 454–458.

Van Toller, S. (1999). Assessing the impact of anosmia: Review of a questionnaire's findings. *Chemical Senses, 24*, 705–712.

Varney, N. R., Pinkston, J. B., & Wu, J. C. (2001). Quantitative PET findings in patients with post-traumatic anosmia. *Journal of Head Trauma Rehabilitation, 16*, 253–259.

Xydakis, M. S., Albers, M. W., & Holbrook, E. H. (2021). Post-viral effects of COVID-19 in the olfactory system and their implications. *Lancet Neurology, 20*, 753–761.

Young, A. A. (2012). Brainstem sensing of meal-related signals in energy homeostasis. *Neuropharmacology, 63*, 31–45.

Yu, Y., de March, C. A., Ni, M. J., et al. (2015). Responsiveness of G-protein coupled odorant receptors is partially attributed to the activation mechanisms. *Proceedings of the National Academy USA, 112*, 14966–14971.

CHAPTER 5

Brain

Outputs and Integration

After reading this chapter, you will be able to:

- Name and give basic principles for studying the living brain.
- Understand the concept of motivation and its application to feeding.
- Identify signals from adipose tissue in regulation of food intake.
- Identify signals from the gut in relation to food intake.
- Describe the role of various subcortical and cortical structures in feeding.

HACKING INTO THE BRAIN

We have seen how some of the involuntary and elective aspects of digestion and feeding are organized in the brain. To find out which brain structures are involved in various components of feeding, it is essential to find effective ways in which to either observe or intervene in brain structure and function (i.e., hacking) in behaving organisms, be they human or animal. In this section, we describe contemporary types of hacking and, briefly, their principles of action, as well as strengths and weaknesses in relation to the goal of understanding the necessary and/or sufficient role of each region and its place in the overall sequence of brain activation.

Functional magnetic resonance imaging (fMRI)

fMRI is a harmless or **non-invasive** way to measure brain activity in humans. It revolutionized hacking the human brain and has been used widely for over 25 years. Instead of measuring electrical activity such as synaptic and action potentials directly, it uses an indirect method that relies upon the premise that electrical activity consumes energy. In the brain, such activity is tightly coupled to utilization of oxygen, carried to the smallest blood vessels of the brain by the iron-containing protein hemoglobin. Oxygen is consumed by stripping oxygen molecules from oxygenated hemoglobin, leaving deoxygenated hemoglobin. These two molecules, oxy- and deoxyhemoglobin, align or spin differently when exposed to high magnetic fields. Through detection of that alignment (using complicated electronics, physics, and math beyond this text), the

DOI: 10.4324/9781032621401-5

relative level of oxygenation of blood in a given location can be assessed: This is often known as the **BOLD** (blood oxygenation level-dependent) **signal** (Figure 5.1, left panel).

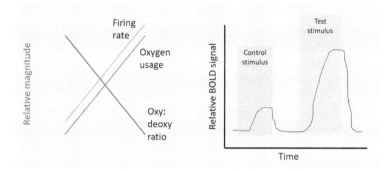

FIGURE 5.1 Left panel shows schematically that, as average local firing rate and resultant oxygen usage increase, the ratio of oxyhemoglobin to deoxyhemoglobin in the local capillary blood vessels decreases. Right panel shows idealized experiment in which a control stimulus causes a small increase above basal in BOLD signal in given voxel(s), and a test stimulus causes a larger increase. The full effects of stimulus onset and offset on BOLD may take several seconds

The bloodstream pumps millions of molecules of oxygenated hemoglobin to the brain every second, and all parts of the brain consume some oxygen, including for purposes other than generating electrical potentials. Repeated measurements of the BOLD signal from discrete cubes of space, or **voxels**, which correspond to a particular part of the brain (no head movement, which would blur the image, can occur), allow dynamic changes in BOLD to be recorded. Because a substantial part of the BOLD signal is due to electrical activity, when the BOLD signal changes, then a net or average change in electrical activity in the voxel occurs over the time frame of the measurement, which is usually a few seconds (Figure 5.1, right panel). By convention, an increase in the reported BOLD signal means increased electrical activity relative to prior or control period(s).

As an illustrative example related to feeding, subjects might be presented successively with two or more images, one of which is of food, or of food of a particular kind, and one of which is not of food. Any difference between these two conditions in BOLD for a given voxel is interpreted as differential processing of the food versus non-food stimuli. One pitfall of this method is that the imaging takes several seconds, whereas changes in electrical activity (and behavior, if relevant) occur much more rapidly; the BOLD signal is an integral across time. Another shortcoming is that each voxel contains thousands of neurons, axons, and synapses, and the resultant signal is the average of all of these. Thus, while fMRI is useful in identifying brain regions of interest, it cannot specify exactly which synapses are active and in what sequence. Nonetheless, it remains one of the best ways available to measure the working human brain.

Chemogenetics

Chemogenetics refers to methods for using genetic modification to allow chemical excitation or inhibition of discrete populations of neurons. This usually involves invasive use of designer receptors exclusively activated by designer drugs (DREADDs; Roth, 2019). The human muscarinic acetylcholine receptor gene has been genetically modified so that it is either excitatory or inhibitory (the mechanism for this is via different G-coupled mechanisms the detail of which need not concern us here). These receptors are introduced into a region or regions of interest in brain, usually in rats or mice, via a harmless virus that acts as a Trojan horse. Once the DREADDs are incorporated and expressed as surface receptors on the neurons of interest, they are inactive or silent until they are engaged by an artificial chemical ligand, usually clozapine-N-oxide (CNO). Depending on the dose, a single CNO injection can provide an adequate stimulus for the DREADDs for several hours, thereby either increasing or decreasing the natural firing rate of the infected cells. When DREADDs are targeted to one phenotype of cell in a region, then the result with CNO allows inference about the normal effect of activation (or inhibition) of that pathway. That might include increasing or decreasing feeding behavior. The method has advantages over older methods that used chemical injection into a region of interest or electrical stimulation because, after the virus injection, no further brain penetration is needed. Also, the reversible effects of CNO last longer than most previous methods, with advantages for the study of feeding across more than one meal, including duration of satiety.

Optogenetics

A relatively recent and powerful tool for functional analysis of brain function is the method of optogenetic stimulation (or inhibition) of neural firing. This method currently is available only for use in mice. Many plants and algae have photosensitive pigments or opsins that are coupled to ion channels and transduce ambient light such as for photosynthesis. The genes encoding these opsins can be inserted, using transgenic methods, into specific brain regions and phenotypes of neurons (for more detail, see www.yout ube.com/watch?v=55meVwea5Ss). When illuminated by an appropriate wavelength of light, delivered via a thin optical fiber into the brain region of interest, neurons expressing the opsin will generate either excitatory (usually via a sodium channel) or inhibitory (usually via a chloride channel) postsynaptic potentials and so become more or less likely to fire, respectively. When there is no light stimulus, the opsin is inactive and has no apparent effect on neural function (Emiliani et al., 2022; Jiang et al., 2017).

One of the first opsins so introduced was channel rhodopsin 2 (ChR2), which is coupled to a sodium channel. Onset of the light (laser) stimulus produces sustained firing in the target cells, and this ceases almost immediately the laser is turned off. The rate (action potentials per second) of the induced firing is, in part, related to the frequency (in hertz) and duration of the laser pulses. The onset and offset of these effects occur within milliseconds, and so the method can be used to measure stimulation-dependent behavior. More recently, channels that are inhibitory and/or have a more prolonged effect have become available and have expanded the horizons of this powerful technology. In a food-related example (see youtube.com/watch?v=7Mmsah0v9Qc), stimulation of the bed nucleus of the stria terminalis (BNST) produced rapid eating in mice that stopped as soon as the laser was turned off.

BRAIN REGIONS INVOLVED IN FEEDING

Many brain regions at multiple levels are involved in the conscious execution of complex behavior such as feeding. The brainstem is the principal input and output region – for example, receiving input from the cranial nerves about location, touch, texture, and taste. This input goes initially to the nucleus of the solitary tract (NTS), which is a bilaterally situated long, skinny nucleus (Figure 5.2). The posterior part receives mostly taste input, and the anterior region receives mostly gut-derived signals. The cranial nerves, including the vagus nerve from the dorsal motor nucleus of the vagus (DMV) that innervates much of the gut, are the output conduits (Figure 5.2).

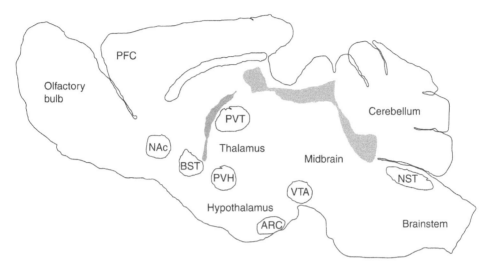

FIGURE 5.2 Schematic diagram of a mouse brain showing the principal structures discussed in the text. This original diagram, based on Figure 102 from Paxinos and Franklin (2001), redrawn and simplified, is a sagittal section slightly to one side of the midline, with the front of the brain facing left. For scale, the actual left-to-right extent shown is about 13 mm or 0.5″. Abbreviations: ARC – arcuate nucleus; BNST – bed nucleus of stria terminalis; NAc – nucleus accumbens; PFC – prefrontal cortex; PVH – paraventricular nucleus of hypothalamus; PVT – paraventricular nucleus of thalamus; NST – nucleus of the solitary tract; VTA – ventral tegmental area. Some areas shown are not on the midline and are shown in projection

Regions such as NST and DMV are heavily connected to more rostral levels of the brain, but it is also the case that they can use this sensory information to drive the motor outputs via local reflexive mechanisms, including the vago-vagal reflex. This conclusion is due to the intact nature of these reflexes in animals with transection of the brain above the brainstem (decerebration). Behavior in these animals is completely dependent on the sensory input: No organized foraging occurs. The taste reactivity test has enabled study of reflexive eating in rats and mice (Grill & Norgren, 1978) and is analogous to taste-related emotive facial expressions shown by newborn humans who have no prior experience with the taste (Forestell & Mennella, 2017).

In one of the first neural models of feeding, Stellar (1954) proposed that both internal chemical (interoceptive) signals and external sensory (exteroceptive) stimuli are integrated by mechanisms excitatory to feeding (i.e., producing hunger) and inhibitory to feeding (i.e., producing satiety). The net outcome from these two hypothetical mechanisms determines when and how much feeding occurs. Contemporary evidence-based theoretical models of feeding typically include a homeostatic or metabolic need component interfacing with an environmentally sensitive reward system and, in some models, an executive control network (Neseliler et al., 2019). Much of what we know about the hindbrain and reward systems has come from work with rats and mice using surgical, chemical, and other procedures that are not feasible in humans. Most of the information about executive control, and to some extent reward, has come from fMRI studies in humans.

The Hypothalamus and Feeding

Stellar's model was built on findings that experimental damage to the ventromedial part of the hypothalamus (VMH) greatly increased food intake and led to extreme obesity in animals. This syndrome has some similarities to the voracious appetite in humans with Frohlich's syndrome, in which tumors invade the VMH. Conversely, lesion of the lateral hypothalamus (LH) caused a syndrome of reduced or absent eating (aphagia) and dramatic weight loss. This led Stellar to propose that the VMH was a satiety center (i.e., damage to it impairs satiety), and the LH is a hunger center (i.e., damage to it impairs expression of hunger).

Today, the arcuate nucleus, which is a small egg-shaped region at the midline base or bottom of the VMH (usually damaged by the aforementioned VMH lesions), is known to be critical in the transduction or sensing of interoceptive, blood-borne hormones related to feeding. Two main types of cells, distinguished by the peptide transmitters that they express, are involved in this transduction. The first of these that we will examine in detail express agouti-related peptide (AgRP), and most if not all of these cells express a second transmitter, neuropeptide Y (NPY). Neurons in the second class express the pro-opiomelanocortin (POMC) gene and produce the transmitter α-MSH that engages melanocortin type 4 receptors (MC4R) in some brain regions.

To get you oriented with the mouse brain, Figure 5.2 is a simplified schematic showing some of the structures we will mention in this section. Let's start with the AgRP neurons in the arcuate nucleus. How do we know they are involved in hunger? One key finding is that progressively more of them are activated as the duration of fasting increases. Activation is often measured by the activity-dependent expression of a gene (*c-fos*) in the nuclei of most cells and subsequent production of a protein called Fos. Fos (and many other proteins) is commonly detected by incubating thin brain slices with an antibody that attaches with high selectivity to the protein of interest and, after a secondary chemical reaction, can be visualized under a microscope. Such immunochemical methods can be "stacked" so that, in this particular example, cells may be reacted sequentially with antibodies to AgRP and Fos, and co-localization would mean that the Fos was induced specifically in AgRP cells. A second key finding is that experimentally stimulating these AgRP cells in non-fasted mice using optogenetics induces immediate feeding, and that ceases as soon as the stimulus is removed. And third, these cells have receptors for leptin, ghrelin, and other metabolic hormones that access them from blood and modulate their activity (Belgardt et al., 2009).

And now things start to get complicated! In mice, there are about 10,000 AgRP neurons in the arcuate nucleus (on the left and right sides). But, they are not all doing the same thing, and it would be massively redundant for a small mouse brain to use this many neurons for the same task. Recent optogenetic findings show that AgRP neurons in different parts of the arcuate nucleus send axonal connections to different parts of the brain and have different functions (Betley et al., 2013; Padilla et al., 2016). The first such connection studied, which we will describe in more detail below, is to the paraventricular nucleus of the hypothalamus (PVH). Betley et al. (2013) estimated that about 30% of arcuate AgRP neurons project to the PVH, and activation of these axonal projections stimulates feeding in the same way as activation of arcuate cell bodies. Slightly less than 20% of the arcuate neurons project to the bed nucleus of the stria terminalis (BST), and they, too, support feeding behavior when stimulated. Some projections to the lateral hypothalamus also support feeding, but several relatively minor (<5%) projections are less or completely ineffective in this regard.

The AgRP arcuate cells projecting to terminals in the PVH have been studied extensively. In addition to using AgRP as a transmitter, these cells co-release neuropeptide Y (NPY) and gamma-aminobutyric acid (GABA) when action potential(s) arrive in the PVH. Tiny injections of NPY or GABA into the PVH of satiated rodents engage receptors on cells in the PVH and stimulate feeding. (At the level of electrical potentials, transmitters can have either an excitatory-depolarizing action or an inhibitory-hyperpolarizing action on cells. In this case, both NPY and GABA electrically inhibit PVH cells but stimulate feeding: Electrical potential change, not direction of change, is the key principle.) AgRP itself has a somewhat different function, blocking activation of MC4R receptors that mediate satiety (see below; that is, they play a "double negative" role vis-à-vis feeding).

Another prominent class of cells in the arcuate nucleus and projecting to the PVH express the proopiomelanocortin (POMC) gene, and one of the protein products from this gene is alpha melanocyte stimulating hormone (α-MSH), which acts as a transmitter in the PVH. It does so by acting on the MC4R receptors, mentioned previously, to inhibit feeding. We have already noted that AgRP blocks the MC4Rs, meaning that it prevents the action of α-MSH at these receptors. These POMC neurons in the arcuate nucleus are modulated by circulating hormonal signals related to energy balance in a manner opposite to the AgRP cells, but, unexpectedly, optogenetic stimulation of POMC cells for up to a few hours does not inhibit food intake. Using a different (chemical) method for selective stimulation of these cells, Zhan et al. (2013) showed that food intake did not decline until the second or third day of treatment. Thus, this feeding inhibitory system seems to work with a delay or longer time-course.

Thus far, we have identified fast-acting hunger and slow-acting satiety mechanisms in the arcuate-to-PVH projections. How would short-term satiation or satiety be represented? To date, at least three answers have been proposed. First, an additional fast-acting satiety projection from arcuate nucleus to PVH has been identified, using glutamate as a transmitter (Fenselau et al., 2017). Second, it has been shown that, as soon as the act of feeding begins, activity of the arcuate AgRP and POMC neurons is reversed (Chen et al., 2015). Third, in addition to the arcuate nucleus, another set of POMC cells is found in the NST: Chemical activation of these cells suppresses food intake in the short term (Zhan et al., 2013), and these authors suggest that POMC cells in the NST inhibit food intake via modulation of short-term mechanisms, such as gut-vagal afferents, while those in the arcuate nucleus mediate longer-term effects (e.g., relating to leptin).

As we stated at the start of this section, our purpose is to give you a "flavor" of the complexity of just one area of the hypothalamus in feeding. Other systems are known to be implicated, but we feel those would not add to the basic concepts about how the brain manages feeding.

FOOD FOR THOUGHT

Food Allergies

Food allergies are part of a more general category of adverse food reactions. Adverse reactions in the toxic category include digestive enzyme defects, such as in lactose intolerance, while those in the pharmacological category include abnormal reactions to agents such as capsaicin or ethanol. Adverse reactions in the non-toxic category are immune-mediated and may be classified into four types, mediated by various immunoglobulins (Ig) of which Type 1, mediated by IgE in response to food allergens, is common; food-induced IgE is often used as a diagnostic measure for this type of food allergy. Also common is Type IV hypersensitivity, caused by T cell responses to specific antigens such as gluten and associated with celiac disease.

In developed countries, IgE-associated food allergy affects 3–8% of children and 1–3% of adults. It has significant effects on an individual's dietary habits and social life. Milk, eggs, wheat, peanuts, nuts, sesame, fish, fruits, and vegetables are common inducers of IgE-associated food allergy. Allergies to foods such as milk, egg, and wheat often are outgrown (patients acquire tolerance), whereas allergies to peanuts, tree nuts, and fish allergies often persist over a lifetime. The prevalence and severity of food allergies seem to be increasing. In addition to genetic factors, a number of environmental, cultural, and behavioral factors affect the frequency, severity, and type of allergic manifestations in patients. One hypothesis for this is related to hygiene: Decreases in family size and improvements in personal hygiene have contributed to the increased prevalence of IgE-mediated allergies. Another hypothesis is that insufficient exposure to natural foods containing dietary and bacterial metabolites might have contributed to increases in inflammatory disorders. Many foods become allergenic because of interaction with the gastrointestinal system, but, with time, the allergen may directly permeate the mucosa and into the bloodstream, and this can also cause allergic responses due to skin contact or inhalation. Some of these responses, which range from eczema to anaphylactic shock, occur soon after exposure, while others may take hours.

There are no good treatments for food allergies, and the most common strategy is avoidance. In addition to avoiding direct ingestion, some food manufacturers now disclose that their factories or equipment may have had prior contact with allergens such as nuts, and some schools ban children from bring their own (unregulated) food items to school. Do you have a food allergy, or do you know someone who does? What behavioral strategies do you/they employ to reduce contact?

Hedonic Mechanisms and Feeding

When you start to consume food, there is often a short warm-up or appetition (Sclafani, 2013) phase during which the rate of intake accelerates to a steady rate. Later, as satiation approaches, eating rate often declines and, when eating stops, it is operationally zero. Aside from nutrient-related mechanisms of hunger and satiety that we discussed previously, the sensory experience of food changes over this time-course. The decrease in the pleasantness and ultimately the acceptability of a given food late in a meal or bout of ingestive behavior is known as negative alliesthesia. In fact, to functionally avoid negative alliesthesia, many cuisines employ both variety and a sequencing of foods that progresses from savory to sweet.

The ventral tegmental area (VTA) contains dopaminergic neurons that project rostrally to the nucleus accumbens and parts of the prefrontal cortex. Berridge and Kringelbach (2015) have conceptualized these dopaminergic systems as one of several distributed brain systems that are especially active during appetitive phases and linked to incentive salience of food or to a state of wanting. In contrast, a state of liking or pleasure is thought to be mediated by a smaller set of loci within these larger systems.

To demonstrate this, Castro and Berridge (2014) used previous observations that neurons in the nucleus accumbens have receptors for opioid peptide transmitters that are released either from local interneurons (consequent to dopamine stimulation) or input from other brain regions. Stimulation of opioid receptors in the nucleus accumbens by micro-injections of opioid agonist (mimicking) drugs is known to increase food intake. In their experiments, rats were surgically implanted with bilateral cannulas (small injection tubes) that, in different rats, were aimed at different parts of the nucleus accumbens. After full recovery from surgery, hedonic liking was assessed by a palatable sucrose solution being slowly infused into the rats' mouths, with appetitive (swallowing) responses being recorded. On separate days, these responses were measured after injection of vehicle (or placebo) or after a single dose of agonists of three subtypes of opioid receptor (mu, kappa, delta). The principal result was that injections into an approximately 1-mm^3 region (about 10% of the total size of the nucleus) of the medio-frontal part of the nucleus accumbens produced a large increase in liking responses when treated with any of the three agents, relative to vehicle. This region was termed a hedonic hotspot. Identical injections into more posterior parts of the nucleus accumbens decreased the liking responses, and this region was termed a hedonic cold spot.

In a subsequent but procedurally similar study examining cortical sites, Castro and Berridge (2017) found that micro-injections of a mu receptor agonist drug into the anterior orbital frontal cortex (part of the PFC, Figure 5.2) and into the posterior insula were consistent with hotspots, and that cortical sites in between were cold spots. Further, by examining patterns of activation (Fos protein) throughout the brain after micro-injections into these cortical hotspots, they were able to demonstrate activation of a circuit linking hotspots in several regions, including the nucleus accumbens. Conversely, injections into the cortical cold spots revealed a circuit linking cold spots in other brain regions. Collectively, these data indicate that reward systems are not homogeneous with respect to liking. We do not have space to contrast the corresponding neuroanatomy of wanting (or food intake), but that also differs from the liking circuitry.

You might be left wondering how the need or hunger-based circuits and signals integrate with the hedonic components, if at all. This is an area of intense investigation, but it is probably important to know that several parts of this "reward" system also contain receptors for hormones such as leptin, ghrelin, and insulin (Ferrario et al., 2016).

QUESTIONS TO ASK YOURSELF

Let's review and apply your knowledge. Take some time to answer these chapter questions.

- What do you understand by the theoretical dual mechanism approach to feeding? Today, which signal molecule(s) best exemplify this approach?
- Describe the discovery and implications of hedonic hotspots and cold spots.

- Does fMRI tell us about real-time activity of single neurons? If not, what are its limitations?
- Describe four main regions of the cerebral cortex that have been implicated in feeding, and in which specific aspect(s)?

GLOSSARY

Agouti-related peptide (AgRP)	A peptide hormone found in neurons in the hypothalamus and other brain regions, generally stimulating food intake.
Alliesthesia	The change in sensory pleasure with continued presentation of a stimulus such as a specified food. Negative alliesthesia is the decline in pleasure/ palatability as ingestion proceeds.
Alpha melanocyte stimulating hormone (α-MSH)	A small peptide cleaved from its POMC parent or precursor and inhibitory to feeding.
Aphagia	Complete absence or loss of feeding when it would normally occur.
Arcuate nucleus	Small bilateral midline structure at the base of the hypothalamus that is prominently involved in transducing blood-borne signals related to feeding.
Bed nucleus of stria terminalis (BST)	A loosely clustered series of neuron groups located around a fiber tract, the stria terminalis, in the limbic system of the brain.
Blood oxygenation level-dependent (BOLD)	The raw signal related to spin of protons in a high magnetic field used to determine metabolic activity of a region in fMRI.
Dietary restraint	Cognitive strategies that people may use to overcome more impulsive eating behaviors, including those relating to amount consumed and particular food types.

Functional magnetic resonance imaging (fMRI)	A method for non-invasive imaging of neural activity in the human brain based on amount of oxygen extracted in unit time for metabolic use (BOLD).
Fos or c-Fos	The product of a gene (*fos*) that is expressed when a neuron is highly activated and, in combination with immunochemistry, can be used to identify activated regions of the brain in thinly sliced tissue with single-cell resolution.
Frohlich's syndrome	A clinical syndrome including symptoms of voracious overeating and eventual obesity due to a tumor encroaching on the medial hypothalamus.
Hedonic hotspots and cold spots	Circumscribed regions in larger areas of the brain that are traditionally thought to be involved in motivation and reward processing. Hotspots (or circuits) have a positive valence in this regard, and cold spots have a negative valence.
Hyperphagia	A term for overeating relative to an established norm.
Immunochemistry	A procedure by which the amount and/or location of a chemical (e.g., a peptide) can be determined, usually in several steps, using an antibody to recognize and bind to that chemical with high specificity.
Incentive salience	The cognitive process that is associated with "wanting" a substance or commodity in the environment. In particular, it motivates appetitive behavior.
Insular cortex	A division of the frontal cortex that is particularly involved in taste processing.
Melanocortin	A member of a group of hormones, including α-MSH, produced from POMC.
Nucleus accumbens	Also known as the ventral striatum, the nucleus accumbens is a region beneath, but contiguous with, the striatum; it is rich in dopamine nerve terminals and is involved in reward processing.
Opioid receptor	One of several classes of receptor the natural ligands of which are endogenous opioids but which are potently engaged

	by specific drugs, including opiates such as morphine.
Orbital frontal cortex (OFC)	The side or lateral divisions of the frontal lobes of the cerebral cortex, thought to be a key integrative area for decision making (e.g., in relation to eating).
Paraventricular nucleus (of the hypothalamus – PVH)	A region of the hypothalamus above or dorsal to the ventromedial region receiving axonal input from (among other regions) the arcuate nucleus.
Pro-opiomelanocortin (POMC)	A peptide (gene transcript) produced in select regions of the brain including the hypothalamus, subsequently cleaved to α-MSH, which is inhibitory to feeding.
Ventral tegmental area (VTA)	A small midline region in the midbrain that contains dopamine-producing cells that project to the nucleus accumbens and are thought to be involved in reward.
Ventromedial hypothalamus (VMH)	The midline and ventral (bottom) region of the hypothalamus; damage (lesions) to this area produces hyperphagia and results in obesity.

REFERENCES

Belgardt, B. F., Okamura, T., & Bruning, J. C. (2009). Hormone and glucose signalling in POMC and AgRP neurons. *Journal of Physiology*, *587*, 5305–5314.

Berridge, K. C., & Kringelbach, M. L. (2015). Pleasure systems in the brain. *Neuron*, *86*, 646–664.

Betley, J. N., Cao, J. F. H., Ritola, K. D., & Sternson, S. M. (2013). Parallel, redundant circuit organization for homeostatic control of feeding behavior. *Cell*, *155*, 1337–1350.

Castro, D. C., & Berridge, K. C. (2014). Opioid hedonic hotspot in nucleus accumbens shell: Mu, delta and kappa maps for enhancement of sweetness "liking" and "wanting." *Journal of Neuroscience*, *34*, 4239–4250.

Castro, D. C., & Berridge, K. C. (2017). Opioid and orexin hedonic hotspots in rat orbitofrontal cortex and insula. *Proceedings of the National Academy of Sciences*, *114*, E9125–E9134.

Chen, Y., Lin, Y.-C., Kuo, T.-W., & Knight, Z. (2015). Sensory detection of food rapidly modulates arcuate feeding circuits. *Cell*, *160*, 829–841.

Emiliani V., Entcheva E., Hedrich R., et al. (2022). Optogenetics for light control of biological systems. *Nature Review Methods Primers*, *2*, 55. doi:10.1038/s43586-022-00136-4

Fenselau, H., Campbell, J. N., Verstegen, A. M. J., et al. (2017). A rapidly acting glutamatergic ARC-PVH satiety circuit postsynaptically regulated by α-MSH. *Nature Neuroscience*, *20*, 42–51.

Ferrario, C. R., Labouebe, G., Liu, S., et al. (2016). Homeostasis meets motivation in the battle to control food intake. *Journal of Neuroscience*, *36*, 11469–11481.

Forestell, C. A., & Mennella, J. A. (2017). The relationship between infant facial expressions and food acceptance. *Current Nutrition Reports*, *6* (2), 141–147. doi:10.1007/s13668-017-0205-y

Grill, H. J., & Norgren, R. (1978). The taste reactivity test. II. Mimetic responses to gustatory stimuli in chronic thalamic and chronic decerebrate rats. *Brain Research, 143* (2), 281–297. doi:10.1016/0006-8993(78)90569-3

Jiang, J., Cui, H., & Rahmouni, K. (2017). Optogenetics and pharmacogenetics: Principles and applications. *American Journal of Physiology Regulatory Integrative Comparative Physiology, 313,* R633–R645.

Neseliler, S., Hu, W., Larcher, K., et al. (2019). Neurocognitive and hormonal correlates of voluntary weight loss in humans. *Cell Metabolism, 29,* 1–11.

Padilla, S. L., Qiu, J., Soden, M. E., et al. (2016). Agouti-related peptide neural circuits mediate adaptive behaviors in the starved state. *Nature Neuroscience, 19,* 734–741.

Paxinos, G., & Franklin, K. B. J. (2001). *The mouse brain in stereotaxic coordinates,* 2nd ed. San Diego: Academic Press.

Roth, B. L. (2019). How structure informs and transforms chemogenetics. *Current Opinion in Structural Biology, 57,* 9–16.

Sclafani, A. (2013). Gut–brain nutrient signaling. Appetition vs. satiation. *Appetite, 71,* 454–458.

Stellar, E. (1954). The physiology of motivation. *Psychological Review, 61,* 5–22.

Zhan, C., Zhou, J., Feng, Q., et al. (2013). Acute and long-term suppression of feeding behavior by POMC neurons in the brainstem and hypothalamus, respectively. *Journal of Neuroscience, 33,* 3624–3632.

CHAPTER 6

Genetics, Epigenetics, and Microbiome

After reading this chapter, you will be able to

- Give examples of monogenic obesity and prevalence in human obesity.
- Understand polygenic obesity and identifying genes.
- Define epigenetics and its implications for obesity.
- Appreciate the gut microbiome and its implications for obesity and other diseases.

We introduce several concepts in this chapter that are linked by what we might consider to be internal or intrinsic factors in relation to obesity. The first concept is genetics, the inherited characteristics that might make one individual more or less prone to develop obesity than another. The second is epigenetics, the study of how gene expression is modified as a result of experience. And the third concerns the genes carried by the trillions of microbiota that live in our gastrointestinal system and participate in utilization of nutrients.

As we go through this chapter, it will become evident that much of the research in the field is devoted to addressing intrinsic factors that contribute to obesity. But, as a widespread population phenomenon, obesity is a relatively recent condition, whereas corresponding genomic changes take tens or hundreds of generations to become entrenched and are thus unlikely to be the sole culprits in obesity. That leaves at least two other possibilities: (1) Intrinsic factors of shorter modification time that either change the expression of, or bypass, our genome; (2) an interaction between genome or specific genes and the environment, the latter having changed rapidly. Finally, it should be emphasized that genes in complex organisms such as mammals do not determine an outcome; instead, they make certain outcome(s) more or less likely given a particular environment (Comfort, 2018). For example, one may have gene(s) favoring fat storage, but lipogenesis cannot occur without adequate food availability.

GENETICS

A Short Primer

Among the most critical and unique functional components of a cell are its proteins: Included among these are those proteins that enable a cell to have shape (structural proteins), to engage in chemical reactions (enzymatic proteins), and to communicate with its outside milieu, including other cells (membrane channels and receptors). Proteins are chains of amino

DOI: 10.4324/9781032621401-6

acids (of which there are 20) linked head-to-tail. The proteins mentioned above are typically several hundred amino acids in length and are folded into complex three-dimensional shapes. The amino acid complement making up these proteins ultimately determines a given protein's unique shape and unique function for a particular cell or cell type.

The essential instructions on how to assemble these proteins, in which cells, in what quantity, and when, are contained in the genome of an organism and coded in molecules of deoxynucleic acid (DNA). Long strands of DNA are coiled together as a double helix and are wrapped around proteins called histones within the nucleus of each somatic cell in an organism. Most organisms are called eukaryotes because their DNA is contained in a nucleus. DNA is constructed from molecules, called nucleotides, joined by chemical bonds in head-to-tail fashion within a strand. One part of each nucleotide is a nitrogenous base of which there are four possibilities (abbreviated to A, C, G, T). These constitute what is essentially a four-letter molecular alphabet, and, like written words, the precise nucleotide sequence imparts a specific "meaning" within the cell. The human genome consists of several billion nucleotides.

Probably only about 2% of the total DNA is involved in protein coding; some of the remaining 98% has other critical functions that we will not address. Genes are segments of DNA that are essential for protein coding: The human genome contains about 20,000 genes, and each gene encodes a specific protein. When a gene is actively making a protein, that gene is said to be expressed. Expression is a two-step sequence (Figure 6.1). The first, transcription, involves making a "working copy" which is called messenger ribonucleic acid (mRNA). The details of this process are beyond the present text, but when, and how many, copies of mRNA are made depend in part on the availability of that gene to the transcription machinery (see the following section on Epigenetics) and the presence of transcription factors that function as molecular switches. Thus, the "on and off" of gene transcription is controlled by several factors inside the cell. Once mRNA is formed, it leaves the nucleus for a process of translation; this is how the sequence of mRNA nucleotides is transformed into a sequence of amino acids, which is like a different molecular language. The "rule" of translation is a triplet code, according to which a sequence of three nucleotide bases (known as a codon) specifies a particular amino acid (a good animation can be viewed at: www.hhmi.org/biointeractive/triplet-code). There are also start and stop codons. The translation machinery effectively locates "start" on the mRNA, then reads off three bases at a time, and so assembles the amino acids into proteins until reaching stop.

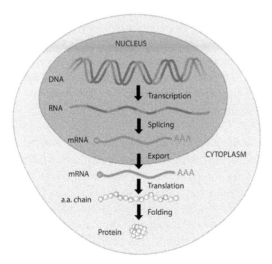

FIGURE 6.1 Sequential steps involved in gene expression, including transcription of DNA into RNA in the nucleus and translation of mRNA into proteins in the cytoplasm

Any given gene can have one or more variants called alleles. Different alleles encode slightly different proteins with usually modestly different functional properties (such as how efficiently an enzyme molecule performs its function). In addition to alleles, which are inherited variants, mistakes or errors of translation can occur, and these are called mutations. These mutations may arise naturally, but modern biology has given us tools to make intentional or directed mutations to specific genes, including so-called "knock-out" or "knock-in" animals – often mice – in which a specific gene is silenced or replaced. Mendelian genetics (so named after Gregor Mendel who, in the 19th century, established the fundamentals of inheritance) refers to a situation in which a particular trait is controlled by a single gene which exists as either dominant or non-dominant alleles. The trait exhibited by offspring is determined by the inherited dominant form. Let's now examine what is known about the gene mutations or alleles that affect body composition or predispose to obesity. Before doing so, we should point out that a given gene may encode a protein that contributes to a physiological process – for example, that of storage of excess food as adipose tissue – or may influence behavioral processes – for example, hunting or gathering skills. Thus, linking a particular gene or gene variant with a state of obesity does not tell us the mechanism (i.e., physiological or behavioral, both of which have many dimensions) of that linkage. Other functional studies, such as injecting the protein product into a donor, are needed to establish mechanism.

Single-Gene Approach and Monogenic Obesity

The traditional approach to genes and obesity was to consider single-gene mutations and then multi-gene (polygenic) mutations. More recently, it has become evident that the single-gene examples are better considered as special cases of the polygenic condition. In particular, because genes encode functional proteins, there are several ways in which a gene could affect the efficiency of that protein and thereby increase or decrease its normal function. In the case of body fat, those effects could include storage or mobilization of fat stores, changes in the signals from fat-derived hormones, and other effects. Twins reared apart show that body mass index (BMI) has a strong (up to 80%) inherited component (Allison et al., 1996; Stunkard et al., 1986). These analyses are statistical correlations determined in part by pairs of twins with similar BMI at the low and high ends of the spectrum – that is, they include both obese and non-obese pairs. To move from these demographic data to determine which genes are involved in the general population is not a simple step. For example, is your scientific question about rare alleles that give rise to large effects on BMI, or is it about commonly occurring alleles that have a small effect on BMI but may have an additive effect with other small-effect alleles in an individual (Gibson, 2015; Hendricks et al., 2017; Speakman et al., 2018)?

One experimental strategy is to study a restricted population that has a high probability of carrying a rare allele; early studies of this type usually focused on children who exhibit very high BMI, on the grounds that such early onset obesity has a high probability of a genetic component. Such studies (e.g., Hendricks et al., 2017) have identified a handful of alleles any one of which has a high penetrance or probability of producing the early-onset obese phenotype. Monogenic obesity is due to a single abnormal gene. A short-cut way of approaching this is to screen DNA for only one or a few genes/alleles in a so-called candidate gene approach, but this "knowing what you are looking for" approach often requires adequate animal models, as discussed below. Over the past decade, enormous advances in our ability to screen entire human genomes and investigate functional linkages has exploded (e.g., Loos & Yeo, 2022).

The strength of animal models is that they allow us to study one factor in relative isolation, an ideal that can rarely be met in a human population. A gene can be rendered non-functional either by a spontaneously occurring mutation or by genetic engineering, often using gene knock-out models. To simplify, in a knock-out organism, the functionality of a gene is interrupted so that it can no longer make a specific protein. In one spontaneously obese mutation in mice, called *ob/ob*, the phenotype or trait (obesity) was found to be the result of a recessive mutation: The obese phenotype arises owing to inheritance of two defective (-/-) copies of the *ob* gene from its parents. This occurs with a one-in-four chance with heterozygous parents who each carry one normal and one defective copy; at the same time, one in four littermates carry two normal copies (+/+). Mice typically have litters of eight or more pups, and so, on average, each litter will have two offspring who will have the -/- genotype and two who will have the +/+ genotype. (The other pups are called heterozygotes, or +/-, but, because the mutant gene is recessive, heterozygotes have more or less normal weight.) Subsequent studies showed the phenotype is caused by a mutation at a single nucleotide base in DNA that results in a premature "stop" codon in translation: The encoded protein is abnormally short and is nonfunctional.

Jeffrey Friedman and his colleagues (Zhang et al., 1994) identified the protein, now called leptin from Greek *leptos*, meaning thin, that is the normal product of this gene. Hence, this genetic mutation is now designated *lep-/-*, and the lean littermates are *lep+/+* (and the heterozygous litter mates are *lep+/-*). The *lep-/-* mice have normal birth weights but start to gain weight early in life; after they are weaned from their mothers, their weight gain is maintained by overeating and low physical activity. These mice also develop type 2 diabetes. In Chapter 5, we met some of the physiological function(s) of leptin, which is produced in rough proportion to the amount of body fat and acts in the brain as a signal to reduce eating. In the absence of this molecular brake, an important constraining mechanism on food intake is lost.

Every chemical signal, such as leptin, requires a receptor to exert its function. Thus, mutations of the receptor for leptin should produce a similar phenotype to *lep-/-*. Another spontaneous mouse mutation, called *db/db* for diabetes, was discovered at about the same time as *ob/ob*. Subsequent investigation showed the genetic mutation was in one type of leptin receptor (*lepRb-/-*) that transports leptin into the brain. Mice with this mutation produce leptin, but it is not able to access the relevant brain regions, resulting in a phenotype comparable in obesity to the *lep-/-* mice.

Are there examples of leptin-related mutations and obesity found in humans? Yes, but they are quite rare. Montague et al. (1997) identified three very obese children who had undetectable blood levels of leptin; the obesity exhibited by these children was reversed by chronic treatment with synthetic leptin. Mutations to the leptin receptor are slightly more common, occurring in up to 3% of early-onset severe obesity. Individuals with these mutations, much like the mice, have normal birth weights but start to gain weight abnormally fast within the first few months of life. They show increased food seeking and overeating at least into adolescence (for a review, see Ramachandrappa & Farooqi, 2011).

A different class of genetic mutations, which are causally associated with an obese phenotype, involves disruption of signaling in the brain mediated by melanocortin type 4 receptors

(MC4R). These receptors can be rendered dysfunctional in mice by gene knock-out (*mc4r-/-*). Since this melanocortin system, like leptin, normally inhibits food intake, impairment of function leads to a phenotype of overeating and eventual obesity. Equivalent loss-of-function mutations in the MC4 receptor in humans are associated with overeating and occur in about 5% of people with early-onset obesity (Ramachandrappa & Farooqi, 2011).

A handful of other alleles, with acronyms such as *ANGPTL6*, *FTO*, and *PACS1* (Hendricks et al., 2017; Pei et al., 2014; Wheeler et al., 2013), have been identified in early-onset obesity, but, unlike for leptin and MC4R, the exact functions of the encoded proteins have yet to be fully elucidated. Together, these monogenic defects account for only about 5% of severe childhood obesity – literally a thin slice out of the immense pie of obesity.

Multiple-Gene Approach and Polygenic Obesity

A potentially more useful but extremely demanding approach is to examine the entire genome for allelic variations and correlate the occurrence of the various alleles with BMI. This is called a genome-wide association (GWA) study and requires sample sizes of many thousands of humans to achieve statistically significant correlations. At the time of writing this chapter, more than 200 different obesity-related genes have been identified from several GWA studies (Speakman et al., 2018). These are most likely commonly occurring variants but each with small effect (Gibson, 2015), and, to achieve significant obesity, an individual would have to have several such allelic variants the effects of which either add up or interact with one another in such a way as to produce an obese phenotype. This is known as polygenic obesity, resulting from the additive or interactive effect of multiple genes.

Given the obvious complexity of this genetic information, you might be asking what the practical utility or significance of knowing which specific gene or genes are causing obesity is – other than the comfort achieved by saying "my genes made me fat"! Well, the hope is that the proteins encoded by the normal gene(s) will be "targetable" by therapeutic drugs. And, while that has been borne out insofar as administration of leptin reverses the *lep-/-* phenotype (i.e., those who are genetically incapable of producing leptin), other targets have as yet proven elusive for useful pharmacological intervention. Further, assuming that any intervention were to be substantially effective, then, because drugs (or other potential types of intervention such as gene therapy) all have risks or side effects and monetary cost, what would be an acceptable threshold BMI for a decision to treat? For these reasons, it is unlikely that gene-based information will be applicable in the foreseeable future except to the extremely obese. In Chapter 12, we will discuss the many other not-genetic strategies and treatments that have been used for weight loss.

EPIGENETICS

Epigenetics refers to changes, sometimes heritable, in gene expression or phenotype caused by mechanisms other than alterations in the nucleotide sequence of DNA. Such changes would not show up in the genetic screens discussed so far. The two well-established epigenetic mechanisms are methylation and histone modification (Figure 6.2). Methylation occurs when a methyl group is added to a specific DNA base(s) and interferes with the transcription of the gene. One of the apparent functions of the FTO gene (which encodes the fat mass and obesity associated protein) is to remove methyl groups from certain gene(s) and so influence the normal balance or ratio of translated proteins in the cell. Another epigenetic mechanism is the potential action of the vast non-coding regions of DNA on transcription of coding regions. One important difference between genetics and epigenetics is the time frame: Epigenetics plays out within the lifetime of an individual and is much more consistent with the time frame for the rapid, population-wide increase in BMI.

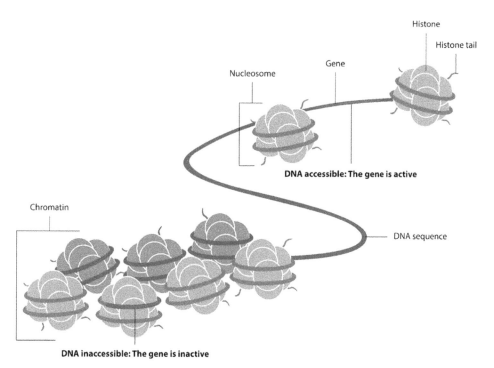

FIGURE 6.2 Illustration of how epigenetic events such as acetylation or methylation affect the unfolding of genes from histone carriers and, hence, whether the DNA in that gene can be expressed

One of the first demonstrations of epigenetic influence came from an examination of Dutch health records: Children who were born in 1940 during the severe war-related famine, with inferred under-nutrition, had higher incidence of overweight or obesity in middle age compared with children born without early-life under-nutrition (Eckel, 2008). This observation spawned controlled animal experiments to test the hypothesis that food restriction during sensitive periods early in life (prenatally and/or early postnatally) would predispose those offspring to be more vulnerable to becoming overweight or obese when food was subsequently plentiful. This concept of developmental programming means that, through stable epigenetic changes, early-life events permanently modify gene expression and thereby lead to different phenotypes in adolescence or adulthood.

Many such animal models also demonstrate genetic or epigenetic interaction with diet. That is, the overeating and obesity only occur with particular diet(s), and these are almost always – you guessed it – high fat. Usually, the animals in question are fed a single diet – for example, high fat in experimental group(s) and low fat in control group(s) – although similar results are often obtained when animals are given access to a variety of foods of varying fat content – a so-called cafeteria diet. Of course, humans almost always have this latter type of diet choice and, at a population-wide level, tend to choose relatively high-fat diets. Thus, although diet is not a controlled factor, many if not most of the humans in the GWA studies mentioned above have diet-related obesity. Since we often impose our own lifestyles on domestic pets (i.e., dogs and cats), it is no surprise that these companion animals are also undergoing an obesity epidemic (Klimentisis et al., 2010).

In mice, there are well-known strain differences in their susceptibility to dietary obesity (West & York, 1998). However, within an ostensibly identical cohort of mice of the B6 strain, Koza et al. (2006) noted substantial individual variability in their propensity to diet-induced obesity. They reasoned that this must be because of individual epigenetically programmed differences and went on to show that the expression of certain genes in fat tissue and in the brain differed among individuals in proportion to their vulnerability to obesity. In rats, it has been shown that propensity to obesity on a high-fat diet is a heritable characteristic. Starting with a commonly used outbred stock strain (Sprague-Dawley), Levin and his colleagues (1997) noticed that some individuals gained more weight than others when fed a moderate-fat diet. He then bred the high-gaining males with high-gaining females for a few generations; most of the resulting offspring then showed a propensity to diet-induced obesity (obesity-prone line). Conversely, when low-gaining males and females were bred for several generations, most of the offspring did not gain much weight on the same diet and so were termed obesity resistant. The concept of dietary resistance provides a different perspective on genes and obesity. The single-gene and GWA approaches referred to earlier are almost all focused on finding alleles or mutations that are associated with human obesity and/or vulnerability to obesity. But there is an assumption that the default condition is lean. If, instead, as we have argued earlier in the book, obesity is a natural biological response to an obesogenic food environment, then it is resistance to obesity that is exceptional and worthy of our attention. Humans probably have additional mechanisms for cognitive resistance available, including body image and dietary restraint (see Chapter 12).

To summarize this section, epigenetic mechanisms operate to modify the expression of the human genome over relatively short periods of time as well as, in some cases, transmission across generations (i.e., resulting in heritable traits).

MICROBIOME

We are not alone. This is not a reference to extraterrestrial life or a movie, but to the trillions of "old friends" that live inside each and every one of us (for a review, see Liang et al., 2018). Humans have been referred to as superorganisms who carry a variety of microorganisms, such as bacteria and fungi, which live and reproduce on our internal and external surfaces. We will restrict this discussion to microorganisms that live in the digestive tract – gut microbiota. A typical human gut contains between 300 and 3,000 different species of commensal microbiota, each with its own genome, and it has been estimated that their total number is 100 trillion. Thus, both the genetic diversity and number of the microbiota exceed the host-specific (viz., human-specific) counterparts by orders of magnitude. Of course, as their name implies, they are very small and collectively weigh about 1 kg. Only within the past few years have we started to appreciate and unravel the implications of the gut microbiome for human health, including variation in BMI.

It should first be recognized that these gut microbiota eat, quite literally, what we eat. The amount of energy they consume is quite small, and they often are able to extract energy from ingested material that we normally cannot digest, such as dietary fiber. But, to some extent, which microbiota flourish and which do not depends in part on the food or diet that we eat. Further, the microbiota are not homogeneously distributed throughout our gut: In general, more and different species inhabit the lower gut or intestine than the upper regions. In general, the number and diversity of bacterial species decreases with high-fat or refined diets. Table 6.1 summarizes some principal species of microbiota and how they change with a high-fat diet. In rodents, some changes are evident within one week of switching from low- to high-fat diets, while more extended exposure to the diet leads to a partial breakdown of the barrier between the lumen of the gut (which is functionally still outside of the human) and body tissue, with subsequent passage of bacterial components into the body. These are believed to precipitate a low-grade inflammatory response as well as decreased signaling from gut to brain via the vagus nerve (Figure 6.3; see also Chapter 5 and Hamilton & Raybould, 2016; Liang et al., 2018).

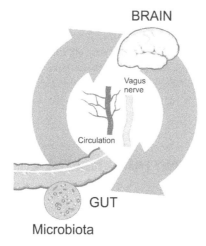

FIGURE 6.3 Representation of how microbiota in the gut can affect the brain via the circulation or vagus nerve, especially in relation to food intake, and how food choices (and other influences of brain origin) affect the microbiota

TABLE 6.1 Select gut microbiota under different dietary conditions		
Diet	*Upper intestine*	*Lower intestine*
Low fat	Clostridiaceae family* Firmicutes Proteobacteria	Prevotella* Bacteriodetes
High fat	Lactococcus* Firmicutes (reduced)	Bacteriodetes* Archaea (reduced)

* Indicates the most abundant species; (reduced) indicates lower levels on a high-fat diet.

Source: Simplified from Figure 4.1 of Hamilton and Raybould (2016).

Mancabelli et al. (2017) performed a meta-analysis of gut microbiomes from individuals from two remaining pre-agricultural or hunter-gatherer civilizations (in Peru and Tanzania) and from several developed/industrialized countries. All of the populations contained 22 species of microbes – the core microbiota – but, significantly, this core represented 82% of all microbiota in the industrialized samples but only 47% in the pre-agricultural samples. On the other hand, 15 "accessory microbiota" accounted for 11% and 40% of the total, respectively. These data suggest that a greater reliance on germ-free food and a lesser reliance on fibrous and/or less processed food, which are often characteristics of urbanized/industrialized diets, is associated with attenuated gut microbiome diversity or number.

What are the consequences of an altered microbiome for metabolism and obesity? Several studies in rodents have shown a relationship between weight change and microbiome. One way in which this can be studied is to perform microbiota transplantation, also known as fecal microbiota transplantation (FMT). This is not quite as gross as it sounds – the bacteria are extracted and purified first! In one such study, starting with germ-free mice (bred in a sterile environment to be devoid of microorganisms), Turnbaugh and colleagues (2006) performed FMT from either obese *lep-/-* or lean *lep+/+* mice, allowed the recipient mice to eat a low-fat diet for two weeks, then examined various physiological end points. Despite the fact that both groups ate exactly the same amount of food, those receiving FMT from obese donors gained twice as much body fat as those receiving FMT from lean donors, an increase estimated to be equivalent to 2% of the total energy consumed during those two weeks. The actual increase in fat tissue in the two groups was 1.3 g versus 0.86 g (about 5% and 3% of total body weight, respectively), and, while that may not sound like a lot, over this short period of time it is (Box 6.1).

BOX 6.1 OF MICE AND HUMANS: THE CUMULATIVE EFFECT OF NUDGES

An adult mouse weighs about 30 g, whereas an adult human weighs about 60 kg – an approximately 2,000-fold difference. A mouse living in the welfare state of a laboratory with all-you-can-eat chow lives about 2 years; modern humans live at least 60 years – approximately 30 times longer. So, is a 2-week experiment showing change in weight of mice (see the text) the equivalent of 30 times 2 weeks (i.e., about a year) in humans, or something different? "Scaling" issues like this don't have any great or universally accepted answers, but one fact on which we should all agree is that long-lived species have much more time over which to accumulate small changes or effects (nudges) than do short-lived species. For example, suppose that a mouse gains 1% body weight per year: Late in life, they would only weigh 2% more than they did as young adults, an insignificant change. But a 20-year-old human weighing 70 kg (150 lbs; BMI perhaps a lean 22 kg/m^2) and thereafter showing a 1% increase per year would, by age 70, weigh 105 kg (225 lbs; BMI classified as obese at 33 kg/m^2). Given that math, do not underestimate the powerful cumulative effect of dietary or other nudges!

The gut microbiota have many functions, including production of small molecules that can either act as receptors in the gut wall or diffuse across the gut wall, thereby affecting the gut–brain signaling in the host. Short chain fatty acids (SCFAs, such as butyric acid) are one class of molecules that are produced by several species of microbiota and are known to affect the gut barrier and nervous and immune systems of the host. These, in turn, can not only affect signaling in and to the adult brain but also, importantly, have developmental consequences. For example, vaginal birth and/or breastfeeding introduce the newborn to a variety of microbiota that populate its gut and have effects on brain growth and maturation. In contrast, caesarean delivery and/or bottle-feeding lead to a markedly different microbiome (Bokulich et al., 2016) with potential effects on early neural development (Liang et al., 2018). FMT as a therapy for an altered or dysfunctional gut microbiome has been used, but prebiotic or probiotic foods sound more attractive! Prebiotics are foods such as dietary fiber that are designed to nourish beneficial microbiota. Probiotics are typically fermented foods such as yogurt designed to introduce specific microbiota to populate or repopulate the gut.

To summarize this section, the gut microbiome is vast, and it changes both developmentally and as a function of diet both within a lifetime (e.g., fat content in one's diet) and as a function of overall lifestyle (e.g., rural versus urban living). Although some of the reported changes may be small (i.e., nudges), cumulated over time they provide a genetic mechanism separate from the host (human genome) that can respond relatively quickly to environmental change.

QUESTIONS TO ASK YOURSELF

Let's review and apply your knowledge. Take some time to answer these chapter questions:

- Distinguish between transcription and translation.
- Explain why, in relation to obesity, epigenetics may occur over a shorter time frame than genetics.
- Discuss the relative merits, and drawbacks or limitations, of the approaches that have been applied to the genetics of human obesity.
- Describe the potential contribution of the microbiome to eating and obesity.
- Distinguish between prebiotic and probiotic interventions.

GLOSSARY

Allele	One of two or more alternative forms (sequences) of a gene that are found at the same place on a given chromosome.
Candidate gene	A gene that has allelic form(s) suspected to be involved in expression of a specific phenotype.

Deoxynucleic acid (DNA)	A self-replicating chemical material that is the main constituent of chromosomes. It exists as two strands that wind themselves into a double helix structure.
Developmental programming	Refers to the concept that events during prenatal and/or early postnatal periods can have lasting effects on the adult phenotype, in part through epigenetic mechanisms.
Epigenetics	The study of changes in phenotype caused by modification of the expression of genes, not by alteration of the genome or genetic code per se.
Expression (gene)	Describes the production or appearance of a characteristic (phenotype, protein) that is due to the transcription and translation of a given gene.
Genetics	The study of heredity and variation of characteristics (e.g., as inherited from parents).
Genome	The complete set of genes and chromosomes present in a cell or organism.
Genome-wide association	Describes a study, usually in very large numbers of subjects, in which genomic characteristic(s) are correlated or associated with one or more phenotypes.
Gut microbiota	Describes the species and amounts of bacterial or other microorganisms that inhabit particular regions of the human gastrointestinal tract, or gut.
Histones	Chemically basic proteins found in the nucleus of cells and around which DNA is wound.
Leptin	A protein (of the class called cytokines) produced by fat tissue that regulates fat storage.
Melanocortins	A class of hormones and/or neurotransmitter molecules that act via specific receptors (MCs) to produce a variety of effects, including inhibiting appetite.
Methylation	A chemical modification (adding methyl group) that, when it occurs in DNA, modifies the binding of DNA to histones and thereby site-specific gene transcription.
Microbiome	Refers to the vast array of microorganisms that are symbiotic with the host (e.g., human being).
Monogenic obesity	Obesity that can be attributed to mutation of a single gene.

Mutation	In genetics refers to alteration of one or more base units in DNA that leads to modification in the functional output of a gene.
Obesity prone (or resistant)	Refers to a genetic background that predisposes an individual to becoming obese (or resisting obesity) when presented with an obesogenic diet such as a high-fat one.
Penetrance	The extent to which particular gene(s) are expressed in the phenotype.
Phenotype	The set of observable characteristics of an individual resulting from (lifelong) interaction of the genome with the environment.
Polygenic obesity	Obesity that is due to the combined or summed effect of several genes, each with small effect.
Prebiotic	In the host organism, a non-digestible food ingredient that promotes the growth of (usually) beneficial microorganisms in the gut.
Probiotic	A food ingredient that introduces specific microorganism(s) to the gut of the host.
Short chain fatty acids (SCFAs)	Organic acids, such as acetic, propionic, or butyric, that function as signal molecules and are manufactured in the intestine by gut microbiota.
Transcription	The process by which a sequence of DNA nucleotides is copied in a template-like fashion into molecules of RNA.
Transcription factor	An intracellular chemical that binds to DNA and initiates transcription.
Translation	The process by which successive triplet sequences of mRNA are assembled into chains of amino acids, as dictated by the specific sequence.
Vagus nerve	A mixed nerve (sensory and motor) that runs to and from nuclei in the brainstem to various organs in the thoracic cavity. Relevant to feeding, various chemical and mechanical sensory signals from the gut activate vagus nerve endings.

REFERENCES

Allison, D. B., Kaprio, J., Korkeila, M., et al. (1996). The heritability of body mass index among an international sample of monozygotic twins reared apart. *International Journal of Obesity and Related Metabolic Disorders, 20*, 501–506.

Bokulich, N. A., Chung, J., Battaglia, T., et al. (2016). Antibiotics, birth mode, and diet shape microbiome maturation during early life. *Science and Translational Medicine, 8*, 343.

Comfort, N. (2018). Genetic determinism rides again. *Nature, 561* (7723), 461–464.

Eckel, R. H. (2008). Obesity research in the next decade. *International Journal of Obesity, 32,* S143–S151.

Gibson, G. (2015). Rare and common variants: Twenty arguments. *Nature Reviews Genetics, 13,* 135–145.

Hamilton, M. K., & Raybould, H. E. (2016). Bugs, guts and brains and the regulation of food intake and body weight. *International Journal of Obesity Supplements, 6,* S8–14.

Hendricks, A. E., Bochukova, E. G., Marenne, G., et al. (2017). Rare variant analyses of human and rodent obesity genes in individuals with severe childhood obesity. *Scientific Reports, 7,* 4394.

Klimentisis, Y. C., Beasley, T. M., Lin, H. Y., et al. (2010). Canaries in the coal mine: A cross-species analysis of the plurality of obesity epidemics. *Proceedings of the Royal Society Series B, 278,* 1626–1632.

Koza, R. A., Nikonova, L., Hogan, J., et al. (2006). Changes in gene expression foreshadow diet-induced obesity in genetically identical mice. *PLOS Genetics, 2,* e81.

Levin, B. E., Dunn-Meynell, A. A., Balkan, B., & Keesey, R. E. (1997). Selective breeding for diet-induced obesity and resistance in Sprague-Dawley rats. *American Journal of Physiology: Regulatory, Integrative and Comparative Physiology, 273,* R725–R730.

Liang, S., Wu, X., & Jin, F. (2018). Gut-brain psychology: Rethinking psychology from the microbiota-gut-brain axis. *Frontiers in Integrative Neuroscience, 12,* 33.

Loos, R. J., & Yeo, G. S. (2022). The genetics of obesity: From discovery to biology. *Nature Reviews Genetics, 23* (2), 120–133.

Mancabelli, L., Milani, C., Lugli, G., et al. (2017). Meta-analysis of the human gut microbiome from urbanized and pre-agricultural populations. *Environmental Microbiology, 19,* 1379–1390.

Montague, C. T., Farooqi, I. S., Whitehead, J. P., et al. (1997). Congenital leptin deficiency is associated with severe early onset obesity in humans. *Nature, 387,* 903–908.

Pei, Y.-F., Zhang, L., Liu, Y., et al. (2014). Meta-analysis of genome-wide association data identifies novel susceptibility loci for obesity. *Human Molecular Genetics, 23,* 820–830.

Ramachandrappa, S., & Farooqi, I. S. (2011). Genetic approaches to understanding human obesity. *Journal of Clinical Investigation, 121,* 2080–2086.

Speakman, J. R., Loos, R. J. F., O'Rahilly, S., et al. (2018). GWAS for BMI: A treasure trove of fundamental insights into the genetic basis of obesity. *International Journal of Obesity, 42,* 1524–1531.

Stunkard, A. J., Foch, T. T., & Hrubec, Z. (1986). A twin study of human obesity. *Journal of the American Medical Association, 256,* 51–54.

Turnbaugh, P. J., Ley, R. E., Mahowald, M. A., et al. (2006). An obesity-associated gut microbiome with increased capacity for energy harvest. *Nature, 444,* 1027–1031.

West, D. B., & York, B. (1998). Dietary fat, genetic predisposition, and obesity: Lessons from animal models. *American Journal of Clinical Nutrition, 67* (Suppl. 3), 505S–512S.

Wheeler, E., Huang, N., Bochukova, E., et al. (2013). Genome-wide SNP and CNV analysis identifies common and low frequency variants associated with severe early-onset obesity. *Nature Genetics, 45,* 513–517.

Zhang, Y., Proenca, R., Maffei, M., Barone, M., Leopold, L., & Friedman, J. M. (1994). Positional cloning of the mouse obese gene and its human homologue. *Nature, 372,* 425–432.

CHAPTER 7

Basic Learning Processes and Eating Behavior

After reading this chapter, you will be able to

- Understand the role of associative learning in eating behavior and its practical implications.
- Know how food preferences and aversions are formed.
- Appreciate that knowing when to start and stop eating is shaped by learning.
- Understand the neurobiology of food learning.

Learning can occur in many ways. Several forms of basic associative learning have been identified in eating behavior research as having particular relevance to the development of food likes and dislikes and the establishment of meal patterns (i.e., amount, timing, and rituals of meals and food selection). The types of learning explored in this chapter are rooted in classical (or Pavlovian) conditioning. This basic form of learning shapes many human and animal behaviors, and the effects can be long-lasting. Before we explore this further, take a moment and imagine going to a movie theater for the premiere of a movie you've been looking forward to seeing. What foods are you likely to want? For some people, it is nearly unthinkable to watch a movie in a theater without eating popcorn or candy. Or to watch a favorite show on Netflix without snacking. Why are these associations so pervasive? Associative learning, as you will see in this chapter, is quite easy to identify and very influential on our eating behaviors.

OVERVIEW OF CLASSICAL CONDITIONING AND ITS TERMINOLOGY

Classical conditioning is a type of basic associative learning in which a stimulus that has previously been neutral (or meaningless) to the animal or person comes to elicit a response that another stimulus naturally elicits. Let's briefly review the research of Ivan Pavlov (Image 7.1), the Russian physiologist who won a Nobel Prize in 1904 for his research on digestion in dogs. Dogs naturally salivate when food – or, in the case of Pavlov's studies, meat powder – reaches their mouths. This is an innate or reflexive response requiring no learning. Pavlov found that his dogs started salivating before the food was delivered to their mouths. For example, they salivated when someone entered the room or neared the food storage area. This salivation, Pavlov realized, was a result of

DOI: 10.4324/9781032621401-7

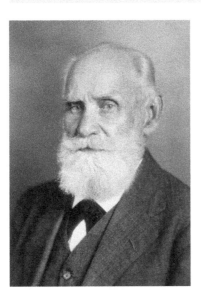

IMAGE 7.1 Nobel-Prize-winning physiologist Ivan Pavlov

learning. The dogs *learned* that, when their handler neared the food storage area, food would soon be delivered. Pavlov conducted many carefully designed studies to more precisely determine the specifics around this type of learning, now known as classical or Pavlovian conditioning. In one well-known example, Pavlov conditioned the dogs to salivate at the sound of a metronome, a clicking device used by musicians to mark rhythm. Metronomes are not usually associated with food, and so salivation at their clicking is certainly not an instinctive behavior.

In formal learning terminology, before the conditioning process begins, meat powder is an unconditioned stimulus (UCS), because dogs naturally salivate at it, salivation is the unconditioned response (UCR), and the metronome is a neutral stimulus (NS) eliciting no salivation (Figure 7.1). After several pairings of the sound of the metronome with the delivery of meat powder, the dogs salivate at the sound of the metronome. The metronome is now the conditioned stimulus (CS), and the salivation is the conditioned response (CR).

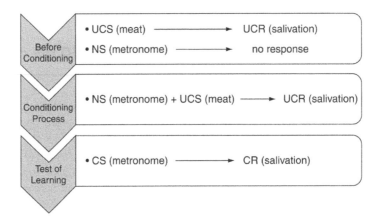

FIGURE 7.1 Schematic diagram illustrating the sequence of events in classical conditioning

Classical conditioning allows animals and people to *predict* the occurrence of future events and to prepare for them physiologically, behaviorally, and/or psychologically. The dogs learned that food was soon to come once they heard the metronome, so they were prepared for it. Physiological changes occurred (hormonal, thermogenic, neurochemical, etc.) so that they were ready to eat and digest the soon-to-arrive food. For many college students, hearing a roommate's rustling potato chip bag triggers a sudden craving for potato chips that can be distracting and irresistible as their bodies, just as those of Pavlov's dogs, prepare for the desired snack. This is clearly the result of a learned association between a particular sound and food.

Marketing of food products is largely based on the principles of classical conditioning. What do you think of when you drive past the "Golden Arches"? Many people experience sudden and overwhelming cravings for cheeseburgers, French fries, milkshakes, and, more recently, McCafé lattes and frappés on seeing the golden M sign associated with a McDonald's restaurant. Are you getting hungry now, too? This is classical conditioning: The pairing of the NS (the golden M sign) with the UCS (tasty food) yielding the UCR (eating and liking), and now the M sign serves as the CS triggering a desire for specific foods (CR). The influences of media, society, and marketing are explored in other chapters, but it is important to bear in mind that, despite its simplicity, associative learning is extremely effective and consequential and can last for one's lifetime.

LEARNING OF POSTINGESTIVE CONSEQUENCES: TASTE AVERSIONS AND PREFERENCES

Taste and Food Aversions

Most people have particular aversions to tastes or foods associated with sickness, even when the person knows that the food is actually safe (Schafe & Bernstein, 1996). If one happens to develop symptoms of the flu (nausea, vomiting) on the same evening that eggplant parmesan was tried for the first time, it is likely that eggplant parmesan will never be tried again, or at least not enthusiastically. The likelihood of an aversion is greater if the flavor or food meets one or more of the following conditions: It is *novel*, it is *less preferred*, it is *distinct*, it is *inconsequential* (not needed in one's diet), and/or it is *unusual* (something one does not typically consume). Examples are licorice and root beer – they have distinct flavors and are bearable to live without. Rats are particularly known to develop long-lasting aversions for flavors associated with gastrointestinal illness. Because rats lack the ability to regurgitate food once it has been ingested, it is essential for their survival that they avoid a food or flavor that previously made them ill (assuming they were lucky enough to survive their first negative experience). So, rats often exhibit one-trial learning, learning the negative association between food or flavor and illness with only one such pairing.

In now classic studies of taste aversion, Garcia and Koelling (1966) showed that rats soon learned to avoid a sweet-tasting liquid (a taste innately liked by rats) when it was followed by an injection of lithium chloride (LiCl) that made them ill. Interestingly, they did not learn to avoid the liquid when they received electric shocks afterward. The rats did, however, learn to avoid the electric shock when it was paired with light and noise (but injection of LiCl paired with light/noise failed to produce such learning). These results indicate that taste is more likely to be associated with visceral illness, and audiovisual cues are associated more with pain. Just like these rats, we (humans) are predisposed to develop particular aversions or avoidances associated with biologically relevant stimuli. This insight into conditioned aversions influenced the ways in which behavioral studies have since been conducted.

Here is a brief overview of a taste aversion procedure:

1   Initial state: UCS (LiCl) = UCR (nausea) and at a different time NS (sweet-tasting liquid) = neutral/positive response (drinking).
2   Learning trials: NS + UCS = UCR (nausea).
3   Acquisition of taste aversion: CS (sweet-tasting liquid) = CR (nausea).

Practical Implications – Animals

Others later applied the newly acquired understanding of learned taste aversions to help ranchers humanely control wolf predation of their livestock (Gustavson et al., 1976). After eating a sheep carcass contaminated with LiCl, wolves no longer preyed on sheep; in fact, they backed away after smelling their potential victims (LiCl induces nausea and vomiting in wolves). Ranchers have since used this method to prevent predation (from wolves, coyotes, crows, etc.) on other types of livestock (e.g., cows, chickens; Nicolaus et al., 1983). Conditioned taste aversion is similarly used to prevent agricultural damage caused by blackbirds and other animals and to protect endangered species (Werner et al., 2008). However, some debate remains around the usefulness of conditioned taste aversion in field conditions (i.e., without experimental controls and manipulation), because the associative learning typically occurs with the use of a carcass rather than live prey.

Practical Implications – Humans

When humans or animals eat a particular food before becoming ill because of a virus or before receiving a drug or radiation treatment that induces visceral illness, they avoid that food in future exposures. This is quite problematic for cancer patients undergoing chemotherapy, a treatment that often causes severe nausea. Many patients experience excessive weight loss because of newly developed food aversions, a condition referred to as *cancer anorexia* (Wisse et al., 2001; Yavuzsen et al., 2009). Unfortunately, many of these patients experience what is known in the learning literature as stimulus generalization, developing aversions not only for the foods consumed prior to their nausea-inducing treatment but also for foods that are similar in taste, appearance, and other qualities.

Efforts have been made to utilize our current understanding of taste aversion learning to prevent or minimize the occurrence of such learning among cancer patients. In a study by Broberg and Bernstein (1987), children who consumed a flavored candy (e.g., coconut or root beer Life Saver) prior to chemotherapy developed an aversion to that flavor but not to normal menu items. The flavored candy served as a "scapegoat" for the development of food aversions following chemotherapy treatment. The flavor to which the patients developed an aversion was inconsequential in their usual diet (most of us can lead healthy, normal lives without consuming coconut or root beer). Thus, the scapegoat aversion helped prevent the unsafe weight loss that often results from conditioned aversions following cancer treatments. Similar scapegoat food aversions have also been useful among adults undergoing chemotherapy (e.g., Andresen et al., 1990; Berteretche et al., 2004).

LEARNING ABOUT FOOD BY EXPERIENCE: INCREASING PREFERENCES

Medicine Effect

Food consumed when we are hungry or deficient in some macro- or micronutrient will be more preferred in subsequent exposures than food consumed when we are sated. And the more severe the deficiency, the greater the food preference we will have. In a classic study by Rozin (1969), rats were fed a diet deficient in thiamine (vitamin B_1). After some weeks (the symptoms of deficiency in thiamine take time to develop), the rats started to reject this diet by eating less and by spilling or spoiling the food. When the deficient rats were given "novel" food that contained the needed thiamine, they sampled it. If more than one novel food was provided, they sampled only one per meal.

The rats quickly came to prefer the food enriched with thiamine. Interestingly, there is no evidence that this preference was guided by the taste of thiamine; instead, other properties of the food (e.g., overall flavor or texture) were what the animals associated with "recovery." This type of learning, known as the **medicine effect**, is an example of a general food learning mechanism. First, deficient animals must become motivated to reject their current food and to overcome neophobia (fear of the new) and try a novel food. Then, they must learn the association between feeling better and the sensory properties that will allow them to recognize that food again in the future. Of course, this is almost the mirror image of the taste or flavor aversion previously discussed, in which animals learn to avoid food that has undesirable postingestive consequences. In common with that mechanism, the learning probably can occur in a single trial. That is, the animal need only eat the good food once to learn that it is safe, and there should be an allowable delay (hours) between eating and the consequence. This is why a strategy of discrete (one at a time) sampling of novel foods is adaptive when one is deficient. The biological rule seems to be something like this: Try one new food and wait and see if it is safe; if so, return to it; if not, try another new food. People who are deficient in vitamins or minerals often engage in pica – eating objects that are not normally considered food, such as soil, paint, or coins, which contain minerals. Some anthropologists believe that cannibalism may have its roots in dietary deficiency (e.g., de Montellano, 1978).

So, how does this feeling better or medicine effect work? It is believed that learning occurs by a process of reinforcement that is mediated by internal reward system(s). It is likely, then, that recovery from deficiencies in trace elements (and perhaps calories, too) uses the same systems. Research indicates that the pleasurable feeling associated with eating good (safe) food and recovery from a deficiency is mediated by the signaling of the neurotransmitter dopamine and endorphins, among others, acting within the reward pathway of the brain (Berridge et al., 2010; Volkow et al., 2003). The neurobiology of food liking and reward is discussed in further detail in other chapters of this book.

Despite our innate liking of the sweet taste, heavily sweetened foods such as candy or sugary beverages are typically not desired when we are truly hungry, at least not to the exclusion of other foods. For example, you would probably not want jelly beans as your only food for dinner. In fact, foods that we normally find appealing, such as a chocolate bar, may seem unappealing or even disgusting when we are energy deficient. Rather, when we are deficient, we tend to seek out and prefer more savory food items. Which types of foods do you prefer after a long day or vigorous workout? In Western culture, pre-ferred foods include sandwiches, meat or pasta dishes, and burgers (Drewnowski, 1997; Drewnowski et al., 1992). In many Asian cultures, the preferred foods are fish and rice. Often, the food preferences shaped by the medicine effect are foods that are of greater nutritional value than the preferences made through other experiences when we are less deficient. This could indicate that the best way to acquire a liking for brussels sprouts or other innately less preferred foods is to consume them when you are very hungry. We'll let you try it out!

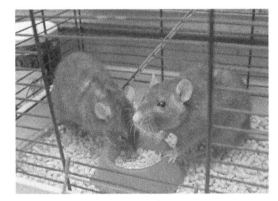

IMAGE 7.2 Rats sampling food

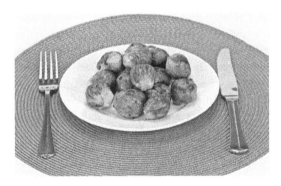

IMAGE 7.3 Brussels sprouts to try

Mere Exposure

Preferences for particular food items or flavors increase with repeated exposure, whether or not the exposure is consciously known about (Bornstein & D'Agostino, 1992). This passive type of learning that shapes eating behavior was first termed the **mere exposure** effect in 1968 by Robert Zajonc (1968). Humans and nonhuman animals are some-what neophobic (wary of novel foods and flavors), yet paradoxically neophilic (liking the new). Unfamiliar foods and flavors can be either beneficial (providing nutrients and calories) or dangerous (containing toxins). As previously described, humans and animals tend to sample new foods and increase consumption with repeated exposure only if the postingestive consequences are positive (or at least not negative). This process results in increased liking and decreased neophobia: The mere exposure effect and reduction of neophobia necessarily co-occur.

As an anecdotal example, most Americans do not consume large portions of sushi (containing raw fish) on their first exposure to that cuisine. Most choose menu options with cooked fish (e.g., the California roll) and gradually increase their liking and consumption of raw sushi over time. Was that your experience?

Mere exposure to new tastes and smells actually begins in utero (Beauchamp & Mennella, 2009). The fetus is exposed to the flavors of foods consumed by the mother and is seemingly more accepting of these otherwise novel flavors when old enough to eat solid foods during infancy. Mennella, Johnson, and Beauchamp (2001) found that, when women consumed carrot juice for three weeks during their third trimester, their infants (six months later) were more accepting of carrot-flavored cereal compared with non-flavored cereal and compared with babies whose mothers did not consume carrot juice, demonstrating that the mere exposure effect on the shaping of food preferences begins prior to birth.

The number of exposures needed to increase liking of novel foods or flavors varies. Foods to which children or adults have been previously exposed or that are similar to familiar items (e.g., trying strawberry yogurt when already familiar with strawberries, or trying blueberry yogurt when already familiar with strawberry yogurt) require fewer exposures than entirely novel or innately less appealing foods (e.g., a novel, bitter-tasting vegetable). So, some foods may be rated as more appealing after just one exposure, whereas others may require many more exposures. Further, for children, mere exposure seems to be more effective in shaping food acceptance and liking than rewards. Wardle et al. (2003) found that children who were exposed to samples of sweet red pepper once a day for almost two weeks increased their liking and intake regardless of receiving a sticker reward for consuming the vegetable.

Flavor–Flavor Associative Learning

Humans have an innate liking of sweet and salty tastes. The sweet taste is associated with energy and nutrient-dense foods, and the salty taste is associated with foods that help maintain fluid and sodium balance. Humans also have an innate aversion to bitter and sour tastes, which are associated with toxins (Birch, 1999). However, many people regularly enjoy bitter or sour foods and beverages such as coffee, tea, beer, broccoli, sour candies, and so on, which seems to defy our innate predispositions. Why is this?

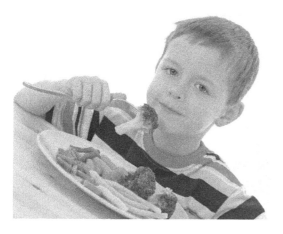

IMAGE 7.4 A boy enjoying broccoli flavored with butter

BOX 7.1 DO FOOD PREFERENCES OF BABIES INCREASE WITH EXPOSURE?

Sullivan and Birch (1994) investigated the liking of novel vegetables in infants who were starting to eat solid foods (aged 4–6 months) and found increased acceptance over the course of ten exposures. Liking of the novel vegetables occurred more quickly in breast-milk-fed infants compared with formula-fed infants, indicating that breast milk "merely exposes" infants to a wider variety of flavors, increasing their liking of novel foods. Studies in rats have shown that the pups quickly prefer flavors they experience through their mother's milk and show preferences for their mother's diet when they start to consume solid food (Galef & Henderson, 1972; Galef & Sherry, 1973).

Pairing a new food or flavor that is not innately preferred with an already liked food or flavor increases the liking of that new food. This is called **flavor–flavor associative learning** (Birch, 1999). Although many adults enjoy coffee, some even preferring it black (without cream or sugar), most are initially exposed to coffee with cream or milk and sweetener. We have an innate liking of cream/milk and the sweet taste. Typically, adults gradually prefer less of the cream/milk and sweetener, but their initial liking of coffee is mediated by flavor–flavor learning. The same applies for tea, often sweetened in first exposures. Similarly, early experience with broccoli often includes cheese or butter sauce (tastes that are innately liked). Despite its bitter taste, the pairing of broccoli with already liked flavors increases liking of it.

It is important to note that flavor–flavor associative learning can also result in conditioned aversions. In other words, the learning can work in reverse. In laboratory experiments, rats given a liked flavor mixed with bitter-tasting quinine demonstrated an aversion for the previously liked flavor, avoiding it even when it was no longer paired with quinine (Rozin & Zellner, 1985). Theoretically, pairing broccoli with cheese, hoping to increase a child's liking of broccoli, could actually create a dislike of cheese! This, however, is typically not the case, as the liking of cheese is greater than the dislike of broccoli for most humans.

Talking Point 7.1 Flavor–Flavor Learning

Have you experienced flavor–flavor learning that increased your preference for a new food? How did you initially experience the food? Do you prefer the food differently now (e.g., maybe less ketchup on your hamburger than you liked as a child)?

BOX 7.2 CAN FLAVOR–FLAVOR LEARNING HAPPEN EASILY?

In a study conducted by Capaldi and Privitera (2008), college student volunteers were given vegetables (cauliflower and broccoli) in three exposure sessions. One vegetable was sweetened with sugar during the exposures, and the other was unsweetened. When subsequently tested with unsweetened vegetables, participants reported a greater liking of the previously sweetened vegetable. So, although the vegetable was no longer sweetened, its taste was preferred because of the association with the sweet taste.

Flavor–Nutrient Associative Learning

Pairing a flavor with calories (or with other needed substances such as vitamins) increases preference. Flavors paired with higher calories will be preferred to those paired with fewer calories (Ackroff & Sclafani, 2006). This **flavor–nutrient associative learning** can result in preference maintained for long durations, even without reinforcement. As with taste avoidance learning, flavor–nutrient learning can occur with a delay of hours between conditioned stimulus (flavor) and unconditioned stimulus (benefit). This type of learning is akin to the medicine effect, in which animals and people learn preferences for foods or flavors associated with feeling good and recovering from a deficit in vitamins, minerals, or calories. However, flavor–nutrient associative learning can occur in a non-deficient state.

Although flavor–nutrient associative learning occurs in sated rats, the results are more robust when the rats (or other animals, including humans) are food deprived. It is easy to assume that the actions of nutrients in the gastrointestinal tract are more reinforcing for hungry than for sated animals. The "incentive value" for a food or flavor consumed when in a deficient state will be higher and will result in an increased appetitive approach to, and intake of, that particular food or flavor (Sclafani, 2004), which is the medicine effect.

Flavor–nutrient learning has been demonstrated in humans. Studies show that flavors associated with nutrients (calories, fat, vitamins, or minerals) are preferred. For example, Johnson and colleagues (Johnson et al., 1991) gave preschool children fixed volumes of distinct flavors of pudding (pumpkin and chocolate-orange) that were either high or low in fat and calories (220 kcal or 110 kcal per serving; 14 g or <2 g fat). The low- and high-fat versions were identical in taste, smell, and appearance. After several exposures to the flavor–nutrient pairing, children consumed less food following consumption of the high-fat, high-calorie pudding (compared with the low-fat, low-calorie pudding), even though, during the test condition, all puddings were of mid-level caloric and fat content. Further, children reported increased liking for the flavor associated with high energy density and no change in preference for the flavor associated with low energy density. These findings suggest that such flavor–nutrient learning shapes food preferences and energy intake. Similar studies (e.g., Booth, 1985) have been conducted in humans of other ages (infants and adults) and in rats, providing evidence that portion size is adjusted based on learned associations with flavors and their energy yield (i.e., flavor–nutrient learning).

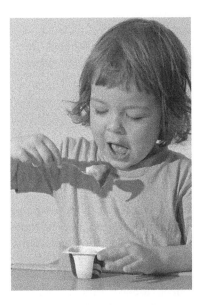

IMAGE 7.5 A girl consuming yogurt

BOX 7.3 DO ANIMALS LEARN ASSOCIATIONS BETWEEN FLAVORS AND NUTRIENTS?

Anthony Sclafani has performed many studies to define the limits of flavor–calorie learning. In one experiment, rats had access to two flavors of Kool-Aid (e.g., grape- or cherry-flavored water with no calories). These flavors were presented in water bottles fitted with contact sensors so that, when the rat licked, a signal was sent to a computer (Drucker et al., 1993). The rats otherwise had ad libitum (i.e., unrestricted) access to food and water. In the one-bottle training trials, they had one flavor per day. Ingestion of one flavor was accompanied by infusion (programmed via the computer) of a caloric solution into the stomach through a surgically implanted tube. Ingestion of the other flavor was accompanied by infusion of water only. After several days of each flavor consequence, the rats were given a two-bottle preference test without any infusions. They strongly preferred the flavor previously paired with calories. Further, when these preference tests were continued without infusions (this is called *extinction*), the preference for the flavor paired with calories remained for weeks. That is, established preferences can be maintained without continued reinforcement. Sclafani and colleagues have also demonstrated similar flavor–nutrient associative learning by pairing Kool-Aid flavors with intragastric infusions of fat (Lucas & Sclafani, 1989) or protein (Pérez et al., 1996).

Talking Point 7.2 Food Preferences

What are some examples of your food preferences and eating behaviors that may have resulted from flavor–flavor *and* flavor–nutrient associative learning?

It is important to note that flavor–flavor and flavor–nutrient associative learning do not typically occur in exclusion of each other outside of the laboratory setting. In real-life situations, preferred flavors are innately liked because they are associated with nutrients (calories, fat, vitamins, or minerals). For example, increased liking of unsweetened peanut butter after pairing it with honey demonstrates both flavor–flavor learning (honey is sweet-tasting and innately liked) and flavor–nutrient learning (honey provides added calories). In fact, even increased liking of coffee after repeatedly consuming it with cream and sugar demonstrates both flavor–flavor and flavor–nutrient associative learning.

LEARNING OF APPROPRIATE FOOD QUANTITY: CONDITIONED SATIETY

Experiments conducted in the 1960s and 1970s routinely demonstrated that both humans and nonhuman animals fail to compensate when a previously consumed food is made either more or less energy dense (Stunkard, 1975). For example, after several exposures of a milkshake-like drink, participants in one study drank their "norm" amount even when the drink was diluted and, consequently, less energy dense and even though they could consume as much as they wanted (Jordan et al., 1966).

Influential researcher A. J. Stunkard proposed that satiety must be a conditioned reflex, a function of learning rather than of physiological satiety cues. Some of the findings regarding flavor–nutrient learning (discussed earlier in this chapter) are consistent with this theory. For example, Johnson and colleagues (1991) found that children consumed less of the flavored pudding that they had learned to associate with higher calories and fat even when it was no longer high in calories and fat. They liked the flavor but learned to regulate calories and stop eating based on flavor cues, supporting the idea that satiety is a conditioned reflex.

How often do you eat three-fourths of a sandwich or cookie? Typically, we completely consume items of defined quantity and have experience with these particular quantities. We can assume that, in early exposures to a sandwich, for example, consumption of one sandwich was followed by comfortable satiety and an adequate level of energy. We also tend to consume entire portions, often completely unaware of how energy dense or dilute they are. For example, many of us consume a "bowlful" of cereal in the morning, regardless of the type of cereal (high or low in calories or other nutrients). Indeed, the popular individual serving bowls of cereals from one commercial source vary between 70 and 130 kcal, and the fat content of the milk you probably add will make even larger differences. We learn, in early experiences with particular foods, what quantities yield satiety, supporting Stunkard's conditioning theory. However, we can easily be "tricked," especially when eating at restaurants, because portion sizes are often larger and more fat and calorie dense than we expect.

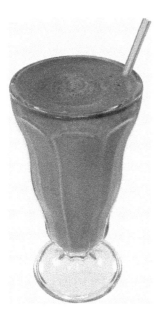

IMAGE 7.6 We tend to consume "norm" amounts of foods such as milkshakes

BOX 7.4 HOW DO RATS KNOW WHEN IT'S MEALTIME?

In a study conducted by Drazen et al. (2006), rats either received food ad libitum (food available all day) or for four hours only per day. The rats in the meal-restricted group soon (within 14 days) learned to anticipate their mealtime and consumed their food much more quickly and robustly. Ghrelin (a hunger-stimulating hormone) levels in the meal-trained rats were significantly higher prior to their anticipated four-hour access to food in comparison with controls as their dark cycle approached (the time during which rats typically consume the most food). Their findings indicate that rats (and presumably humans) have learned physiological responses in anticipation of mealtimes.

LEARNING ABOUT WHEN TO EAT: CONDITIONED HUNGER

If satiety is conditioned, is hunger also conditioned? Consider the frequent long lines at many delis and cafeterias at lunchtime. Why do so many of us eat at similar times of the day, such as lunch around noon in particular? Perhaps we all have similar energy and nutrient needs at the same time of day. Does this seem logical, given that many of us wake at different times in the morning, exert varying amounts of energy early in the day, have different metabolic rates, and consume varied calories and nutrients (or none at all) for breakfast? It is more likely that our "hunger" for lunch at noon is a result of learning that this is mealtime. Because of our learned expectation of consumption of food at lunchtime, physiological changes occur (e.g., insulin and ghrelin levels rise; blood glucose drops) that intensify our hunger (see Box 7.3).

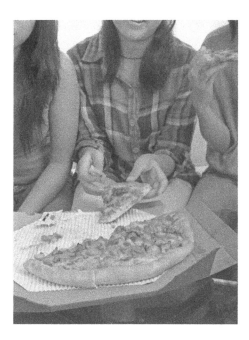

IMAGE 7.7 Pizza with friends

BOX 7.5 DO FOOD CUES TRIGGER EATING EVEN IN THE ABSENCE OF HUNGER?

In experiments conducted in the 1980s by Weingarten (e.g., 1984), food was delivered to rats following a buzzer and light stimulus. After several days of conditioning, rats ate when exposed to the buzzer and light stimulus, despite the fact that they were not food deprived in the test condition.

When rats are placed on a meal schedule (something analogous to breakfast, lunch, and dinner), rather than allowed food ad libitum, they consume the most in the meal that precedes the longest between-meal interval (i.e., dinner). One might expect the opposite, that they eat the most following the longest stretch of deprivation. The fact that this is not the case is quite interesting, and much like with human eating patterns, suggesting that they have learned to anticipate the longest interval without food access and consume more in advance of it. It seems likely that eating behavior (ours and that of rats) is largely attributed to learning to anticipate and prevent future disruptions to physiological homeostasis (Woods, 2009).

In addition to time-of-day cues, other stimuli associated with food also trigger hunger and eating. As mentioned, we tend to think of and crave particular food items on seeing certain corporate logos. After conditioning, Pavlov's dogs salivated at the sound of a metronome. Animals and people quickly associate food with the stimuli surrounding the experience with the food (physical, visual, olfactory, and auditory cues; mood; etc.), and later encounters with these stimuli trigger hunger, even when there is no physiological need for food. Food-associated cues are increasingly ubiquitous in Western society, and their impact on eating (and overeating) is tremendous.

INFLUENCE OF LEARNED CONTEXTUAL CUES

Have you ever noticed feeling hungry when you enter the place in which you typically eat meals or snacks? People and animals tend to consume more food when they are in places that they have learned to associate with food. This helps explain the frequent "mindless" behavior of grabbing a soda out of the refrigerator or snack from the kitchen when passing by, even in the absence of thirst, hunger, or a planned intention to consume anything.

Contextual cues, such as sights, smells, and sounds, are non-food stimuli that we quickly learn to associate with food. This type of learning is simply classical conditioning, which, as mentioned earlier, is basic but effective. Birch et al. (1989) examined the impact that a physical setting has on a child's eating. In this study, preschool children were exposed to two playrooms that were similar in appearance and had similar contents (toys, etc.), but in one room they received snacks regularly and in the other room they were never fed. On the test day, both rooms were "baited" with snacks, and half the children were sent to play in one room and half to the other. The group sent to the playroom in which they had experienced snacks before started eating/snacking sooner and ate more than the group sent to the room in which they had not previously experienced snacks. This indicates a powerful influence of social and environmental learning on readiness to eat and/or amount consumed, and this is established early in life.

Talking Point 7.3 Contextual Cues

Are there specific foods that you associate with particular places or other cues? How about the movie theater, as discussed in the opening paragraph of this chapter? A local bakery or coffee shop? Grandma's house? A football or baseball game? Write down some of these associations and see how your list compares with your classmates' lists.

Rats, too, demonstrate increased eating as a result of learning about physical or contextual cues. Rats eat more quickly and ingest larger amounts when placed in cages previously associated with food, especially if the food to which they were previously exposed was palatable (e.g., cookies; Boggiano et al., 2009). Further, rats and people eat more of palatable and bland food when they are exposed to contextual cues associated with palatable food. It seems that we (rats and humans) feel hungrier when exposed to food-related conditions or places. Learned contextual cues can be more influential on hunger and eating than the actual taste of food (an unconditioned stimulus).

In a study of college students and staff, Ferriday and Brunstrom (2008) found that the *sight* and *smell* of pizza were more associated with increased consumption of pizza and other foods than was the *taste* of pizza. How could this be? Exposure to contextual cues associated with a pleasurable experience such as consumption of palatable food activates the brain's reward pathways and areas associated with wanting and motivation (Berridge et al., 2010). This powerful activation can drive the appetitive behavior toward the desired food. Further, physiological changes (e.g., increase in insulin, decrease in blood glucose) intensify hunger when we are exposed to cues associated with particular foods, explaining the difficulty many people have in resisting foods on exposure to those cues.

CONDITIONED IMMUNE SYSTEM ACTIVITY

Efforts have been made to utilize classical conditioning techniques to boost immune system functioning, particularly among clinically ill patients (Exton et al., 2000). Initially, researchers realized that immune system functioning weakens when patients enter the hospital or treatment facility where they receive chemotherapy, a consequence of associative learning. This, however, only puts patients at greater risk for the negative physiological side effects of chemotherapy and the toll it takes on the immune system and overall health (although the benefits of such treatment usually outweigh the risks). In one study, as an example of these experiments, patients consumed particular flavors of sherbet and afterward received an adrenaline injection (which boosts immune system activity and overall physical feeling). After several pairings, the patients' immune systems were more active following consumption of the sherbet, even when it was no longer followed by the adrenaline injection (Exton et al., 2000).

NEUROBIOLOGY OF FOOD LEARNING

The neurobiology associated with *conditioned* taste aversions and preferences is different from that associated with *innately* disliked and liked tastes (which were mentioned in earlier chapters). The brain regions associated with *learned* taste dislikes and likes include those associated with memory, emotion, and reward (see Figure 7.2). It seems obvious that emotional memory (e.g., disgust) is important in preventing an organism from re-exposing itself to a dangerous food or flavor, as the lack of this recall ability could result in fatality. And pleasant experiences with particular foods, such as warm soup on a chilly night or a substantial pasta dish following an exhausting soccer game, should be remembered so that those positive experiences can be repeated. These types of emotional memories require an intact hippocampus. Severe damage to the hippocampus disrupts the ability to form new explicit memories (i.e., memories that can be consciously recalled). Amnesic patients with hippocampal damage will consume a second meal soon after eating a first meal if it is presented to them, and often a third meal as well, indicating that physiological satiety signals are not sufficient to regulate their food intake (Rozin et al., 1998). It seems, rather, that *memory* of food intake (type and amount of food) is more important in making subsequent food choices (Benoit et al., 2010).

In addition to the hippocampus, other brain regions associated with emotional memory are important in the establishment of conditioned taste aversions and preferences. Establishing a learned food aversion is unpleasant (often including nausea and vomiting) and can be considered frightening and upsetting. The amygdala, a brain region associated with various motivated and emotional behaviors, including fearful and aggressive responses, plays an important role in the formation of learned taste aversions. It seems, though, that different regions within the amygdala function differentially in the *establishment* of a conditioned taste aversion compared with the *avoidance response* in future exposures (Reilly & Bornaovalova, 2005; Yamamoto, 2006). Further, regions of the amygdala communicate differently with the nucleus accumbens and other brain reward circuitry following exposure to a liked versus disliked taste, which may not be surprising as the neurobiology of conditioned taste preferences and conditioned taste aversions serve different functions. Avoiding harmful foods and flavors is important for the survival of any animal, and thus brainstem anatomy and physiology shared among many species, including reptiles and mammals, likely underlie the basic ability to form conditioned taste aversions. Further, conditioned taste aversions in animals under anesthesia when exposed to the CS–US pairing have been demonstrated (Yamamoto, 2006); this does not occur for conditioned preferences. Conditioned taste preferences (again, these are learned and shaped by experience and are not necessarily innate preferences) are influenced by social and cultural factors (e.g., parents, friends, local cuisine, expectations, accessibility). Although these are extremely important aspects of our eating behaviors, they are not as essential as learning to avoid what may kill us. Brain regions that have more recently evolved or grown in relative size (e.g., the forebrain) may be of greater importance in the formation of conditioned taste preferences compared with conditioned aversions. The involvement of the forebrain, and specifically reward circuitry, in eating behavior is of recent interest as it relates to the concept of excessive and problematic food liking and the possibility of food addiction, discussed in Chapter 10.

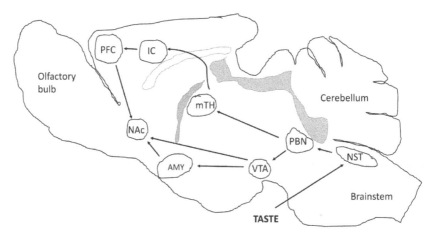

FIGURE 7.2 Brain regions important for the processing of taste information and the development of conditioned taste aversions are shown in this figure of the rodent brain. (Note that this is similar to Figure 6.1 but with the key pathways indicated by arrows.) Key: NST – nucleus of the solitary tract; PBN – parabrachial nucleus; VTA – ventral tegmental area; AMY – amygdala; mTH – medial thalamus; IC – insular gustatory cortex; NAc – nucleus accumbens; PFC – prefrontal cortex

The neurobiology of feeding has been explored in other chapters, and, therefore, the focus of the remaining discussion in this chapter is on the neurobiology of conditioned taste aversions.

Within the brainstem, the nucleus of the solitary tract (NST) and the parabrachial nucleus (PBN) are the first and second brain relay nuclei, respectively, for taste and gastrointestinal information. Rats with lesions on the PBN do not acquire conditioned taste aversions despite their demonstrated capacity to maintain the ability to process taste and visceral information. And any previously learned taste aversion is abolished by a lesion in this region. The association between taste and gastrointestinal information occurs in the PBN and not in the NST, an integration that is seemingly necessary for the formation of conditioned taste aversion. Taste and gastrointestinal information from the PBN is relayed to the medial thalamus and then to the gustatory insular cortex in the frontal cortex. In parallel fashion, the same information projects from the PBN to the amygdala. Severe damage to the gustatory insular cortex (or gustatory cortex), the medial thalamus, or areas within the amygdala (specifically, the basolateral amygdala) can prevent a human or animal from forming a conditioned taste aversion or from retaining the learned association. Although many other regions are likely involved (e.g., hypothalamic nuclei), as the brain circuitry of eating behavior is complex and involves multiple pathways, the PBN, medial thalamus, basolateral amygdala, and gustatory insular cortex are of particular importance for the formation and maintenance of conditioned taste aversions (Yamamoto, 2006; Yamamoto & Ueju, 2011).

QUESTIONS TO ASK YOURSELF

Let's review and apply your knowledge. Take some time to answer these chapter questions.

1 Use classical conditioning terminology (UCR, UCS, etc.) to briefly diagram and describe an example of how classical conditioning has shaped one of your food preferences or aversions.
2 What are the four ways in which food preference can be increased by experience? Give examples of each. Do you think that satiety is conditioned? What is the scientific evidence for this? Describe some evidence in your own eating behavior that supports or refutes this theory.
3 What are some of the learned cues that trigger hunger? Why does this occur?
4 What brain regions are most important for learned food preferences and aversions?

GLOSSARY

Amygdala	A forebrain region associated with raw emotion, particularly fear and aggression.
Conditioned response (CR)	A learned response to a previously neutral stimulus.

Conditioned stimulus (CS)	A previously neutral stimulus that comes to elicit the response of an unconditioned stimulus.
Flavor–flavor associative learning	Increased liking of a flavor that is associated with a flavor that is already or innately liked.
Flavor–nutrient associative learning	Increased liking of a flavor associated with nutrients, usually calories.
Gustatory insular cortex	The primary taste cortex; allows for perception of taste.
Hippocampus	A forebrain region involved in the formation of memories.
Medicine effect	Increased liking of a food associated with recovery from illness.
Mere exposure effect	Increased liking of food resulting from repeated exposures to the food.
Neophobia	Fear of the new (for the purposes of this text, fear of new food or flavors).
Neutral stimulus (NS)	A stimulus that elicits no response.
Nucleus accumbens	A forebrain region associated with pleasure and reinforcement.
Nucleus of the solitary tract (NST)	A brainstem region to which taste information from the tongue projects.
Parabrachial nucleus (PBN)	A brainstem region that receives taste information from the NST.
Pica	The appetite for items that are generally not considered food (e.g., dirt).
Stimulus generalization	The response to stimuli that are similar to the conditioned stimulus.
Unconditioned response (UCR)	An unlearned response to a stimulus.
Unconditioned stimulus (UCS)	A stimulus that triggers an unlearned response.

REFERENCES

Ackroff, K., & Sclafani, A. (2006). Energy density and macronutrient composition determine flavor preference conditioned by intragastric infusions of mixed diets. *Physiology & Behavior, 89* (2), 250–260.

Andresen, G. V., Birch, L. L., & Johnson, P. A. (1990). The scapegoat effect on food aversions after chemotherapy. *Cancer, 66,* 1649–1653.

Beauchamp, G. K., & Mennella, J. A. (2009). Early flavor learning and its impact on later feeding behavior. *Journal of Pediatric Gastroenterology and Nutrition, 48,* S25–S30.

Benoit, S. C., Davis, J. F., & Davidson, T. L. (2010). Learned and cognitive controls of food intake. *Brain Research, 1350,* 71–76.

Berridge, K. C., Ho, C. Y., Richard, J. M., & DiFeliceantonio, A. G. (2010). The tempted brain eats: Pleasure and desire circuits in obesity and eating disorders. *Brain Research, 1350,* 43–64.

Berteretche, M. V., Dalix, A. M., d'Ornano, A. C., Bellisle, F., Khayat, D., & Faurion, A. J. S. C. (2004). Decreased taste sensitivity in cancer patients under chemotherapy. *Supportive Care in Cancer, 12,* 571–576.

Birch, L. L. (1999). Development of food preferences. *Annual Review of Nutrition, 19* (1), 41–62.

Birch, L. L., McPhee, L., Sullivan, S., & Johnson, S. (1989). Conditioned meal initiation in young children. *Appetite, 13* (2), 105–113.

Boggiano, M. M., Dorsey, J. R., Thomas, J. M., & Murdaugh, D. L. (2009). The Pavlovian power of palatable food: Lessons for weight-loss adherence from a new rodent model of cue-induced overeating. *International Journal of Obesity, 33* (6), 693–701.

Booth, D. A. (1985). Food-conditioned eating preferences and aversions with interoceptive elements: Conditioned appetites and satieties. *Annals of the New York Academy of Sciences, 443* (1), 22–41.

Bornstein, R. F., & D'Agostino, P. R. (1992). Stimulus recognition and the mere exposure effect. *Journal of Personality and Social Psychology, 63* (4), 545–552.

Broberg, D. J., & Bernstein, I. L. (1987). Candy as a scapegoat in the prevention of food aversions in children receiving chemotherapy. *Cancer, 60* (9), 2344–2347.

Capaldi, E. D., & Privitera, G. J. (2008). Decreasing dislike for sour and bitter in children and adults. *Appetite, 50* (1), 139–145.

de Montellano, B. R. O. (1978). Aztec cannibalism: An ecological necessity? *Science, 200* (4342), 611–617.

Drazen, D. L., Vahl, T. P., D'Alessio, D. A., Seeley, R. J., & Woods, S. C. (2006). Effects of a fixed meal pattern on ghrelin secretion: Evidence for a learned response independent of nutrient status. *Endocrinology, 147* (1), 23–30.

Drewnowski, A., Kurth, C., Holden-Wiltse, J., & Saari, J. (1992). Food preferences in human obesity: Carbohydrates versus fats. *Appetite, 18,* 207–221.

Drewnowski, A. A. (1997). Taste preferences and food intake. *Annual Review of Nutrition, 17* (1), 237.

Drucker, D. B., Ackroff, K., & Sclafani, A. (1993). Flavor preference produced by intragastric polycose infusions in rats using a concurrent conditioning procedure. *Physiology and Behavior, 54,* 351–355.

Exton, M. S., von Auer, A. K., Buske-Kirschbaum, A., Stockhorst, U., Göbel, U., & Schedlowski, M. (2000). Pavlovian conditioning of immune function: Animal investigation and the challenge of human application. *Behavioural Brain Research, 110* (1), 129–141.

Ferriday, D., & Brunstrom, J. M. (2008). How does food-cue exposure lead to larger meal sizes? *British Journal of Nutrition, 100,* 1325–1332.

Galef, B. G., & Henderson, P. W. (1972). Mother's milk: A determinant of the feeding preferences of weaning rat pups. *Journal of Comparative and Physiological Psychology, 78* (2), 213–219.

Galef, B. G., & Sherry, D. F. (1973). Mother's milk: A medium for transmission of cues reflecting the flavor of mother's diet. *Journal of Comparative and Physiological Psychology, 83* (3), 374.

Garcia, J., & Koelling, R. A. (1966). Relation of cue to consequence in avoidance learning. *Psychonomic Science, 4* (3), 123–124.

Gustavson, C. R., Kelly, D. J., & Sweeney, M. (1976). Prey-lithium aversions I: Coyotes and wolves. *Behavioral Biology, 17,* 61–72.

Johnson, S. L., McPhee, L., & Birch, L. L. (1991). Conditioned preferences: Young children prefer flavors associated with high dietary fat. *Physiology & Behavior, 50* (6), 1245–1251.

Jordan, H. A., Wieland, W. F., Zebley, S. P., Stellar, E., & Stunkard, A. J. (1966). Direct measurement of food intake in man: A method for the objective study of eating behavior. *Psychosomatic Medicine, 28* (6), 836–842.

Lucas, F., & Sclafani, A. (1989). Flavor preferences conditioned by intragastric fat infusions in rats. *Physiology & Behavior, 46* (3), 403–412.

Mennella, J. A., Johnson, A., & Beauchamp, G. K. (2001). Prenatal and postnatal flavor learning by human infants. *Pediatrics, 107* (6), 88–97.

Nicolaus, L. K., Cassel, J. F., Carlson, R. B., & Gustavson, R. (1983). Taste-aversion conditioning of crows to control predation on eggs. *Science, 220,* 212–214. doi:10.1126/science.220.4593.212

Pérez, C., Ackroff, K., & Sclafani, A. (1996). Carbohydrate- and protein-conditioned flavor preferences: Effects of nutrient preloads. *Physiology & Behavior, 59* (3), 467–474.

Reilly, S., & Bornaovalova, M. A. (2005). Conditioned taste aversion and amygdala lesions in the rat: A critical review. *Neuroscience and Biobehavioral Reviews, 29,* 1067–1088.

Rozin, P. (1969). Adaptive food sampling patterns in vitamin deficient rats. *Journal of Comparative and Physiological Psychology, 69* (1), 126–132. doi:10.1037/h0027940

Rozin, P., Dow, S., Moscovitch, M., & Rajaram, S. (1998). What causes humans to begin and end a meal? A role for memory for what has been eaten, as evidenced by a study of multiple meal eating in amnesic patients. *Psychological Science, 9* (5), 392–396.

Rozin, P., & Zellner, D. (1985). The role of Pavlovian conditioning in the acquisition of food likes and dislikes. *Annals of the New York Academy of Sciences, 443* (1), 189–202.

Schafe, G. E., & Bernstein, I. L. (1996). Taste aversion learning. In E. D. Capaldi (ed.), *Why we eat what we eat: The psychology of eating* (pp. 31–51). American Psychological Association. doi.org/10.1037/10291-002

Sclafani, A. (2004). Oral and postoral determinants of food reward. *Physiology & Behavior, 81* (5), 773–779.

Stunkard, A. (1975). Satiety is a conditioned reflex. *Psychosomatic Medicine, 37* (5), 383–387.

Sullivan, S. A., & Birch, L. L. (1994). Infant dietary experience and acceptance of solid foods. *Pediatrics, 93,* 271–277.

Volkow, N. D., Wang, G. J., Maynard, L., et al. (2003). Brain dopamine is associated with eating behavior in humans. *International Journal of Eating Disorders, 33,* 136–142.

Wardle, J., Herrera, M., Cooke, L., & Gibson, E. (2003). Modifying children's food preferences: The effects of exposure and reward on acceptance of an unfamiliar vegetable. *European Journal of Clinical Nutrition, 57* (2), 341–348.

Weingarten, H. P. (1984). Meal initiation controlled by learned cues: Basic behavioral properties. *Appetite, 5* (2), 147–158.

Werner, S. J., Kimball, B. A., & Provenza, F. D. (2008). Food color, flavor, and conditioned avoidance among red-winged blackbirds. *Physiology & Behavior, 93* (1–2), 110–117.

Wisse, B. E., Frayo, R. S., Schwartz, M. W., & Cummings, E. (2001). Reversal of cancer anorexia by blockade of central melanocortin receptors in rats. *Endocrinology, 142* (8), 3292–3301.

Woods, S. C. (2009). The control of food intake: Behavioral versus molecular perspectives. *Cell Metabolism, 9* (6), 489–498.

Yamamoto, T. (2006). Brain regions responsible for the expression of conditioned taste aversions in rats. *Chemical Senses, 32,* 105–109.

Yamamoto, T., & Ueji, K. (2011). Brain mechanisms of flavor learning. *Frontiers in Systems Neuroscience, 5,* 76–85.

Yavuzsen, T., Walsh, D., Davis, M. P., Kirkova, J., Jin, T., LeGrand, S., Lagman, R., Bicanovsky, L., Estfan, B., Creema, B., & Haddad, A. (2009). Components of the anorexia–cachexia syndrome: Gastrointestinal symptom correlates of cancer anorexia. *Supportive Care in Cancer, 17,* 1531–1541.

Zajonc, R. B. (1968). Attitudinal effects of mere exposure. *Journal of Personality and Social Psychology Monographs, 9* (2p2), 1.

CHAPTER 8

The Development of Eating Behaviors

After reading this chapter, you will be able to

- Understand the effects of prenatal exposure to nutrients and flavors.
- Appreciate the impact of early postnatal experience with food and the advantages of breastfeeding.
- Identify evidence for and against the theory that children can regulate their own energy and nutrient needs.
- Understand the influence of external factors (parents, media, portion sizes, etc.) on the eating behaviors of children.
- Provide parents, caregivers, and policy makers with ideas for instilling healthy eating behaviors for children.

Significant changes in eating behavior occur in the first few years of life – from suckling, to being spoon fed, to eating independently. New tastes and smells are encountered, and likes and dislikes are formed. Infants and toddlers learn what foods are socially acceptable, how much should be eaten, and when. Eating patterns established during the early years shape future eating behaviors. Because the obesity rate is increasing in countries around the world, it is important to understand the impact of eating practices established in the first few years of life so that parents, caregivers, and policy makers can improve the food environment of young children, better preparing them for lifelong healthy eating. We know that infants innately like sweet tastes and dislike bitter and sour tastes. This biological predisposition helps us, from birth, identify and consume foods associated with more calories and avoid those that could be dangerous. This served our ancestors well in a world with scarce food supplies, but it puts us at an increased risk for obesity in an environment containing an overabundance of sweet-tasting foods with calories exceeding our needs. In this chapter, we explore biological predispositions that we have at birth, and even before birth, and the sociocultural influences (parents, friends, culture, and media) that further shape our eating behaviors during our early years.

DOI: 10.4324/9781032621401-8

ONTOGENY OF HUMAN FEEDING: PRENATAL EXPERIENCE

Fetal brain development is impacted by the food, drink, and other substances that the mother ingests, particularly during critical periods. Maternal malnutrition is correlated with low birth weight, lower intelligence, reduced motor coordination, and other lifelong impairments (Lechtig et al., 1975). We know that alcohol consumption during pregnancy can result in fetal alcohol syndrome, a condition associated with abnormal facial features, mental retardation, and poor motor coordination (Mattson & Riley, 2006). As with the effects of maternal malnutrition, fetal alcohol syndrome and other developmental disorders associated with a toxic uterine environment result in permanent alterations to neurodevelopment. Even disruptions to sodium balance are linked to lifelong changes, such as altered connectivity between specific brain regions and altered gene expression. For example, it has been shown that early-life sodium depletion (e.g., from mothers vomiting often during pregnancy or infants eating a low-salt diet) increases salt preference during adulthood (Crystal & Bernstein, 1995; Curtis et al., 2004). Early sodium depletion increases levels of the circulating hormones aldosterone and angiotensin; these elevations may have permanent or so-called *organizational* effects within the developing nervous system. Also, children born to mothers who are either over- or underweight while pregnant are at increased risk for being overweight, likely because of organizational changes within the developing brain (Black et al., 2008; Cripps et al., 2005; Herring et al., 2012). These are referred to as epigenetic changes, meaning that the DNA sequence (building blocks of genes) is unchanged, but *expression* of genes is altered (this and other genetic concepts are reviewed in Chapter 6).

BOX 8.1 WHAT'S THE EVIDENCE FOR ORGANIZATION EFFECTS?

Statistics from the Dutch famine during the winter of 1944–1945 (due to severe food rationing in the Netherlands during World War II) reveal that individuals exposed to prolonged famine conditions during early prenatal development were at increased risk for obesity, diabetes, cardiovascular problems, and other health issues later in life (Roseboom et al., 2006). Before and after the famine, food was plentiful for most people. It seems that those exposed to energy and nutrient restriction during critical periods of brain organization developed heightened "starvation-resistance" circuitry. So, when these individuals entered an environment with food abundance rather than scarcity, they had increased desire to eat, a reduced ability to regulate energy needs, and more efficient energy storage, making them more likely to overeat and become obese. Similar effects have been found in other human and rodent studies (Levin, 2006).

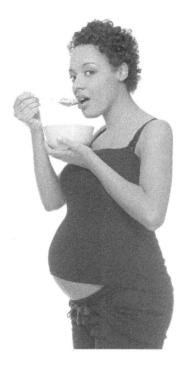

IMAGE 8.1 An expectant mom eating healthfully

You are probably familiar with the adage that expectant mothers can "eat for two," but is overconsumption during pregnancy a good idea? Until recent decades, food and nutrient scarcity was a threat to the developing child, and so pregnant women, with added energy needs, were encouraged to eat heartily. In our current Western environment of food abundance, the advice given to women in earlier decades is no longer applicable. In fact, consuming beyond their energy needs puts pregnant women at increased risk for gestational diabetes, preeclampsia (gestational high blood pressure), and other medical problems that can complicate pregnancy and the health of the child. Further, children born to mothers who gained excessive weight during pregnancy have higher body fat percentages (thus, higher leptin levels) and are at increased risk for obesity later in life compared with children born to mothers who gained a healthy amount of weight during pregnancy (Cripps et al., 2005; Herring et al., 2012).

Results of recent studies indicate that junk food consumption (i.e., foods high in energy and low in nutrients) during pregnancy predisposes children for heightened junk food cravings, which increase the likelihood of unhealthy weight. However, in studies of early human development, it is difficult to distinguish prenatal and postnatal influences. For example, children born to mothers who consume large amounts of junk food during pregnancy are often raised in homes where unhealthy food is eaten, making it difficult for researchers to determine the impact of the prenatal experience only. To address this issue, Bayol and colleagues (2007) conducted a study using a rat model, which allows for greater control over the variables. The design of their study is outlined in Figure 8.1.

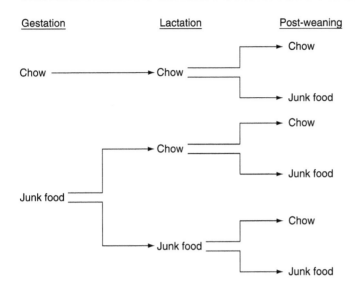

Gestation   Lactation   Post-weaning

FIGURE 8.1 The design of the "junk food" diet study

Source: Recreated from Bayol et al. (2007).

The junk food diet included doughnuts, cookies, candy bars, potato chips, cheese, and muffins in addition to standard rat chow. As expected, pregnant rats on the junk food diet consumed more energy and gained more weight compared with rats eating only chow. Although their consumption of sugar, fat, and salt increased, their intake of protein decreased compared with the control animals. So, the development of the fetal brains was impacted not only by overconsumption of energy but also by inadequate consumption of protein. Further, the offspring of dams (mothers) consuming the junk food diet demonstrated enhanced liking and preference for the junk food diet post-weaning compared with controls. All newly weaned rats demonstrated a liking for the junk food diet, but those exposed prenatally and during lactation selectively preferred foods high in sugar and fat over foods containing protein or fiber. Offspring exposed to the junk food diet during gestation and lactation but then fed only chow after weaning did not demonstrate overconsumption of chow. It seems that early exposure to highly palatable, energy-dense food creates an enhanced taste preference for tasty, high-calorie, high-fat food, which serves as a predisposition for obesity.

BOX 8.2 CAN BABIES SMELL AND TASTE BEFORE BIRTH?

Mennella and colleagues (2001) had groups of pregnant women consume either water or carrot juice during three weeks of their last trimester and then water or carrot juice during the first two months of breastfeeding. When the babies were about six months and already eating some baby foods such as rice cereal, they were videotaped as they tried carrot-flavored cereal for the first time. Mennella's group found that babies exposed to carrot juice flavors either prenatally in amniotic fluid or postnatally in breast milk were more accepting of this otherwise novel food than were babies of mothers who consumed only water during these times. These findings indicate that food flavors are detected in amniotic fluid, and that this early exposure influences food preferences after birth. Further, flavor exposure early in life through breast milk also enhances liking of a wider range of foods, preparing a baby for the cuisine of his or her environment.

BOX 8.3 DOES EXPOSURE AFFECT INTAKE?

Sullivan and Birch (1994) studied the first acceptance of solid foods in infants age four–six months. This was an in-home study in which mothers fed their infants a novel vegetable puree on ten occasions (e.g., one per meal per day). Intake was measured and videotaped. Over the exposure period, infants doubled their intake of novel foods from 30 g to 60 g. This was likely both a mere exposure effect and a decline of neophobia. Interestingly, this increase across exposures was much greater in breastfed compared with formula-fed infants. Sullivan and Birch hypothesized that breastfed infants experience an array of food flavors in their mothers' milk that enhances their acceptance of other novel foods, as previously discussed, better preparing them to accept a wider range of foods including fruits and vegetables.

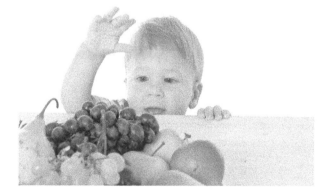

IMAGE 8.2 This boy is choosing fruit for a snack

Although it is relatively easy to understand how changes in hormones or nutrients in a mother's blood would be transmitted to the fetus, some questions about prenatal exposure to tastes and other sensory stimuli remain. We know that a fetus can hear, which is why some expectant mothers read stories or play music for their developing babies.

The fetus is also exposed to tastes and smells, and these exposures seem to contribute to post-birth preferences. Fetuses show swallowing behavior at approximately three months, which becomes more vigorous in the following months. They are swallowing amniotic fluid. The fetus also has mature taste cells at this early time of gestation (~four weeks; Mistretta & Bradley, 1975), though it is not known when the taste pathway to the cortex for processing of taste information becomes functional.

Mennella and colleagues (1995) found that amniotic fluid contains food flavors. They asked pregnant women who were undergoing amniocentesis (sampling of amniotic fluid) for other reasons to consume either a garlic or placebo pill about one hour before the procedure. The researchers then paired up the samples (forming five pairs of garlic and non-garlic samples) and asked a "smell panel" to judge which one of the pair contained garlic. In four of the five pairs, most judges were able to correctly pick out the garlic sample. Smell panels in other studies have similarly detected cumin and curry. This indicates that flavors are transmitted into amniotic fluid and can potentially stimulate smell or taste receptors in the fetus. This early exposure can actually influence the acceptance of flavors by infants.

EARLY POSTNATAL EATING: FROM SUCKLING TO EATING SOLID FOODS

Infants have an innate preference for sweet tastes: Newborns will suck much more vigorously at a sweet-tasting artificial nipple than at a neutral-tasting nipple. This is even evident in premature infants, although the overall vigor of the response is less (Tatzer et al., 1985). This indicates that detection of and preference for sweet tastes are innate and mature well before birth. Newborns also respond with displeasure to bitter and sour tastes, indicating innate aversions to these potentially dangerous tastes (Birch, 1999). Are all primary taste preferences and aversions innate? Maybe not. Using similar artificial nipple-sucking methods, newborns were indifferent to salt compared with water. Instead, the preference for salt appears at approximately four months after birth (Beauchamp et al., 1994, 1986). Experience does not seem to play a role (after all, amniotic fluid is largely a salt solution). Rather, maturation of central taste systems underlies this effect. Thus, the chemosensory world of newborns, while rich, differs from that of adults presented with the same tastes. Recent findings indicate that chemoreceptors in the enteric nervous system provide important sensory information for infants (see Chapters 4 and 5 and Mayer [2011] for a review of gut–brain communication).

A newborn is able to discriminate his or her mother's breast and underarm odors from those of other mothers (measured by the time spent orienting to the mother for breastfeeding). Newborns, either by prenatal exposure or, more likely, by rapid postnatal learning, are able to learn to seek a complex olfactory stimulus that is predictive of food and shelter. There is evidence that, by a few weeks of age, infants are able to detect food flavors in their mother's milk (Beauchamp & Mennella, 2009). Novel flavors (such as garlic and vanilla) produce more vigorous suckling, indicating that the novelty has been detected. Adult smell panels can also detect garlic and vanilla in mothers' milk (Savage et al., 2007).

To address early-life taste and smell abilities, some researchers have investigated whether or not babies can detect alcohol in breast milk. In one study, mothers drank a test beverage (orange juice) that was normal on one occasion and "spiked" with a small amount of alcohol on another occasion (Mennella, 2001). They breastfed their infants three to four hours after consuming the beverage. Infants consumed significantly less of their mother's milk on the alcohol day compared with the non-alcohol day. This indicated that the infants not only detected the alcohol but also disliked it (alcohol has a bitter taste). It is important to note that this study does not unequivocally prove it is the taste of alcohol in the milk that resulted in a decreased consumption; the mothers' breath or underarm odors could also have been affected, or the mothers' supply of breast milk could have been reduced.

BREAST VERSUS BOTTLE (FORMULA) FEEDING

There is something of a debate among neonatologists (and parents) regarding the benefits of "natural" versus "artificial" milk for infants, and it is our hunch that their positions in the debate reflect complex belief systems that transcend babies and milk. Breast milk has immunological properties, providing some protection from early-life illnesses, and it is associated with a reduced risk for obesity and other health problems (Field, 2005; Gartner et al., 2005; Kramer & Kakuma, 2012); furthermore, breastfeeding facilitates an emotional bond between mother and child. The American Academy of Pediatrics currently recommends exclusive breastfeeding for approximately the first six months and support for breastfeeding with appropriate complementary foods for two years, as long as mutually desired by mother and child (Meek et al., 2022). However, recent survey results indicate that about 20% of babies born in the U.S. were breastfed exclusively for their first six months (Victora et al., 2016). Although research unequivocally suggests that breastfeeding is advantageous for the infant (and mother), some parents decide to formula feed for a number of reasons, including convenience, health problems, a desire or financial need to return to work, insufficient milk production, or the mother's need to take medication that could be harmful to the baby. Importantly, both breast-milk-fed and formula-fed infants grow up fit and well, and so a parent's choice about which type of feeding may ultimately come down to personal preference. Let's review some of the main findings around breast versus bottle (formula) feeding.

Because breastfed infants are exposed to flavors from the mother's diet, their chemosensory exposure is more varied than that of formula-fed infants, as the flavor of formula is unchanging. There is some evidence that this better prepares infants for acceptance and liking of novel foods and flavors (Forestell & Mennella, 2007; Hausner et al., 2009; Sullivan & Birch, 1994). As previously described in this chapter, Mennella and colleagues (2001) found that, when breastfeeding mothers consumed carrot juice (consequently exposing their infants to that flavor through breast milk), their infants demonstrated increased acceptance and enjoyment of carrot flavor in infant cereal. This is an example of the *mere exposure effect*, meaning that preferences for foods and flavors increase with repeated exposures. Breastfed infants have the opportunity to experience a wider variety of flavors and develop more food preferences (and reduced neophobia [fear of new tastes]) than formula-fed infants. And this experience is correlated with a higher consumption of fruits and vegetables in childhood. Breastfeeding is often done "on demand"; that is, the infant is fed whenever he or she fusses. The infant then suckles for as long (and ingests as much) as desired. This arrangement allows the infant to control both meal size and interval between meals. In these demand-fed infants, by approximately two months of age, meal size (measured by weight gain during a suckling episode) correlates with the length of the preceding interval since their last suckling. The first nursing episode in the morning is the largest and follows the longest episode (sleep) without feeding (Matheny et al., 1990). (Although infants at this age are typically not sleeping through the entire night, they may sleep for up to six hours, usually their longest bout in a 24-hour period.) In contrast, by about age six months, their meal size correlates with the interval that follows the breastfeeding. This correlation seems to be driven by the fact that the last nursing episode in the evening is the largest (and these infants do now typically sleep through the night). They *apparently* (but would not be able to tell us in words for another year or two!) are anticipating the period of deprivation.

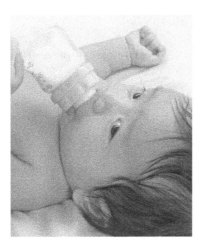

IMAGE 8.3 Baby consuming formula from a bottle

In contrast, formula-fed infants are usually not fed on demand; they are fed a "bottleful" (i.e., a fixed maximum meal size) and may not be fed immediately when they start fussing. Parents and caregivers often adhere to a relatively fixed schedule when bottle-feeding and, thus, may attempt to delay the onset of a meal. Consequently, meal taking (timing and amount) is relatively more imposed by the parents and/or caregivers. Research reveals no correlation between the intervals before or after the meal under these conditions. Perhaps bottle-fed babies are not given the full opportunity to either learn or determine these natural or normal meal size–interval relationships.

The consumption process is more passive for bottle-fed infants (i.e., they have less control over the amount and timing of meals) and requires less effort compared with breastfeeding, leading to frequent overfeeding of infants consuming formula. These conditions seem to interfere with their ability to self-regulate calorie consumption and possibly put formula-fed infants at greater risk for obesity later in life (Savage et al., 2007).

Results of several studies indicate that, in general, breastfeeding is associated with a decreased risk of being overweight later in life, decreased blood cholesterol and blood pressure, and a reduced risk of developing type 2 diabetes relative to formula-fed babies (Arenz et al., 2004; Owen et al., 2005; Plagemann & Harder, 2005). Further, longer durations of breastfeeding (e.g., nine months compared with one month) are linked to reduced risks of unhealthy high weights later (Gillman et al., 2001; Harder et al., 2005). The mechanism by which breastfeeding may protect from weight-related problems could be its facilitation of early self-regulation of energy intake, which then could persist later in life. Or the mechanism(s) could be related to the nutritional properties (hormones, peptides, or nutrients) of breast milk compared with formula. For example, maternal levels of circulating leptin, a hormone associated with satiety, correlate with levels of leptin in breast milk. Some evidence indicates that this early leptin exposure may contribute to energy and weight regulation (Miralles et al., 2006). Additionally, formula-fed infants consume larger amounts of protein and generally gain weight more rapidly than breastfed infants, possibly "programming" them for weight-related problems later in life (Cripps et al., 2005; Singhal & Lanigan, 2007).

Adding Solid Foods to the Diet

Typically, solid foods are introduced to complement breast milk or formula at around four to six months, the age at which infants have developed the motor coordination for swallowing food. Rice cereal mixed with breast milk or formula is often a first "solid" food (food is more soggy than solid in the early exposures). Later, pureed meats, fruits, and vegetables are added. Babies have an innate preference for the sweet-tasting (and more energy-dense) fruits and veggies, such as pureed bananas, sweet potatoes, applesauce, and peaches, and an aversion for the bitter foods, such as pureed green beans or spinach. As discussed earlier in this chapter, repeated exposure to initially disliked foods effectively increases the liking and acceptance of those foods. Around seven to nine months, finger foods are added, requiring the fine motor coordination of a pincher grasp.

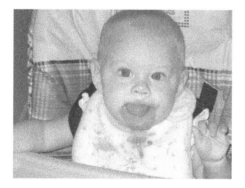

IMAGE 8.4 This baby is learning to eat solid foods. It's a messy learning process!

Over time, the ratio of solid food to breast milk or formula increases, and often, by age one or two years, a child's diet no longer includes breast milk or formula. So, in a relatively short period of time (from about six months in age to one year), a baby learns to accept a spoon, move food to the back of the mouth, and safely swallow it (in earlier months, babies reflexively spit food out, which often results in a mess!); then, to pick up foods and chew them before swallowing; and, lastly, to use a spoon independently (or, at least, start to). These are important developmental milestones that depend on physical ability and readiness, cognitive processing, and guidance from parents or caretakers. It is during this time that children are introduced to cultural norms and also to family norms regarding eating behavior, including mealtimes, foods associated with particular meals, meal and snack size, table manners, proper use of utensils, and so on. Certainly, these are not well understood or mastered at age one year, but a foundation for what will be considered "normal" eating behavior in a particular culture is established. Thus, a parent's role in these early months and years is tremendously influential.

NOT NEEDING A BOTTLE BUT STILL NEEDING GUIDANCE: EATING IN EARLY CHILDHOOD

One important job that parents and caregivers have is ensuring that infants and young children are receiving proper nutrition (calories and nutrients) to grow well and maintain health. This is sometimes a difficult task because babies and very young children cannot always communicate specific desires or needs. For example, a crying toddler may want more juice or cereal; may be tired, sick, or hurt; or may want a particular toy that is out of reach. Parents are often good guessers as to the child's needs, but clearly there is room for error. In our current culture, this error often is overfeeding or feeding foods that give comfort, usually food that is high in calories and fat, when a child cries. These attempts at meeting needs or soothing an upset child can establish an emotional link with food early in life, increasing the likelihood that, as the child grows past infancy, he or she will continue to eat for emotional rather than hunger needs. In the next section, we explore evidence that infants and children have some ability to regulate their food (energy) needs, but this ability is decreased as children become older and more aware of environmental cues.

Can Infants and Young Children Self-Regulate Energy Needs?

The question of whether or not infants and young children can innately regulate calorie and nutrient needs has been long debated. In the early 1900s, the philosophy among pediatricians was that children should be fed specific and regulated diets. It was assumed that, without parental guidance, children would choose unhealthy ratios of macro- and micronutrients. Thus, parents were advised to exercise an authoritarian approach to eating, leading to commonly used phrases such as "clean your plate." A landmark study by pediatrician Clara Davis (1939) challenged this thinking. She studied 15 newly weaned infants for several months in an institutional setting. Initially, all of the solid foods were novel. In this institution, meals were served at fixed times, but the infants had their choice of what to select (10–12 choices were available at each meal) and how much of each to eat. Davis maintained records of food choices and amounts consumed for several years (up to 4.5 years for two of the children).

An important finding was that children consumed only a few food items at a meal, typically two or three items. Also, children went on what Davis called "food jags," eating only one or two foods for several days in a row. However, over time, those preferences changed so that, overall, children selected a diet that contained approximately 17% of calories as protein, 35% as fat, and 48% as carbohydrate, healthy ratios of macronutrients for children. Lastly, despite large individual differences in feeding habits, all of the children grew well and were deemed healthy. Davis interpreted her data as support for an "innate self-selection mechanism," which was in striking contrast at the time to the leading philosophy among pediatricians. Davis advocated allowing children to self-select food items and amounts. Following the publication of her findings, pediatricians and parents began loosening controls on children's eating with the new understanding that children had the innate ability to self-regulate energy and nutrient needs.

Are you surprised by Davis's findings? Let's examine some of the details of her study a bit more. The food choices for infants and toddlers in Davis's study included beets, spinach, fruit, oatmeal, potatoes, milk, fish, and meat (liver, brains, beef, kidneys, lamb).

Do those menu options sound very appealing to you? Do you think that a typical American four-year-old would excitedly choose a dinner of liver and beets? Probably not! So, would the results of Davis's study have been the same if she used today's typical kids' menu options? Imagine offering a child all-you-can-eat chicken nuggets, French fries, cookies, pizza, ice cream, and candy every day for years. It is very likely that the child will eat beyond his or her energy needs and not regulate vitamin and mineral levels. Unfortunately, this scenario is the reality in our current environment. We have easy access to highly palatable foods and a poor ability to self-regulate caloric intake under these conditions. Perhaps if our only options were items like those in Davis's study, we (children and adults) would be much better at maintaining healthy weights. So, despite the groundbreaking results of Davis's study at the time, the innate ability to self-regulate energy seems to work well only in an environment with less palatable and less calorie- and fat-dense foods than those prevalent in modern Western society.

EXPERIMENTAL STUDY OF CALORIC REGULATION IN CHILDREN

Some research suggests that infants and young children (~two months to three years) have internal controls for caloric regulation, and that these controls are less effective in older children. For example, Fomon et al. (1975) found that six-week-old infants consumed more of dilute (~5 kcal/ml) than dense (~10 kcal/ml) formula. However, over time, they did not achieve perfect caloric compensation. That is, the volume consumed of the half-strength formula was not double that of the high-strength formula. Recall what you read earlier in this chapter about formula feeding (or bottle-feeding) in general: It is an externally imposed regimen of size and time, and, although these are young infants, they presumably already have had a lot of prior bottle-feedings. Thus, these infants may already have learned about portion size and average caloric yield, and so their adaptation to this caloric manipulation may be compromised or limited by prior experience. Other findings indicate that overall energy intake remains constant when solid foods are added to the diets of breastfed babies, meaning that the infants compensate for the added calories by consuming less breast milk (Savage et al., 2007).

Evidence shows that preschoolers exhibit at least short-term (within-meal) caloric compensation. A protocol used by Birch and her colleagues in several studies for over 20 years involved giving a calorically disguised first course (which serves as a preload) followed about 30 minutes later by a self-selected second course (e.g., lunch). Birch found that, after a low-calorie preload, the selected meal was calorically larger than after a high-calorie preload. This study design demonstrates short-term caloric adjustment. Interestingly, but perhaps not surprisingly, caloric regulation is poorer in overweight children (Birch & Fisher, 2000; Johnson & Birch, 1994). To quantify the precision of regulation, Birch's group developed the compensation index, a measurement of the difference in caloric intake at the second course divided by the caloric difference in the preload. An index of +1 indicates perfect compensation, and an index of 0 indicates no effect of the preload (i.e., no compensation). They and others have used the compensation index as a mechanism for quantifying energy compensation in studies of children's eating.

BOX 8.4 DO CHILDREN RECOGNIZE CALORIES?

Birch et al. (1990) found that children demonstrated conditioned flavor preferences based on caloric density. Novel drink flavors were used in these trials, and the drinks were either high in calories (155 kcal/150 ml) or low (less than 5 kcal/150 ml). (A low-calorie sweetener was used to reduce calories.) The children consumed the beverage and were then allowed to consume additional snacks as desired (milk, cheese, fruit, cookies). The trials actually substituted for the children's regularly scheduled morning snack, thus not interfering with normal meals or routines. At the end of the study, the children reported increased liking of both flavors, a function of the mere exposure effect. However, they had greater liking of the flavor associated with higher calories, both rating it higher and consuming it when given a choice between the flavors. Additionally, the children consumed fewer snacks after consumption of the flavor associated with high calories, indicating learned energy regulation.

Does caloric compensation occur over a longer period of time? Birch et al. (1991) measured 24-hour intakes of children (ages two to five years) over a six-day period. The children received the same menus each day. Like Davis, Birch found that intake at individual meals was highly variable. In contrast, 24-hour energy intakes were relatively constant. This implies meal-to-meal adjustments of intake for longer-term caloric regulation. However, menu options in this study, as in Davis's, were relatively nutritious items (e.g., turkey sandwiches, fruit, and yogurt) compared with the calorie-dense and nutrient-poor foods found in many restaurants, homes, and schools in our current Western culture.

In a subsequent study to directly manipulate this situation, children were again studied over several days, but, on some days, 14 g of dietary fat (~130 kcal, which is more than 10% of the total mean caloric intake) were substituted by a zero-calorie fat substitute ("fake fat" – chemically modified fat molecules that cannot be broken down in the gut and absorbed). For example, muffins were baked with fake fat on low-calorie/fat days and with butter on high-calorie/fat days, but the muffins and other manipulated foods were otherwise as similar as possible in appearance and taste. The results again showed high variability between meals, but daily energy intake was constant, regardless of whether fake or real fat was offered (Birch et al., 1993). This shows that children are able to compensate for the low-fat version by eating more of other foods, even when they are not aware of the manipulation. What are the implications? This study not only demonstrated caloric regulation in children, it also helped explain the general lack of success that many dieters have when exchanging their regular snacks for low-fat versions. It is likely that adult dieters compensate for the calories and fat grams by consuming more of other foods.

Following a large meal, children tend to regulate calories by eating fewer food items in a second meal, but they do not regulate calories by reducing the amount of each item consumed in the next meal. Children tend to choose their preferred foods in the second meal and eliminate the less preferred, which are often the more nutritious foods (Birch et al., 1993). And different children have different preferred foods. Fisher and Birch (1995) found that, when children were allowed to self-select their foods (over a six-day period), their percentage of calories taken from fat varied greatly among them (from 25% to 41% of calories from fat). Some children consistently chose a high-fat diet, and some a low-fat diet, despite having the same choices. Not surprisingly, the children with the highest preference for fat had the highest body mass index (BMI) and also the heaviest parents (based on BMI; Fisher & Birch, 1995; Johnson & Birch, 1994). These results indicate the importance of familial factors in establishing dietary intake and choice in children, although the findings do not discriminate between genetic and environmental influences.

EXTERNAL INFLUENCES ON CHILDREN'S' EATING: DISRUPTIONS IN ENERGY SELF-REGULATION

Taken together, studies of caloric and nutrient regulation, from Davis's in the 1930s to many conducted in recent decades, indicate that infants and young children have some ability to regulate energy needs, both within and across meals. However, this regulation is imperfect and becomes blunted with age. Self-regulation of energy need is disrupted by the external influences to which older children are exposed, including food attractiveness and palatability, eating behaviors of peers, media, and parental behaviors and attitudes. Thus, with age, children are more likely to eat in response to external cues rather than internal physiological hunger cues.

Parenting Styles, Attitudes, and Weights

Parenting styles and approaches to children's eating have been found to impact food choices and calorie and fat regulation among children. Children of authoritarian parents (parents who are controlling, set strict rules, and expect obedience) have a reduced ability to regulate calorie needs (Johnson & Birch, 1994). Further, the more authoritarian the parents, the poorer a child's ability to regulate. This parenting style, in contrast to permissive and authoritative styles, is associated with behaviors such as demanding that the child eat particular foods while forbidding others, without regard for the child's needs or preferences. A permissive parenting style is associated with few parental regulations or controls. Regarding eating behavior, permissive parents tend to let children have what they want when they want it. These conditions require the child to make his or her own decisions, which typically leads to consumption of the tastiest, most easily available foods (as the child is limited to whatever is in the home or at school).

Authoritative parenting is the happy middle ground between authoritarian and permissive parenting. Authoritative parents provide structure and guidelines but explain the reasons for them and allow flexibility when warranted. This parenting style regarding eating includes behaviors such as encouraging a nutritious diet and explaining the benefits of a healthy lifestyle, but not forcing children to eat foods that are disliked. Rather, an authoritative parent is likely to offer healthy food options that children can select from. Children of authoritative parents have increased eating of healthy foods (fruits and vegetables) and reduced eating of junk foods compared with children of authoritarian parents (Patrick et al., 2005).

Children of parents who restrict or forbid certain foods, a behavior often associated with the authoritarian style, are more likely to overeat in the absence of hunger, to have higher BMI, and to suffer with body image dissatisfaction and eating disorders during ado-lescence. This effect is most pronounced among daughters of restrictive mothers (Birch et al., 2003; Johnson & Birch, 1994). When foods are labeled "forbidden," children have reduced ability to control their eating of those foods when given access (perhaps at a friend's house). Researchers have also shown that, when food is used as a reward or bribe (e.g., "if you clean your room you can have a cookie"), the liking of that food increases. And, interestingly, promising a treat for eating a disliked food (e.g., "you can have ice cream if you eat your spinach") actually increases the liking of the treat and worsens the aversion for the disliked food (Birch et al., 1982; Savage et al., 2007). Essentially, all of these examples (restricting, forbidding, using food as a reward) focus attention on **external cues** and decrease a child's responsiveness to internal cues of hunger or satiety.

Homes of authoritative parents have more frequent availability of fruits, vegetables, and dairy and less availability of junk food compared with homes of authoritarian parents. Thus, children of authoritative parents are more frequently exposed to and offered healthy foods. Further, authoritative parents are more likely to model the con-sumption of healthy foods. So, in addition to parenting style, children of authoritative parents are influenced by mere exposure and modeling (two learning principles) that further enhance their liking of healthy foods. Researchers have found that children of parents who eat more fruits and vegetables and drink more milk at home are more likely to like and consume the same foods even when they are not at home (see Savage et al. [2007] for a more thorough review).

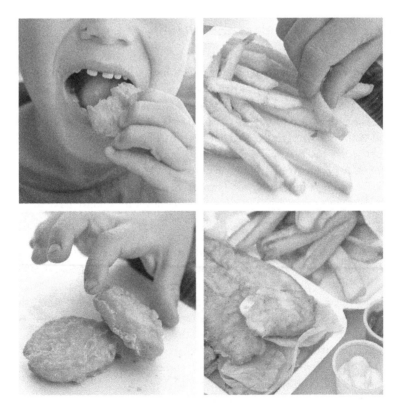

IMAGE 8.5 Unhealthy kids' meal options

Talking Point 8.1

How would you advise parents to monitor children's food choices? Consider both Davis's findings and the rising number of overweight children in Western countries. Revisit this question after you complete the chapter; you may have additional ideas or you may consider some modifications to your initial advice.

Parents' food choices and BMIs are also correlated with those of their children (Johnson & Birch, 1994). Parents who consume more junk food have high BMIs, as do their children. And children of parents who themselves have difficulty controlling their eating also have poorer ability at regulating energy needs. These effects are more pronounced among girls, particularly obese girls. Can you think of explanations for these correlations? Perhaps the effect is due to shared genes. Certainly, genes do predispose individuals to deposit fat in particular places in their body and to metabolize energy at varying rates (see Chapter 6). But do you think that shared genetics is the only explanation? It is probably not, given the rapid rise in the obesity rate. Shared environment is also a likely explanation. Parents and children in these homes are eating many of the same foods, often those high in fat and calories. Parents model eating of these types of foods, whereas eating of healthy fruits and vegetables is not frequent in these homes.

Obesity is seen among people of all levels of socio-economic status (SES), but the highest incidence is among people with low SES, including poverty conditions. What is interesting and paradoxical about this situation is that people in this group have both the highest rates of reported hunger and the highest rates of obesity. How could this be? Low-SES families often have reduced access to fresh fruits and vegetables but convenient access to junk food, which is typically high in calories and fat and low in nutritional value. Some low-SES communities in Western society have recently been considered to be in "food deserts," areas characterized by limited accessibility to nutritional foods. Limited exposure to healthy foods (i.e., they are infrequently accessible, and their consumption is rarely modeled) increases the likelihood that children will have unhealthy diets and weight problems later in life.

Talking Point 8.2

Research indicates that children of authoritative parents not only have healthier eating habits but also tend to have higher self-esteem and greater success in life compared with children of permissive or authoritarian parents. So, why do you think that the authoritative style is not used by all parents?

SOCIAL INFLUENCES

With age, children are increasingly influenced by their peers' behaviors, and this applies to eating behavior too. Children are more likely to sample a novel food when consumption of that food is modeled by an adult or peer (Hendy & Raudenbush, 2000). Studies have shown that children will modify their food preference when they observe that a peer has a different preference (Addessi et al., 2005). As an example, Birch (1980) found that preschool-age children would quickly select the fruit that the other children around them chose, even when the fruit that they typically preferred was available.

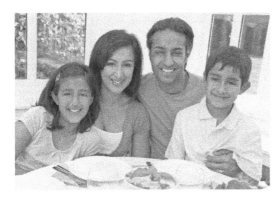

IMAGE 8.6 Parents are early models of eating behavior

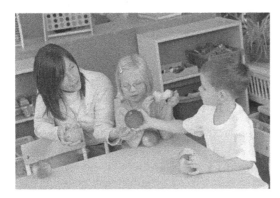

IMAGE 8.7 Children are influenced by the food preferences of others

The effects of education about food seem to be age related. In a study involving jelly bean flavors, some familiar and others novel (e.g., grape, kiwi, watermelon, coffee, and Dr. Pepper), preschool-age children (three to six years old) were told positive associations (e.g., "Grape is Winnie the Pooh's favorite flavor") for some flavors and not others. In a second phase, children were asked to rate the hedonic value (using smiley, neutral, or unhappy faces) of the flavors. Exposure to positive information had an effect on the hedonic rating of the flavors, but only for the children older than 4.5 years (Lumeng & Cardinal, 2007). This supports the theory that children are more impacted by external cues with age. It seems that the relatively slow maturation of areas of the brain associated with memory (e.g., hippocampus, frontal cortex) contribute to this effect of age.

FOOD AVAILABILITY AND PORTION SIZES

As discussed in other chapters, the current food environment of Western culture is obesogenic, meaning that food is easily available, energy dense, highly palatable, and heavily (or strategically) marketed. Further, portion sizes have increased progressively, leading to increased caloric intake. Studies have shown that children and adults eat more when they are served larger portions and generally do not compensate by eating less of other foods (Fisher et al., 2007, 2003). Significant elevations in energy intake over a 24-hour period were found when portion sizes of entrees and snacks were doubled. Fisher and colleagues (2007) found that portion size and **energy density** have additive effects. Either factor alone increased overall energy intake, but together they had an enhanced impact on energy intake. Although this information is perhaps not surprising, it is important to have this type of empirical evidence, as many of the foods that we are exposed to, particularly in restaurants, are both in large portions and high in energy density.

Total caloric intake is also related to feeding frequency (Garcia et al., 1990a, 1990b). In one study, children were fed two scheduled meals per day but additionally could request and receive snacks. They requested food frequently and ate a mean of 13.5 times per day. Children who ate more snacks consumed more calories per day; that is, snacks did not detract from main meal size. (So much for the mother's adage that too much snacking will spoil your appetite for dinner!) Of course, this implies that caloric compensation is weak, contrasting with Birch's findings. These results also indicate that frequent offering of food leads to increased eating. This information, paired with the results of the Fisher et al. (2007) study, illuminates how problematic our modern food environment has become for children. They are exposed to large portions of foods high in energy density and offered foods frequently while they are in the early process of establishing patterns of meal sizes and frequency.

MEDIA

Marketers in the food industry base much of their work on the central tenets of classical conditioning. A seminal aim in advertising is to create positive associations between a branded food item, a store, or restaurant, and the customers. It is estimated that more than $14 billion is spent on advertisements for U.S. food products (UConn Rudd Center for Food Policy and Health, 2017). And food and beverage advertisements account for about 25% of advertisements aired during children's television programming. Commercials depicting happy children singing and eating a particular food item lead to associations in the minds of children and parents between consumption of that food and positive experiences. As an example, McDonald's has been one of the most successful businesses at associating its brand and food items with positive experiences. Its kids' meal is the "Happy Meal," the Ronald McDonald clown makes appearances at children's birthday parties, and the restaurants often have indoor play areas. These are among the powerfully effective marketing tools used by McDonald's (and other food businesses as well) to instill lifelong positive associations with their food items.

Robinson and colleagues (2007) demonstrated this effect. Preschool children were asked to taste familiar food items (hamburgers, chicken nuggets, and French fries from McDonald's, and carrots, milk, and apple juice from a grocery store). The children tasted two identical samples of each food, one in McDonald's packaging and the other in unmarked wrapping. The children overwhelmingly preferred the food items in the branded packaging, even the carrots, which are not currently offered on McDonald's menu. We should add that it is not our intent to vilify any one brand or even class of foods, because all food companies are engaging in more or less the same behavior.

Another study similarly demonstrated the preference that four- to six-year-old children have for snacks branded with popular cartoon characters (Scooby Doo, Dora the Explorer, or Shrek). Children both selected the cartoon-branded snacks more often and preferred the tastes of the branded snacks compared with the same snacks in unbranded packaging (Roberto et al., 2010).

Other studies have shown increased food consumption, particularly of sweet snacks, after viewing food advertisements compared with non-food-related advertisements on television (Halford et al., 2004). Because many nutrient-poor and energy-dense snacks (e.g., candies, fruit roll-ups, cookies, sugary cereals) are frequently marketed to children with popular cartoon characters, instilling preferences for healthier foods is increasingly difficult. A group of researchers analyzed the nutritional content of food depicted in television shows aimed at children aged five and younger (Radnitz et al., 2009). They found that unhealthy foods were shown about twice as often as healthy foods, and that the characters on these shows frequently endorsed consumption and overconsumption of unhealthy food.

Overweight children are influenced by external influences and marketing to a greater extent than normal-weight children. In a study by Formon et al. (2009), normal-weight children consumed fewer calories when a meal was branded, but overweight children consumed significantly more calories when the meal was branded versus non-branded. Their findings indicate that overweight children are more likely to recognize marketed food items and eat more when food is associated with marketed brands. Halford et al. (2004) also found that obese children were more likely than normal-weight children to recognize food advertisements; further, the amount of snacks consumed was correlated with familiarity with the advertisement. This associative learning may put overweight children at a greater risk for obesity and associated health problems in a media-saturated environment. Further, in cities and countries where food-related commercials have been limited or eliminated during times of television programming for children, there is consistent reduction in sales and, consequently, consumption of unhealthy snack foods (Taillie et al., 2019)

Implications for Instilling Healthy Eating Behaviors in Children

Prenatal and early postnatal food and flavor experiences prepare children for the variety of foods that they will encounter in their culture. Exposure to healthy foods during this early time in life enhances children's acceptance of otherwise novel foods. This helps minimize "picky" eating of only heavily processed foods that are high in fat and calories and low in nutrients (e.g., foods often found on restaurant menus for children such as chicken nuggets and hot dogs). Children enter the present food environment with a better predisposition for healthy living when exposed to fruits and vegetables rather than excessive junk food during prenatal (through amniotic fluid) and early postnatal (through breast milk) months. When infants begin consuming solid foods, parents should be patient with the process and continue to offer nutritious foods repeatedly, as acceptance and liking of novel foods (especially bitter-tasting vegetables) can take many exposures. Results of studies of children's eating behavior revealed that the most frequently consumed vegetable among toddlers is French fries, if they consume any vegetables at all (Fox et al., 2004; Moding et al., 2018). Clearly, parents and caregivers too infrequently prioritize the need for early exposure to a healthy variety of foods.

As children grow, parents and caregivers should encourage them to focus on their internal hunger and satiety cues and minimize the focus on external cues by refraining from using phrases such as "you must clean your plate." Parents should also be mindful of their own eating behaviors, both for their own health and as models for their children. Children's consumption of healthy fruits, vegetables, and dairy is correlated with their parents' consumption of the same foods. After extensive research into children's eating behaviors, Birch and Fisher (2000) suggested that parents should provide children with a variety of balanced foods at each meal, but be nondirective about what items and how much are eaten. The argument (like Davis's) is that children will come to focus on their own internal controls ("listen to what their bodies are telling them"), select a nutritionally adequate diet, and be less prone to obesity or eating disorders as teens or adults. This may be especially important in girls, as the loss of internal compensation in obese girls (and the reason that led to their obesity) may reflect this externalization of control by an authoritarian parenting style regarding eating.

Finally, as a society, we need to seriously consider the impact that our current food environment has on the health of the current and next generations. The obesity rate has increased dramatically in the past 30 years and, unfortunately, continues to rise. Childhood obesity rates have also risen, and data from the Centers for Disease Control and Prevention (2007) indicate that one in three children born in the year 2000 or more recently will develop type 2 diabetes (a disorder typically associated with unhealthy eating and weight). The economic burden of the preventable health problems associated with obesity is staggering. The rates of diabetes are predicted to double by 2030, and the associated health costs are expected to be $622 billion (Rowley et al., 2017). Further, obesity (or unhealthy weight) is correlated with psychological dysfunction. Overweight children are at a much greater risk for developing depression during adolescence and adulthood. These mental and physical health issues negatively impact quality of life – and much of this can be prevented by a healthy lifestyle, which includes healthy eating.

So, whereas parents certainly share responsibility for the health of their children, our culture needs to change so that healthy eating is of greater importance. School lunches, for example, should include fresh fruits and vegetables and healthy ratios of micro- and macronutrients. Many children are not provided with healthy food options at home; thus, school may be the only environment in which some children have at least one daily exposure to healthy foods. This affords children the opportunity to overcome neophobia of novel foods and increases the likelihood that they will make healthy food choices as adults. Children exposed only to foods such as pizza, French fries, and chicken nuggets will continue to choose only those foods later in life, and this is a pattern associated with poor health. Certainly, the inclusion of regular exercise in physical education classes, playtime, and sports is another way that schools and communities can promote healthy living.

Talking Point 8.3

If children are more likely to eat snacks with popular cartoon characters on the packaging, then don't you think that this type of marketing could help increase consumption of healthy fruits and veggies? Why do you think this tactic is not frequently used? (Hint: Consider costs.)

Something else for you to think about: In 2007, the Department of Health and Human Services (HHS) and the Ad Council teamed up with DreamWorks studios to launch a healthy eating ad campaign featuring characters from the *Shrek* movie series. Maybe you enjoyed these movies during childhood. Within months, members of children advocacy groups objected, some conducting letter-writing petitions in opposition. In the public service advertisements, *Shrek* characters encouraged children to "get up and play." However, the Ad Council also teamed up with for-profit companies, including Kraft Foods, General Mills, Kellogg's, Coca-Cola, and Pepsico, among others. So, soon after the initiation of the campaign to combat childhood obesity, the *Shrek* character branding could be found on more than 70 food products, most of which were heavily processed, high in sugar, and low in nutrients, and many contained added green dye for effect. Some of the food products included Snicker's candy bars, pop-tarts, chocolate chip cookies, M&M candies, frozen waffles and pancakes, Twinkies, and several types of sugary cereals. The initiative started with good intent, but the involvement of for-profit companies steered the efforts far from promoting healthy food choices for children. You may want to watch the documentary *Fed Up* (released in 2014) for more information on ideas and failures by policy makers and the consequences for children's health.

Talking Point 8.4

Do you think, both at theoretical and practical/ethical levels, that you could use the compensation index as a diagnostic test for children at risk for later eating disorders and try to reeducate them and their parents?

QUESTIONS TO ASK YOURSELF

Let's review and apply your knowledge. Take some time to answer these chapter questions:

- Describe at least three pieces of evidence that demonstrate the effects of prenatal experience on eating behavior later in life.
- How might breastfeeding enhance healthy eating among children later in life? Explain.
- Describe Dr. Clara Davis's study and her conclusions. What do you think about her findings in light of our current food environment?
- How do parenting styles and parents' eating behaviors and weight influence children's eating behaviors and weight? Are gender and/or socio-economic status contributing factors?
- What is the evidence of the impact of peer influence and media on children's eating behavior? Does weight contribute to this? Explain.

GLOSSARY

Authoritarian parenting	A style characterized by control, strict rules, and expectations of obedience.
Authoritative parenting	A style that encourages a child's independence but provides guidelines and structure.
Compensation index	A measurement of the difference in caloric intake at the second course divided by the caloric difference in the preload; an index of +1 indicates perfect compensation, and an index of 0 indicates no effect of the preload (i.e., no compensation).
Energy density	The amount of energy in a given weight of food.
External cues	Stimuli in the environment (e.g., sight and smell of food, eating behavior of others, attractiveness of food).
Permissive parenting	A style characterized by few rules or limits.
Portion size	The amount of allotted food.

REFERENCES

Addessi, E., Galloway, A. T., Visalberghi, E., & Birch, L. L. (2005). Specific social influences on the acceptance of novel foods in 2–5-year-old children. *Appetite, 45*, 264–271.

Arenz, S., Rückerl, R., Koletzko, B., & Von Kries, R. (2004). Breast-feeding and childhood obesity – a systematic review. *International Journal of Obesity Related Metabolic Disorders, 28*, 1247–1256.

Bayol, S. A., Farrington, S. J., & Stickland, N. C. (2007). A maternal "junk food" diet in pregnancy and lactation promotes an exacerbated taste for "junk food" and a greater propensity for obesity in rat offspring. *British Journal of Nutrition.* doi:10.1017/S0007114507812037

Beauchamp, G. K., Cowart, B. J., Mennella, J. A., & Marsh, R. R. (1994). Infant salt taste: Developmental, methodological, and contextual factors. *Developmental Psychobiology, 27* (6), 353–365.

Beauchamp, G. K., Cowart, B. J., & Moran, M. (1986). Developmental changes in salt acceptability in human infants. *Developmental Psychobiology, 19*, 17–25.

Beauchamp, G. K., & Mennella, J. A. (2009). Early flavor learning and its impact on later feeding behavior. *Journal of Pediatric Gastroenterology and Nutrition, 48*, S25–S30.

Birch, L. L. (1980). Effects of peer models' food choices and eating behaviors on preschooler's food preferences. *Child Development, 51*, 489–496.

Birch, L. L. (1999). Development of food preferences. *Annual Review of Nutrition, 19* (1), 41–62.

Birch, L. L., Birch, D., Marlin, D. W., & Kramer, L. (1982). Effects of instrumental consumption on children's food preference. *Appetite, 3*, 125–134.

Birch, L. L., & Fisher, J. O. (2000). Mothers' child-feeding practices influence daughters' eating and weight. *The American Journal of Clinical Nutrition, 71* (5), 1054–1061.

Birch, L. L., Fisher, J. O., & Davison, K. K. (2003). Learning to overeat: Maternal use of restrictive feeding practices promotes girls' eating in the absence of hunger. *American Journal of Clinical Nutrition, 78* (2), 215–220.

Birch, L. L., Johnson, S. L., Andresen, G., Peters, J. C., & Schulte, M. C. (1991). The variability of young children's energy intake. *The New England Journal of Medicine, 324* (4), 232–235.

Birch, L. L., Johnson, S. L., Jones, M. B., & Peters, J. C. (1993). Effects of a nonenergy fat substitute on children's energy and macronutrient intake. *The American Journal of Clinical Nutrition, 58* (3), 326–333.

Birch, L. L., McPhee, L., Steinberg, L., & Sullivan, S. (1990). Conditioned flavor preferences in young children. *Physiology & Behavior, 47* (3), 501–505.

Black, B. E., Allen, L. H., Bhutta, Z. A., et al. (2008). Maternal and child undernutrition: Global and regional exposures and health consequences. *The Lancet, 371* (9608), 243–260. doi:10.1016/S0140-6736(07)61690-0

Centers for Disease Control and Prevention. (2007). 2007 national diabetes fact sheet. Retrieved from www.cdc.gov/diabetes/pubs/figuretext07.htm

Cripps, R. X., Martin-Gronert, M. X., & Ozanne, S. X. (2005). Fetal and perinatal programming of appetite. *Clinical Science, 109* (1), 1–12.

Crystal, S. R., & Bernstein, I. L. (1995). Morning sickness: Impact on offspring salt preference. *Appetite, 25,* 231–240.

Curtis, K. S., Krause, E. G., Wong, D. L., & Contreras, R. J. (2004). Gestational and early postnatal dietary NaCl levels affect NaCl intake, but not stimulated water intake, by adult rats. *American Journal of Physiology – Regulatory, Integrative and Comparative Physiology, 286,* R1043–1050.

Davis, C. (1939). Results of the self-selection of diets by young children. *The Canadian Medical Association Journal, 41,* 257–261.

Field, C. J. (2005). The immunological components of human milk and their effect on immune development in infants. *The Journal of Nutrition, 135* (1), 1–4.

Fisher, J. A., & Birch, L. L. (1995). Fat preferences and fat consumption of 3- to 5-year-old children are related to parental adiposity. *Journal of the American Dietetic Association, 95,* 759–764.

Fisher, J. O., Liu, Y., Birch, L. L., & Rolls, B. J. (2007). Effects of portion size and energy density on young children's intake at a meal. *American Journal of Clinical Nutrition, 86,* 174–179.

Fisher, J. O., Rolls, B. J., & Birch, L. L. (2003). Children's bite size and intake of an entrée are greater with large portions than with age-appropriate or self-selected portions. *American Journal of Clinical Nutrition, 77,* 1164–1170.

Fomon, S. J., Filmer, L. J., Thomas, L. N., Anderson, T. A., & Nelson, S. E. (1975). Influence of formula concentration on caloric intake and growth of normal infants. *Acta Paediatrica Scandanavia, 64,* 172–181.

Forestell, C. A., & Mennella, J. A. (2007). Early determinants of fruit and vegetable acceptance. *Pediatrics, 120,* 1247.

Formon, J., Halford, J. C. G., Summe, H., MacDougall, M., & Keller, K. L. (2009). Food branding influences ad libitum intake differently in children depending on weight status. *Appetite, 53,* 76–83.

Fox, M. K., Pac, S., Devaney, B., & Jankowski, L. (2004). Feeding infants and toddlers study: What foods are infants and toddlers eating? *Journal of the American Dietetic Association, 104* (Supplement 1), S22–S30.

Garcia, S. E., Kaiser, L. L., & Dewey, K. G. (1990a). Self-regulation of food intake among rural Mexican preschool children. *European Journal of Clinical Nutrition, 44* (5), 371–380.

Garcia, S. E., Kaiser, L. L., & Dewey, K. G. (1990b). The relationship of eating frequency and caloric density to energy intake among rural Mexican preschool children. *European Journal of Clinical Nutrition, 44* (5), 381–387.

Gartner, L. M., Morton, J., Lawrence, R. A., et al. (2005). Breastfeeding and the use of human milk. *Pediatrics, 115* (2), 496–506.

Gillman, M. W., Rifas-Shiman, S. L., Camargo, J. C. A., et al. (2001). Risk of overweight among adolescents who were breastfed as infants. *Journal of the American Medical Association, 285* (19), 2461–2467.

Halford, J. C., Gillespie, J., Brown, V., Pontin, E. E., & Dovey, T. M. (2004). Effect of television advertisements for food on food consumption in children. *Appetite, 42* (2), 221–225.

Harder, T., Bergmann, R., Kallischnigg, G., & Plagemann, A. (2005). Duration of breastfeeding and risk of overweight: A meta-analysis. *American Journal of Epidemiology, 162* (5), 397–403.

Hausner, H., Nicklaus, S., Issanchou, S., Mølgaard, C., & Møller, P. (2009). Breastfeeding facilitates acceptance of a novel dietary flavour compound. *Clinical Nutrition, 29* (1), 141–148.

Hendy, H. M., & Raudenbush, B. (2000). Effectiveness of teacher modeling to encourage food acceptance in preschool children. *Appetite, 34* (1), 61–76.

Herring, S. J., Rose, M. Z., Skouteris, H., & Oken, E. (2012). Optimizing weight gain in pregnancy to prevent obesity in women and children. *Diabetes, Obesity, & Metabolism, 14* (3), 195–203. doi:10.1111/j.1463-1326.2011.01489

Johnson, S. L., & Birch, L. L. (1994). Parents' and children's adiposity and eating style. *Pediatrics, 95* (5), 653–661.

Kramer, M. S., & Kakuma, R. (2012). Optimal duration of exclusive breastfeeding. *Cochrane Database of Systematic Reviews,* (8), Art. No.: CD003517. doi:10.1002/14651858.CD003517.pub2

Lechtig, A., Habicht, J., Delgado, H., Klein, R. E., Yarbrough, C., & Martorell, R. (1975). Effect of food supplementation during pregnancy on birthweight. *Pediatrics, 56* (4), 508.

Levin, B. E. (2006). Metabolic imprinting: Critical impact of the perinatal environment on the regulation of energy homeostasis. *Philosophical Transactions of the Royal Society B: Biological Sciences, 361* (1471), 1107–1121.

Lumeng, J. C., & Cardinal, T. M. (2007). Providing information about a flavor to preschoolers: Effects on liking and memory for having tasting it. *Chemical Senses, 32,* 505–513.

Matheny, R. J., Birch, L. L., & Picciano, M. F. (1990). Control of intake by human-milk-fed infants: Relationships between feeding size and interval. *Developmental Psychobiology, 23* (6), 511–518.

Mattson, S. N., & Riley, E. P. (2006). A review of the neurobehavioral deficits in children with fetal alcohol syndrome or prenatal exposure to alcohol. *Alcoholism: Clinical and Experimental Research, 22* (2), 279–294.

Mayer, E. A. (2011). Gut feelings: The emerging biology of gut-brain communication. *Nature Reviews Neuroscience, 12* (8), 453–466.

Meek, J. Y., Noble, L., & Section on Breastfeeding. (2022). Policy statement: Breastfeeding and the use of human milk. *Pediatrics, 150* (1), e2022057988.

Mennella, J. A. (2001). Regulation of milk intake after exposure to alcohol in mothers' milk. *Alcoholism: Clinical and Experimental Research, 25* (4), 590–593.

Mennella, J. A., Jagnow, C. P., & Beauchamp, G. K. (2001). Prenatal and postnatal flavor learning by human infants. *Pediatrics, 107,* 88–94.

Mennella, J. A., Johnson, A., & Beauchamp, G. K. (1995). Garlic ingestion by pregnant women alters the odor of amniotic fluid. *Chemical Senses, 20* (2), 207–209.

Miralles, O., Sanchez, J., Palou, A., & Pico, C. (2006). A physiological role of breast milk leptin in body weight control in developing infants. *Obesity, 14,* 1371–1377.

Mistretta, C. M., & Bradley, R. M. (1975). Taste and swallowing in utero: A discussion of fetal sensory function. *British Medical Bulletin, 31* (1), 80–84.

Moding, K. J., Ferrante, M. J., Bellows, L. L., Bakke, A. J., Hayes, J. E., & Johnson, S. L. (2018). Variety and content of commercial infant and toddler vegetable products manufactured and sold in the United States. *The American Journal of Clinical Nutrition, 107* (4), 576–583.

Owen, C. G., Martin, R. M., Whincup, P. H., Davey Smith, G., Gillman, M. W., & Cook, D. G. (2005). The effect of breast-feeding on mean body mass index throughout life: A quantitative review of published and unpublished observational evidence. *American Journal of Clinical Nutrition, 82,* 1298–1307.

Patrick, H., Nicklas, T. A., Hughes, S. O., & Morales, M. (2005). The benefits of authoritative feeding style: Caregiver feeding styles and children's food consumption patterns. *Appetite, 44,* 243–249.

Plagemann, A., & Harder, T. (2005). Breast feeding and the risk of obesity and related metabolic diseases in the child. *Metabolic Syndrome and Related Disorders, 3* (3), 222–232.

Radnitz, C., Byrne, S., Goldman, R., Sparks, M., Gantshar, M., & Tung, K. (2009). Food cues in children's television programs. *Appetite, 52,* 230–233.

Roberto, C. A., Baik, J., Harris, J. L., & Brownell, K. D. (2010). Influence of licensed characters on children's taste and snack preferences. *Pediatrics, 126,* 88–93.

Robinson, T. N., Borzekowski, D. L., Matheson, D. M., & Kraemer, H. C. (2007). Effects of fast food branding on young children's taste preferences. *Archives of Pediatric Adolescent Medicine, 161* (8), 792–797.

Roseboom, T., Rooij, S., & Painter, R. (2006). The Dutch famine and its long-term consequences for adult health. *Early Human Development, 82,* 485–491.

Rowley, W. R., Bezold, C., Arikan, Y., Byrne, E., & Krohe, S. (2017). Diabetes 2030: Insights from yesterday, today, and future trends. *Population Health Management, 20* (1), 6–12.

Savage, J. S., Fisher, J. O., & Birch, L. L. (2007). Parental influence on eating behavior. *Journal of Law and Medical Ethics, 35,* 22–34.

Singhal, A. A., & Lanigan, J. J. (2007). Breastfeeding, early growth and later obesity. *Obesity Reviews, 8,* 51–54.

Sullivan, S. A., & Birch, L. L. (1994). Infant dietary experience and acceptance of solid food. *Pediatrics, 93,* 271–277.

Taillie, L. S., Busey, E., Stoltze, F. M., & Dillman Carpentier, F. R. (2019). Governmental policies to reduce unhealthy food marketing to children. *Nutrition Reviews, 77* (11), 787–816.

Tatzer, E., Schubert, M. T., Timischl, W., & Simbruner, G. (1985). Discrimination of taste and preference for sweet in premature babies. *Early Human Development, 12* (1), 23–30.

UConn Rudd Center for Food Policy and Health. (2017). Food marketing. Retrieved from http://uconnrud dcenter.org/research/food-marketing/

Victora, C. G., Bahl, R., Barros, A. J., França, G. V., Horton, S., Krasevec, J., Murch, S., Sankar, M. J., Walker, N., & Rollins, N. C. (2016). Breastfeeding in the 21st century: Epidemiology, mechanisms, and lifelong effect. *The Lancet, 387* (10017), 475–490.

CHAPTER 9

Social Influences on Eating

After reading this chapter, you will be able to

- Understand the meaning and determinants of cuisine.
- Appreciate the influences of "food rules."
- Distinguish indirect versus direct influences on eating.
- recognize and critically consider the direct influences of others on our eating behavior
- appreciate that the provider (person or company) carries meaning.

Food often plays a central role in social gatherings, such as family meals, parties, or holiday events. Imagine attending a friend's birthday or graduation party, or visiting a relative for a holiday such as Thanksgiving, and finding that no food was being served. That would likely be a disappointing surprise! Not only is food associated with social gatherings, but specific food items are often linked with particular holidays or occasions. For example, most of us anticipate that cake will be served at a birthday party. What foods do you expect or associate with other holidays or events? Have you ever wondered why this is? For example, why is eggnog often consumed during winter, but not during other seasons? In this chapter, we will explore the broader contextual or institutional influences that shape our eating behavior, such as cuisine and religion, and then the more immediate influence of other people on eating and food choice.

CUISINE

What constitutes cuisine, and how can we distinguish one cuisine from another? Do particular foods and preparations come to mind when you think of Chinese cuisine? What about when you think of Indian or Mexican cuisine? With each, you probably think of distinctly different foods, flavors, and preparations. According to influential researcher and cultural historian Paul Rozin,

> cuisines are defined by the basic ingredients they employ (e.g., rice, potatoes, fish), the characteristic flavors (flavor principles) employed (e.g., a combination of chili pepper with either tomato or lime for Mexico; a varied mixture of spices called 'curry' for India), and particular modes of food preparation (e.g., stir-frying for China).
>
> (Rozin, 1996a, p. 236; Image 9.1)

DOI: 10.4324/9781032621401-9

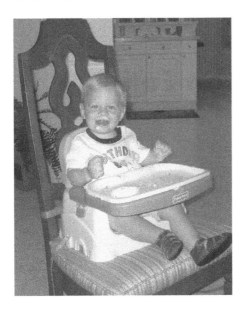

IMAGE 9.1 Boy enjoying cake on his first birthday

Additionally, cuisine is influenced by cultural rules about which foods should be served with what and when. For example, in many Western cultures, it is socially acceptable and normal to have cereal with milk, toast with butter, and coffee with creamer for breakfast. However, the serving of this meal at dinnertime would be considered odd, as would pairing the foods differently (e.g., coffee with butter instead of creamer). But the serving of the same meal for breakfast at a home in Japan would not be considered the social norm; Japanese people typically eat rice and fish for breakfast.

Anthropologists regard cuisines as a reflection of adaptive (in a Darwinian evolutionary sense) choices for a particular environment. According to this widely accepted view, if a cuisine was maladaptive in some nutritional sense, then the culture practicing it would have become extinct. It is not a goal of the field of psychology to assess the optimality of a given cuisine for the environment in which it evolved; rather, psychology provides an account of human behavioral mechanisms that allow learning and perpetuation of adaptive eating behaviors. An example of an adaptation is the consumption of milk or milk products in many cultures, despite lactose intolerance among adults. Lactase is a digestive enzyme that is required to break down lactose, the sugar present in milk; although all healthy infants express this enzyme, the amount of the enzyme drops to very low levels after infancy in most ethnic groups of the world (e.g., those indigenous to Asia, Africa, the Americas). Lack of this enzyme makes adults lactose intolerant: Lactose is not absorbed from the stomach, and this makes people feel ill. These cultures have either largely rejected milk products or use fermented/cultured products (yogurt, cheese, etc.). The reason that fermentation works is that specific bacteria outside the body do what our digestive systems can no longer perform in adulthood – namely, splitting lactose into a digestible molecule (lactic acid). Thus, lactose-intolerant individuals are able to eat products containing this "processed" lactose and receive beneficial energy and nutrients. There are many other examples around the world of food procurement facilitated by human ingenuity. We recommend Rozin (1996a) for additional evidence of cuisine as a social adaptive mechanism of survival.

DETERMINANTS OF CUISINE

What factors contribute to the determination of ingredients, flavors, and preparation associated with particular cuisines? The first is availability (Figure 9.1). Cuisines largely consist of ingredients and flavors that are accessible and relatively inexpensive in terms of cost and effort to procure. This concept of behavioral economics is explored more thoroughly in other chapters. The mode of preparation typically also depends on what is available in that culture (e.g., tools and technology). Not all available foods and flavors will be adapted as part of a local cuisine; those that are most innately appealing (e.g., energy dense, sweet or salty tasting) are more likely to be incorporated into a cuisine than those that are less attractive (e.g., low in energy yield, bitter or bland tasting).

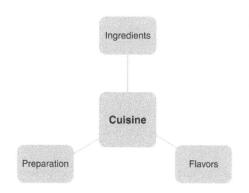

FIGURE 9.1 Determinants of cuisine

A second important determinant of cuisine is the nutritional completeness of the ingredients. Because no natural food source provides all of the nutrients needed for an omnivore's adequate nutrition, combinations of foods are important. For example, served alone, beans, rice, and corn provide inadequate sources of protein, but, when served in pairs (beans and rice, beans and corn), they are complementary and provide adequate protein. This is why these combinations are staples in many Central and South American cultures where they are relatively easily grown, procured, and stored.

A third category contributing to the determination of cuisine comprises beliefs and attitudes, and these require social learning and the direct or indirect influence of others. This category includes religious beliefs and cultural attitudes, cultural food rules, perception of risk associated with particular foods, and attitudes about health. These will be discussed individually.

Religious Beliefs and Cultural Attitudes

The Hindu reverence for the "sacred cow" stems from the early belief in Indian culture that cows are an important self-renewing source of high-energy food (milk) and a symbol of life that should not be killed (Simoons, 1961). Consequently, beef is not eaten in Hindu cuisine. In fact, most Hindu Indians are vegetarians; none eat beef, and virtually all consider the taste or consumption of beef "disgusting" (Rozin & Fallon, 1987). Anthropologist Marvin Harris theorized that the prohibition of meat eating by Hindus is nutritionally adaptive: Cows are more useful as a dairy resource (in fermented products of course!) than as a meat resource. That is, a cow can provide many more important protein and fat calories in its lifetime from its milk than from its meat (Harris et al., 1966).

Harris also suggested that consumption of dog meat is taboo in Europe and North America because dogs are more useful as hunters or herders or are valuable as companions; in regions with little game and, as a consequence, no need for hunting or herding animals, dogs are considered acceptable as food, and in some areas are even considered delicacies (Harris & Ross, 1987). Regardless of the origin of these beliefs and attitudes about cows or dogs, they are set by the culture and not by any one individual's experience.

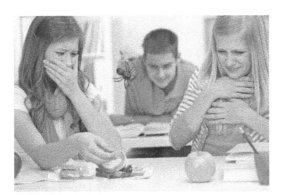

IMAGE 9.2 Contagion and disgust

How likely are you to eat a sandwich that a bug just crawled across? Despite how unappealing insects may be to you as food (or contaminants of food), they are widely consumed in many non-European cultures (DeFoliart, 1999). Insects such as caterpillars, termites, and locusts are frequently consumed in Africa and Asia, as these contain relatively high amounts of protein and other nutrients. And, importantly for inclusion in a local cuisine, they are easily available in the environment. So, why do we (Westerners) consider them disgusting as food? There is no clear-cut answer, except for the simple explanation that they did not become part of our cuisine.

Our cultural attitude is that insects are not food. Rozin conducted an interesting experiment to demonstrate the pervasiveness of this concept. He asked volunteers to consume juice into which a cockroach had just been dipped. (The juice had been previously consumed and liked by the volunteers.) The volunteers rejected it, despite knowing that the cockroach was dead and sterilized and thus could not actually contaminate the drink. Would you drink the juice if it were offered to you? What would be your rationale if you refused the drink? Rozin reported that volunteers' explanations included "it's a cockroach!" (Rozin, 1996a; Rozin et al., 1986). In other words, the *idea* of a roach or insect, despite its cleanliness following sterilization, elicits a feeling of disgust that is a result of social learning. (Trust us, this attitude is not innate. Just ask any parent, and you will be assured that one- and two-year-olds have no qualms about picking up and putting in their mouths nearly anything, including insects!)

Culturally Determined Food Rules

Cultural food rules dictate the time of day at which specific foods are considered appropriate, which foods should be served with which other foods, and how they should be eaten (e.g., with fingers, a fork, chopsticks). As previously mentioned, cereal for breakfast is considered normal according to American food rules, but it is generally unacceptable for dinner (or, at least, unexpected). We will highlight a few other cross-cultural comparisons of food rules. In the U.S., salad is often served as a first course for dinner, whereas it is usually served after the main dish, as a third course, in France. In Japan, the dishes, or courses, of the dinner meal are traditionally all served at once rather than in the sequential process that is typical in Western cultures. Americans typically consume French fries by picking them up with fingers. However, it is regarded as inappropriate to do the same with other potato preparations, such as roasted or baked potatoes. None of these food rules (and there are many) is inherently superior to any others, as they all allow for healthful eating. They are the result of social learning and not of biological necessity.

Perception of Risk

In the early 2000s, there was mass media concern about mad cow disease, technically called bovine spongiform encephalopathy (BSE). This is a progressive and fatal neurological disease in cattle; neurological problems can result among people who consume contaminated beef, particularly if it contains nervous system tissue. In the U.S., although no human health problems were linked to contaminated beef, consumption of beef declined significantly for a few months in 2003 following the first report of an infected cow. This occurred nationwide (not just in areas near the location of the infected cow in the U.S.) and was accompanied by increased consumption of other meats such as chicken and pork (Schlenker & Villas-Boas, 2009). In cases like this and others, when the perception of risk associated with a particular food is high, the incorporation of it in the diet of that society decreases. Of course, this often makes good sense, particularly when other food options exist with fewer perceived risks. In the case of beef, the perceived risk was short-lived, and so it was not removed from the American cuisine. However, if risk associated with a particular food persists, whether it's actual or simply perceived, that food is eliminated from a culture's cuisine. Presumably, this is an explanation for the relative absence of dairy in Asian cuisine (as a result of lactose intolerance among that population).

Another example of a societally inflicted risk involves medication and juice. In today's world, health-promoting drugs are frequently taken, for example, to stabilize mood or reduce blood pressure. Many drugs are inactivated and broken down in the intestine and liver by a particular enzyme (in the P450 family). Grapefruit juice contains compounds called *furanocoumarins* that can interfere with this enzyme's actions. Thus, the metabolism and, hence, effectiveness of many drugs (including statins, antidepressants, and others) are potentially affected by grapefruit. Prescribing physicians routinely recommend that patients do not eat grapefruit, even though these drugs do not have a uniformly high risk of adverse interaction (see Bailey et al. [2012] for a review). The risk is sometimes that the drug would be more effective, but the idea of taking lower doses of the drug with grapefruit does not seem to have caught on. As a result of this risk that is passed down by physicians, sales of grapefruit juice have dropped, and grapefruit hybrids (e.g., pomelos) are being developed that have lower levels of furanocoumarins.

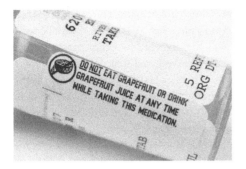

IMAGE 9.3 Example of a warning label on a container of prescription medication

Attitudes about Health

In modern Western cultures with food abundance, concerns about personal appearance and, in particular thin appearance, are common. Attitudes about food and health are also different in these cultures compared with more traditional cultures and less Westernized cultures. Nonetheless, despite the obesity epidemic, Americans are more likely than people in European countries and Japan to rate all fats as "harmful to health," despite known benefits of some fats (e.g., omega-3 fatty acids) in moderation. Americans also exhibit more anxiety and guilt about eating (Rozin et al., 1999). Rozin and colleagues have theorized that this heightened concern with healthy eating contributes to stress- and emotion-related overeating and, thus, reduces our ability to moderate our food intake.

DIRECT VERSUS INDIRECT INFLUENCES

Eating behaviors, including food combinations, portion sizes, and timing of meals or snacks, are a culmination of a lifetime of experience. Starting in infancy, our parents and caregivers teach us what items are appropriate as food, how much we should eat, and when. Some of this teaching is direct or explicit (e.g., a parent's directive to "clean your plate"), and other teaching is more incidental or passive (e.g., modeling of parents' eating behaviors or exposure to flavors through breast milk). We will discuss other examples of the direct influence of others on our eating behavior in the next section, but first we will consider the combination of direct and indirect factors that shape cuisine and adherence to the associated food rules within a culture.

Indirect Influences

Indirect influences are those that are effective even in the absence of other people, although they most likely first developed in the presence of others. As a case in point, most of you are unlikely to consume the beverage contacted by an insect such as a roach previously discussed, regardless of whether or not other people are around. This is because you learned at an early age that roaches are not food, that they contaminate food and should be avoided. Likewise, as a consequence of social learning, Hindu Indians neither consume, nor want to consume, beef, either when alone or in the presence of others.

What about portion sizes? How do you know how much of any particular food item to choose or consume when making your own selections? We typically consume food in amounts with which we are familiar. For example, you might have a sandwich, apple, and can of soda for lunch because this is a meal of which you have had prior positive experiences (e.g., no one laughed at you because this is a socially "normal" meal in Western culture, you felt appropriately satiated, and you didn't get sick). The sandwich may be relatively low in fat and calories, the apple quite small, and the soda calorie free; or the sandwich could be dense in fat and calories, the apple large, and the soda more than 100 calories. Yet people typically consume such items in their entirety. Food and portion selections such as these occur with or without the presence of others, though earlier in life we learned of them from others (Nestle et al., 1998).

Availability, as previously discussed, is an important influence on our food selection, and this is largely an indirect influence. Availability of food is both a *determinant* and a *consequence* of cuisine. Upon being adopted as a staple in a particular cuisine, that food becomes much more accessible than foods that are not part of the cuisine. For instance, if you were to crave fish and rice for breakfast while visiting Japan, you would be in luck, because those are the items you are most likely to find in restaurants, markets, and perhaps in the home in which you are a guest. You would be less fortunate, though, if you desired pancakes and bacon, as those items are not as frequently available. And the converse would be true in the U.S.: Pancakes and bacon are often on the menus for breakfast at restaurants, and the ingredients are available in most grocery stores. Our desire for particular foods is shaped by experience, but our consumption of those foods is limited by our access, and this applies whether or not others are around us.

a
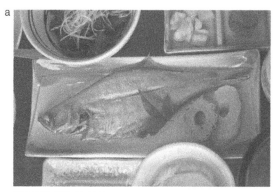

b
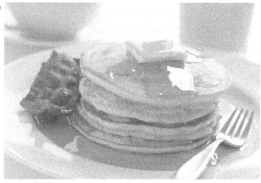

IMAGE 9.4 A AND B Typical Japanese and American breakfasts

Direct Influences of Others

Direct influences are those that require the actual presence of others. It is known that people tend to eat more when in a group (De Castro, 1990). However, overconsumption, including binge eating, often occurs in isolation (Stice et al., 2000). Thus, whereas social gatherings often facilitate food consumption, social constraints may at the same time promote healthy eating behavior. This has even been demonstrated in laboratory rats. Rats normally avoid novel foods but are more likely to consume a novel food and choose healthy ratios of macronutrients in the presence of a rat who is demonstrating these behaviors than rats tested alone (Galef et al., 1985, 1990; Galef & Wright, 1995).

As omnivores, we are able to consume an incredibly wide range of food items, and we need to consume a variety of foods to obtain optimal nutrition. However, our natural attraction to new foods (neophilia) juxtaposes with our fear of potential dangers of new foods (neophobia); this is known as the **omnivore's paradox** (Fischler, 1980). Cultural beliefs, traditions, and rules provide guidance around which foods to eat, how much, and when, allowing a society to manage the omnivore's paradox. Thus, group or commensal food consumption allows for the sharing of these practices and the continuance of them among generations, keeping societies safe from danger and adequately nourished. Evidence suggests that cultures in which meals are consumed in group (e.g., family) settings have lower obesity rates and longer life expectancies than cultures in which individuals eat alone (e.g., Veugelers & Fitzgerald, 2005).

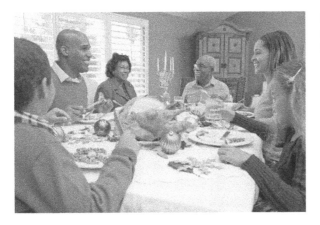

IMAGE 9.5 Commensal eating contributes to healthy food consumption

Food sharing is associated with increased levels of oxytocin, a neurotransmitter associated with social bonds in humans and other mammals (Wittig et al., 2014). Oxytocin has also been found to enhance trust and memories of positive social situations (Guastella et al., 2008; Kosfeld et al., 2005), which suggests that commensal food consumption and food sharing facilitate social bonds and pleasant memories. Further, oxytocin reduces the consumption of palatable snacks, such as cookies, helping to promote healthful eating and reduce overconsumption (Ott et al., 2013).

French sociologist Claude Fischler and others have surveyed people from the U.S. and several Western European countries regarding attitudes to food, meals, and health (see

Rozin's [2005] review of this research). French people, compared with Americans, feel that the quality of the food, drink, and company of others (essentially the meal *experi-ence*) is more important than the quantity of the food. Further, the French spend more time per day consuming their meals (two hours compared with one hour for Americans), consume a diet higher in fat, *and* have lower obesity rates. This is considered the "French paradox" (Drewnowski et al., 1996; Renaud & de Lorgeril, 1992). It seems that, in post-industrial societies, such as the U.S., rules of eating are loosening, and even vanishing, perhaps because meals are often eaten in isolation, reducing the opportunity for the sharing of food rules and healthy practices. Food delivery services are more common than they have ever been, adding convenience to eating meals alone. Further, portion sizes are typically larger in countries such as the U.S.. Fischler (1980, 1988) and others (e.g., Rozin et al., 2003) consider this lack of proper management of the omnivore's paradox to be a contributing factor to rising obesity.

It is known that we tend to copy the intake of others, closely matching the amount that the people around us are eating; this trend persists despite either extreme hunger or fullness (Herman et al., 2003, 2005). We also tend to eat more when served food in large containers (Marchiori et al., 2012) and we are prone to mindless eating when distracted – for example, when watching television – and consequently underestimate our overall food consumption (Ogden et al., 2013).

These findings support Fischler's (2011) belief that commensal eating helps maintain food consumption at, or constrain it to, appropriate levels. Eating in groups reduces the risk of overconsumption because of the awkwardness associated with deviation from social norms and may, in some cases, promote healthier food choices.

WHY DO WE EAT PREVIOUSLY DISLIKED FOODS?

Children develop many food preferences on the basis of social-affective context; for example, foods eaten by parents, older siblings, or peers or food items associated with fictional superheroes, smiling faces, and so on are often preferred. The acquired chili pepper preference in some cultures is an example of this socially mediated food liking. Spicy, "hot" foods are innately disliked because they activate pain receptors in the mouth (Caterina et al., 1997). However, as children are slowly introduced to chili peppers with adult approval and encouragement, they come to like them (this is particularly evident in the Mexican culture; Rozin, 1996a).

You may have had a similar experience with coffee. Can you recall your first sip of black coffee? It probably tasted bitter and gross. The addition of sweetener and creamer made it taste much more appealing. Typically, the amount of sweetener and creamer preferred by coffee drinkers decreases, and over time people enjoy a bitter-tasting beverage that they previously disliked. The role of associative learning in chan-ging this type of food or flavor preference is discussed in other chapters. However, if coffee tasted disgusting to you on your first exposure and you had no other positive associations with it, then why would you ever try coffee again? The fact is that coffee has many appealing associations in our culture – the smell of the kitchen on a relaxed morning, the vibe at popular coffee houses, the availability of Wi-Fi, studying with friends late into the night, and so on. Thus, we have a social motivation to overcome our innate dislike of the bitter taste and we are reinforced for doing so, all resulting from direct influences of others.

FOOD ASSOCIATIONS WITH THE PROVIDER

Most of us have a fondness for foods made by familiar people (especially loved ones), served at particular restaurants, or associated with certain brands. Can you think of any examples of this that apply to your food preferences? Perhaps your grandmother's apple pie is your favorite. We feel connections to the handlers, providers, or brand associations of the food we eat. Grandma's pie is better because it was made by grandma; particular cookies are better than others because they are branded in packaging with which we have positive associations. These associations are emotionally and psychologically rooted. Rozin (1996b) and anthropologists before him refer to this as the **law of contagion**, meaning that, once two things have been in physical contact, that contact remains an influence, even after the physical bond is broken (to the point of nostalgia!). So, food prepared by people whom we like carries their "essence" and is preferred; conversely, food prepared by enemies or people we find unappealing will not be desired or enjoyed. In other cultures, such as the Hindu Indian culture, the law of contagion pertaining to human handlers is more evident as people are often acutely aware of the handler's identity and social status. In Western culture, we are often detached from the original sources of our food; thus, many of our food associations are with companies and logos rather than with individuals. We prefer food branded with the essence of companies with which we have positive associations to those with which we have unpleasant associations. Even at very young ages, children prefer branded over non-branded foods (Roberto et al., 2010; Robinson et al., 2007), and this certainly persists into adulthood. Interestingly, our perception that certain branded foods taste better is associated with altered neural activity in areas of the brain associated with memory (McClure et al., 2004).

BOX 9.1 ARE WE NEUROLOGICALLY AFFECTED BY FOOD LABELS?

Coke and Pepsi sodas are chemically nearly identical; however, many soda drinkers have strong allegiance to, and preference for, one over the other. McClure et al. (2004) used fMRI technology to compare brain activity of people who consumed Coke and Pepsi in a blinded condition (i.e., the participants didn't know which soda they were receiving) with that of people who were "brand-cued" (i.e., they were exposed to the familiar Coke or Pepsi labeling before consuming the beverage). In the blinded condition, brain activity was most intense in areas of the prefrontal cortex associated with decision making and reward. However, in the cued condition, increased activity was seen in the hippocampus (associated with memory) and part of the prefrontal cortex associated with bias. These results help explain why food or drink from liked sources (people or companies) seems to taste better; altered brain activity affects perception.

MEDIA'S INFLUENCE

Media messages are ubiquitous, including television commercials, magazine advertisements, billboards, and internet messages among other forms. As discussed in the previous chapter, children reliably prefer foods with television or movie characters portrayed on the packaging. Children also prefer and consume more of foods endorsed by celebrities, and these are typically not fresh fruits and vegetables (Boyland et al., 2013). Further, there is a correlation between the number of television advertisements viewed per hour, especially those marketing unhealthy foods, and BMI for children (Lake & Townshend, 2006). The food industry and lobbyists have deep pockets. As an example of the contrast in funding between promotion of healthy food and that of unhealthy processed food, for every $1 that the World Health Organization spends on improving health, the food industry spends over $500 promoting processed foods. And the processed food business is a multi-billion-dollar industry. In one year, the revenue of ten of the largest corporations (e.g., PepsiCo, General Mills, Coca Cola, Nestlé) is over $1 billion dollars per day (Monteiro & Cannon, 2019). So, there is little motivation on the part of for-profit businesses to monitor or limit the marketing of their products to the widest possible audience, which includes children. The products produced by these companies include baby formula, snack foods, sweetened drinks (sodas and energy drinks), and breakfast foods.

Adult food and beverage choices are also influenced by media. In the mid-1900s, carbonated beverages were infrequently consumed, especially when compared with consumption of milk and water. By 2000, this trend had reversed, with frequent consumption of carbonated beverages and other sugary drinks, and this change has been largely attributed to marketing and media (Kearney, 2010).

Several decades ago, Quebec imposed legislation that banned advertisements for toys and fast food aimed at children under 13 years of age in all forms of media. Years later, fast food consumption among households was compared between those in Quebec and those in different areas of Canada without the ban, and it was found that fast food consumption was significantly lower in Quebec (Dhar & Baylis, 2011). Importantly, Quebec's childhood obesity was lower than rates in other parts of Canada. These results demonstrate both the strong influence media can have on our eating choices and the ability of regulations to blunt this influence. Several other countries in Europe and around the world have since adopted similar policies (Liu et al., 2020).

CONCLUDING REMARKS

Despite our largely similar, biologically predisposed taste preferences, aversions, and physiology, eating behaviors vary widely around the world. Cuisines and food rules, both of which have tremendous influence on our eating, endure within a culture only if they allow for the survival of its population. We learn of what is normal in our culture and establish our eating behaviors early in life with the guidance of parents and caregivers. As we age, the influence of others on our eating continues. In fact, most of our eating occurs in the presence of others. Research indicates that, if the food consumption of those around us is healthy (appropriate portions and ratios of macronutrients), our eating is likely to be healthy as well. Conversely, when eating alone without the healthy model, societal food rules loosen, and we are likely to consume beyond our energy needs. The issues discussed in this chapter, including the role of media, are important for policy makers and advocates of a healthier society to consider as they illuminate some of the challenges in improving eating behaviors.

QUESTIONS TO ASK YOURSELF

Let's review and apply your knowledge. Take some time to answer these chapter questions:

1 What is cuisine, and what factors determine it?
2 Discuss indirect influences on eating behavior.
3 Discuss direct influences on eating behavior.
4 What are the benefits of commensal eating and food sharing?
5 What influence do media have on eating behavior?

GLOSSARY

Commensal food consumption	Eating in groups.
Cuisine	A style of cooking usually associated with a particular culture.
Direct influence	Eating behavior influenced by the presence of others.
French paradox	The French spend more time per day consuming their meals, consume a diet higher in fat, *and* have lower obesity rates.
Indirect influence	Eating behavior influence that does not require the presence of others (e.g., religion, known food "rules").
Lactose intolerance	Too little of the enzyme needed to break down lactose, leading to discomfort and illness upon consuming dairy.
Law of contagion	Contact between two people or objects results in a lasting connection.
Omnivore's paradox	The contradiction between omnivores' liking of new food and fear of new food.

REFERENCES

Bailey, D. G., Dresser, G., & Arnold, J. M. O. (2012). Grapefruit-medication interactions: Forbidden fruit or avoidable consequences? *Canadian Medical Association Journal.* doi:10.1503/cmaj.120951

Boyland, E. J., Harrold, J. A., Dovey, T. M., Allison, M., Dobson, S., Jacobs, M. C., & Halford, J. C. (2013). Food choice and overconsumption: Effect of a premium sports celebrity endorser. *The Journal of Pediatrics, 163* (2), 339–343.

Caterina, M. J., Schumacher, M. A., Tominaga, M., Rosen, T. A., Levine, J. D., & Julius, D. (1997). The capsaicin receptor: A heat-activated ion channel in the pain pathway. *Nature, 389 (6653),* 816–824.

De Castro, J. M. (1990). Social facilitation of duration and size but not rate of the spontaneous meal intake of humans. *Physiology & Behavior, 47,* 1129–1135.

DeFoliart, G. R. (1999). Insects as food: Why the Western attitude is important. *Annual Review of Entomology, 44 (1),* 21–50.

Dhar, T., & Baylis, K. (2011). Fast-food consumption and the ban on advertising targeting children: The Quebec experience. *Journal of Marketing Research, 48 (5),* 799–813.

Drewnowski, A., Henderson, S. A., Shore, A. B., Fischler, C., Preziosi, P., & Hercberg, S. (1996). Diet quality and dietary diversity in France: Implications for the French paradox. *Journal of the American Dietetic Association, 96 (7),* 663.

Fischler, C. (1980). Food habits, social change, and the nature/culture dilemma. *Social Science Information, 19 (6),* 937–953.

Fischler, C. (1988). Food, self, and identity. *Social Science Information, 27 (2),* 275–292.

Fischler, C. (2011). Commensality, society and culture. *Social Science Information, 50,* 528–548.

Galef, B. G., Jr., Attenborough, K. S., & Whiskin, E. E. (1990). Responses of observer rats (Rattus norvegicus) to complex, diet-related signals emitted by demonstrator rats. *Journal of Comparative Psychology, 104 (1),* 11–19.

Galef, B. G., Jr., & Wright, T. J. (1995). Groups of naive rats learn to select nutritionally adequate foods faster than do isolated naive rats. *Animal Behaviour, 49 (2),* 403–409.

Galef, J. B., Jr., G., Kennett, D. J., & Stein, M. (1985). Demonstrator influence on observer diet preference: Effects of simple exposure and presence of a demonstrator. *Animal Learning & Behavior, 13,* 25–30.

Guastella, A. J., Mitchell, P. B., & Mathews, F. (2008). Oxytocin enhances the encoding of positive social memories in humans. *Biological Psychiatry, 64 (3),* 256–258.

Harris, M., Bose, N. K., Klass, M., et al. (1966). The cultural ecology of India's sacred cattle. *Current Anthropology, 7(1),* 51–66.

Harris, M., & Ross, E. B. (1987). *Food and evolution: Toward a theory of human food habits.* Philadelphia: Temple University Press.

Herman, C. P., Koenig-Nobert, S., Peterson, J. B., & Polivy, J. (2005). Matching effects on eating: Do individual differences make a difference? *Appetite, 45,* 108–109.

Herman, C. P., Roth, D. A., & Polivy, J. (2003). Effects of the presence of others on eating: A normative interpretation. *Psychological Bulletin, 129,* 873–886.

Kearney, J. (2010). Food consumption trends and drivers. *Philosophical Transactions of the Royal Society of London B: Biological Sciences, 365 (1554),* 2793–2807.

Kosfeld, M., Heinrichs, M., Zak, P. J., Fischbacher, U., & Fehr, E. (2005). Oxytocin increases trust in humans. *Nature, 435 (7042),* 673–676.

Lake, A., & Townshend, T. (2006). Obesogenic environments: Exploring the built and food environments. *The Journal of the Royal Society for the Promotion of Health, 126 (6),* 262–267.

Liu, W., Barr, M., Pearson, A. L., Chambers, T., Pfeiffer, K. A., Smith, M., & Signal, L. (2020). Space–time analysis of unhealthy food advertising: New Zealand children's exposure and health policy options. *Health Promotion International, 35 (4),* 812–820.

Marchiori, D., Corneille, O., & Klein, O. (2012). Container size influences snack food intake independently of portion size. *Appetite, 58 (3),* 814–817.

McClure, S. M., Li, J., Tomlin, D., Cypert, K. S., Montague, L. M., & Montague, P. R. (2004). Neural correlates of behavioral preference for culturally familiar drinks. *Neuron, 44,* 379–387.

Monteiro, C. A., & Cannon, G. J. (2019). The role of the transnational ultra-processed food industry in the pandemic of obesity and its associated diseases: Problems and solutions. *World Nutrition, 10* (*1*), 89–99.

Nestle, M., Wing, R., Birch, L., DiSogra, L., Drewnowski, A., Middleton, S., & Economos, C. (1998). Behavioral and social influences on food choice. *Nutrition Reviews, 56* (*5*), S50–S74.

Ogden, J., Coop, N., Cousins, C., Crump, R., Field, L., Hughes, S., & Woodger, N. (2013). Distraction, the desire to eat and food intake. Towards an expanded model of mindless eating. *Appetite, 62,* 119–126.

Ott, V., Finlayson, G., Lehnert, H., Heitmann, B., Heinrichs, M., Born, J., & Hallschmid, M. (2013). Oxytocin reduces reward-driven food intake in humans. *Diabetes, 62* (*10*), 3418–3425.

Renaud, S., & de Lorgeril, M. (1992). Wine, alcohol, platelets, and the French paradox for coronary heart disease. *The Lancet, 339* (*8808*), 1523–1526.

Roberto, C. A., Baik, J., Harris, J. L., & Brownell, K. D. (2010). Influence of licensed characters on children's taste and snack preferences. *Pediatrics, 126,* 88–93.

Robinson, T. N., Borzekowski, D. L., Matheson, D. M., & Kraemer, H. C. (2007). Effects of fast food branding on young children's taste preferences. *Archives of Pediatric Adolescent Medicine, 161* (*8*), 792–797.

Rozin, P. (1996a). Social influences on food preferences and feeding. In E. D. Capaldi (ed.), *Why we eat what we eat: The psychology of eating* (pp. 233–263). Washington, DC: American Psychological Association.

Rozin, P. (1996b). Towards a psychology of food and eating: From motivation to module to model to marker, morality, meaning, and metaphor. *Current Directions in Psychological Science, 5* (*1*), 18–24.

Rozin, P. (2005). The meaning of food in our lives: A cross-cultural perspective on eating and well-being. *Journal of Nutrition Education and Behavior, 37,* S107–S112.

Rozin, P., & Fallon, A. E. (1987). A perspective on disgust. *Psychological Review, 94* (*1*), 23–41.

Rozin, P., Fischler, C., Imada, S., Sarubin, A., & Wrzesniewski, A. (1999). Attitudes to food and the role of food in life in the U.S.A., Japan, Flemish Belgium and France: Possible implications for the diet-health debate. *Appetite, 33,* 163–180.

Rozin, P., Kabnick, K., Pete, E., Fischler, C., & Shields, C. (2003). The ecology of eating smaller portion sizes in France than in the United States help explain the French paradox. *Psychological Science, 14* (*5*), 450–454.

Rozin, P., Millman, L., & Nemeroff, C. (1986). Operation of the laws of sympathetic magic in disgust and other domains. *Journal of Personality and Social Psychology, 50* (*4*), 703–712.

Schlenker, W., & Villas-Boas, S. B. (2009). Consumer and market responses to mad cow disease. *American Journal of Agricultural Economics, 91* (*4*), 1140–1152.

Simoons, F. J. (1961). *Eat not this flesh: Food avoidances in the Old World.* Madison: University of Wisconsin Press.

Stice, E., Telch, C. F., & Rizvi, S. L. (2000). Development and validation of the Eating Disorder Diagnostic Scale: A brief self-report measure of anorexia, bulimia, and binge-eating disorder. *Psychological Assessment, 12* (*2*), 123–131.

Veugelers, P. J., & Fitzgerald, A. L. (2005). Prevalence of and risk factors for childhood overweight and obesity. *Canadian Medical Association Journal, 173* (*6*), 607–613.

Wittig, R. M., Crockford, C., Deschner, T., Langergraber, K. E., Ziegler, T. E., & Zuberbühler, K. (2014). Food sharing is linked to urinary oxytocin levels and bonding in related and unrelated wild chimpanzees. *Proceedings of the Royal Society B, 281* (*1778*), 1–10.

CHAPTER 10

Mood and Food, Cravings, and Addiction

After reading this chapter, you will be able to

- Describe the connections between mood and eating behavior.
- Understand the effect of stress on eating.
- Provide the biological and psychological explanations for food cravings.
- Appreciate and understand a basis for an addiction model of overeating.

Have you ever headed straight to the freezer for some ice cream after a particularly stressful day? Have you ever eaten far more chips than you intended to eat while nervously studying for an upcoming exam? Mood plays an interesting role in eating behavior, which can be problematic and associated with unhealthy eating habits. Some people report cravings for the foods that seem to comfort them or, at least temporarily, improve their mood. A *craving* is characterized by an intense and prolonged desire or yearning for a specific food item or type. Food cravings are very common (especially among women), but some people claim that these cravings are intrusive and are resolved only by the consumption, and at times overconsumption, of the craved food. The cycle of powerful craving followed by compulsive consumption is similar to that seen among drug addicts. The idea that palatable food can be addictive has received much attention and has also spawned debate. Perhaps, as with drug addiction, some people are more prone to becoming addicted to palatable food and, consequently, have a difficult time regulating their intake. In this chapter, we explore the mood–food connection and the neurobiological evidence for food addiction.

THE MOOD–FOOD CONNECTION

Which types of food do you typically prefer when you are feeling down or stressed? Frequently craved "comfort foods" include cookies, chips, pasta, pizza, ice cream, and candy (especially chocolate!). What do these foods have in common, and why are they among the most desired foods when we're depressed or tense? These foods are quite diverse, but one common feature is that they contain a lot of carbohydrates; we often refer to these foods as "high carb," although they usually also contain quite a lot of fat. Maybe the commonality in macronutrient composition is what makes these foods craved. Or, maybe these foods are just the tastiest, so of course they would be preferred.

DOI: 10.4324/9781032621401-10

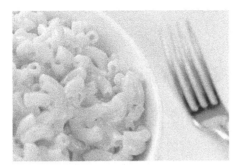

IMAGE 10.1 Carbohydrate-rich foods are frequent choices when our mood is low

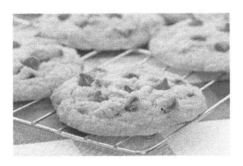

It could instead be that these foods were our favorites during childhood, and we feel comforted by them when we're having a bad day. All of these are reasonable explanations for our comfort food preferences associated with a depressed mood. Let's first consider the explanation that relates to postingestive consequences – macronutrients – because that is not as intuitive as the taste or experience explanations.

Talking Point 10.1 When Do You Eat?

Do you eat differently when you're feeling down? What foods do you tend to consume more or less of when your mood is low? Compare your list with your classmates' lists.

A Biological Explanation for Carbohydrate (Sugar) Craving?

Depression is believed to be associated with reduced activity of the neurotransmitter **serotonin** (e.g., Parsey et al., 2006), although other neurotransmitters are likely also involved. One of the pillars of this theory of depression is that the most effective antidepressant medications work primarily by increasing synaptic levels of serotonin in the brain. Carbohydrate consumption also boosts serotonin activity in the brain, though the mechanism is different from that of antidepressants. **Tryptophan** (a diet-derived amino acid) is the raw material for a two-step synthesis of serotonin (5-HT) in the neuron. It is one of six large neutral amino acids (LNAAs; see Table 2.1 for additional information) that all compete for the same molecular carrier to get across the blood–brain barrier and into the brain. So, 5-HT synthesis in the brain ultimately depends on the ratio of tryptophan to all LNAAs in the blood. (If you think of the molecular carriers as boats and the LNAAs as potential passengers, and there being many more passengers than seats in the boats, then you'll get the picture.) It turns out that **insulin** in the blood stream increases the tryptophan/LNAA ratio and so increases the net amount of tryptophan getting into these molecular "boats." Because carbohydrates, especially those high in glycemic index, increase insulin secretion to a greater extent than proteins or fats, carbohydrate consumption has the greatest impact on 5-HT synthesis relative to the other macronutrients. The theory is, then, that carbohydrate-dense foods elevate 5-HT and so have an antidepressant or mood-elevating effect, at least among people who identify themselves as "carbohydrate cravers" (this is the *medicine effect*; Corsica & Spring, 2008; Lieberman et al., 1986; Wurtman & Wurtman, 1995). This association is probably learned very early in life, leading some people to continue to desire these types of foods when mood is low, using food as a form of self-medication (Wurtman & Wurtman, 1995). The effect of carbohydrate consumption on 5-HT activity may take hours, whereas the mood-elevating effect is very rapid. This evidence supports the impact of learning of the medicine effect and also the idea that the *expectation* that our mood will be enhanced actually enhances our mood (i.e., a placebo effect). This same effect of expectation/placebo usually occurs with other medications. For example, we typically feel relief from headaches soon after taking medication, before it has its physiological effect (Barrett et al., 2006). These examples are a result of learning through experience.

Stress and Eating

Most people eat differently when they are stressed (Zellner et al., 2006). Stress has diverse causes and descriptions, and so more precise terms have been introduced. *Eustress* is stress that is associated with positive experiences, and *distress* is stress associated with negative experiences; these can be thought of as being at opposite ends of a stress continuum. However, despite our polar opposite reasons for feeling stressed (from encountering a bear in the woods, to hearing your professor announce a pop quiz, to walking into a surprise party), our bodily response is quite similar. When we perceive a situation as stressful, our **hypothalamic–pituitary–adrenal (HPA) axis** is activated, triggering an increase in blood pressure, heart rate, and breathing and also the release of the hormones adrenaline and cortisol that perpetuate the elevated physiological state. Typically, hunger is suppressed with short-term exposure to a severe stressor (such as the bear in the woods). However, longer-term exposure to non-life-threatening stressors (e.g., preparing for final exams) is more associated with increased eating.

IMAGE 10.2 Eating behavior changes with stress

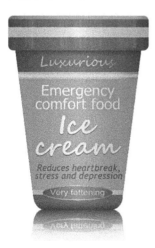

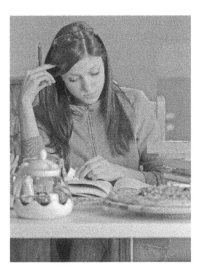

IMAGE 10.3 Eating behavior changes with stress

Talking Point 10.2 What Do You Eat?

Do you think that you eat more when you're "stressed"? What types of foods do you typically consume more or less of in this state?

The foods that we eat more of when we are stressed are "comfort" or "junk" foods, and not healthy foods (Dallman et al., 2005; Zellner et al., 2006). It has been demonstrated that even people who feel less hungry when stressed eat more of their calories as high-energy and high-fat comfort foods. So, for some people, overall eating may decrease, but the ratio of unhealthy to healthy foods consumed increases (Gibson, 2006). Further, most increased food consumption associated with stress is in the form of snacks rather than meals. Most students tend to snack on high-energy, fat-dense foods such as chips and candy when studying, and many adults report similar junk food preferences when stressed (e.g., Dallman et al., 2005; Oliver & Wardle, 1999). Cantor and colleagues (1982) found that people working on an information-processing (tracking) task consumed more snacks than when they were not performing the task. And the more difficult the task (presumably, the more stressful), the more snacks consumed.

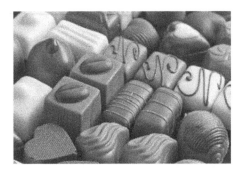

IMAGE 10.4 Why is chocolate often craved?

Other research indicates that women are more prone than men to this type of stress-induced palatable-food consumption (e.g., Zellner et al., 2007). Rats and mice, like humans, also selectively consume more energy- and fat-dense food when experiencing stress (Foster et al., 2009).

When we (humans and rodents) are stressed, it seems that external factors, particularly the attractiveness and palatability of food, have an increased influence on our food intake. Like eating associated with a depressed mood, stress-induced eating may also be explained by the pleasurable and mood-enhancing activity of serotonin, dopamine, opioids, and other chemicals, which reinforce the eating behavior (Gibson, 2006). Thus, people living in environments with chronic stress are more likely to overeat in the absence of physiological hunger, making them more likely to become overweight or obese.

Stress seems to impact eating for another reason. Activation of the HPA axis also triggers secretion of **glucocorticoids**, which are hormones with several associated functions including elevated emotional state, increase in insulin secretion, and changes in dopamine and serotonin activity. It seems that stress-induced glucocorticoid release and the cascade of other chemical changes work to additively alter eating behaviors, including the desire to eat, the motivation to obtain and consume food, and the pleasure experience of eating the food (Dallman, 2010; Dallman et al., 2005). Eating behavior then reduces stresses, at least temporarily, reinforcing the behavior. This can become a habitual pattern for some people. And, because the foods preferred when we are stressed are palatable high-energy junk or comfort foods rather than more healthful foods such as fruits and veggies, this habit is likely to lead to unhealthy weight gain (Dallman, 2010).

Talking Point 10.3 Stress Points

How might a downturn in the economy affect eating behaviors? Might the effects of feeling stuck in a bad job, dealing with a break-up, or grieving for a loved one be similar?

FOOD CRAVINGS

Elsewhere in this book, we have talked about specific appetites. For example, salt appetite is well documented and is triggered initially by a physiological need for sodium. However, most of the substances that we crave are not specific molecules; for example, it would sound odd to say, "I really need some tryptophan today." Further, craved foods are rarely single macronutrients (e.g., pure sugar), but are instead specific food commodities that are mixtures of many ingredients. So, a critical question is whether or not cravings for specific commodities have an underlying need basis. Surveys indicate that most people experience cravings – about 70% of young men and nearly 100% of young women (Weingarten & Elston, 1991). Cravings vary in intensity but are typically characterized by a strong desire for a particular food. Often, but certainly not always, cravings are followed by the consumption of the desired food. The availability or proximity of the commodity and/or an individual's level of dietary restraint contribute largely to whether or not the food will be consumed, but typically the craving is satisfied only by consumption of the craved food item. Physiological hunger is not a necessary precondition for food craving. Often, foods craved and consumed (or overconsumed) are high in carbohydrate and fat and are neither essential nor high in nutritional quality (e.g., chocolate is the most frequently craved food in Western society [Hallam et al., 2016]). In contrast, when we are physiologically hungry, we tend to desire more nutritious and savory-tasting foods, such as a pasta dish, a turkey sandwich, or steak and potatoes. And, when truly hungry, we are more accepting of a variety of foods.

One group of researchers (Pelchat & Schaefer, 2000) found that participants on a monotonous but nutritionally complete diet for several days had large increases in cravings. (They consumed a nutritional supplement beverage and water only.) This further supports that food craving and unhealthy snacking are not necessarily due to hunger or nutritional need. Rather, mood and desire for dietary variety have more documented links with cravings than with physiological hunger. Cravings are also influenced by age (they decrease with advanced age), culture, and hormone fluctuations (particularly among women; Hallam et al., 2016; Pelchat, 1997; Zellner et al., 1999).

Craving-related eating, particularly when it occurs frequently, increases the risk of binge eating, which in turn is associated with bulimia nervosa, binge eating disorder, and obesity. The pattern of craving, consuming, overconsuming, feeling good, then feeling guilty, leading to repetition of the cycle is similar to that seen among drug abusers. Drug and food cravings can both be powerfully triggered by exposure to associated stimuli (e.g., sight of drug paraphernalia or a candy bar wrapper). The shared neurobiology involved in food craving and drug abuse is discussed later in this chapter.

Is Chocolate Special?

Many desired and craved snacks contain chocolate, which is carbohydrate (sugar) dense but also contains fat and protein and some bioactive ingredients and micronutrients. In light of the fact that chocolate is the most craved food in Western society (Zellner et al., 1999), two questions have arisen: Is chocolate special, and, if so, why? Some researchers believe that the bioactive substances in chocolate (specifically in cocoa, a major ingredient in chocolate) trigger a mood-enhancing release of neurotransmitters within the brain. Among the proposed mood-elevating, and possibly addictive, substances are caffeine (a stimulant), theobromine (structurally similar to caffeine but with a far lower stimulating effect), anandamide (binds pleasure-inducing cannabinoid receptors), phenylethylamine (similar to amphetamine, triggers dopamine activity within the brain reward pathway), and tryptophan (increases serotonin synthesis).

In a study of chocolate craving (Michener & Rozin, 1994), self-identified chocolate cravers were given five small sealed boxes that appeared identical but, in fact, each contained a different item: Milk chocolate, white chocolate (similar in texture to milk chocolate, but without the bioactive substances found in cocoa), cocoa capsules (these have the bioactive ingredients but none of the sensory aspects of chocolate), placebo capsules, or nothing. Participants were told to open one box at random whenever they craved chocolate and consume the contents. (Which box would you hope to open if you were a participant?) They were asked to rate perceived intensity of the chocolate cravings before and 90 minutes after eating the contents. The results showed that only milk chocolate consumption reduced the craving for chocolate. The finding that cocoa alone did not reduce craving indicates that the bioactive substances have little or no role in chocolate craving (i.e., no specific biological deficit caused the craving, the alleviation of which reduced craving). In fact, participants preferred the white chocolate to the cocoa capsules, indicating that the taste, smell, and additional sensory components of chocolate consumption are more important than bioactive ingredients. Additional evidence against the role of chemical-enhancement as the basis for chocolate craving or addiction comes from food-use studies that show that dark chocolate (which contains the highest amounts of cocoa and, thus, the highest levels of the bioactive substances) is less preferred and less consumed than either milk chocolate or chocolate-coated sweets that contain lesser amounts of the chemicals. (Try eating baker's chocolate – just awful!) Furthermore, the amounts of the bioactive compounds mentioned previously that actually cross the blood–brain barrier and have any effect within the brain are likely very small.

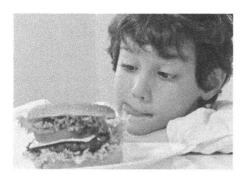

IMAGE 10.5 This boy is eyeing some tasty food

Talking Point 10.4 Do You Crave?

Do you ever experience food cravings? Which foods do you most often crave? Do your cravings occur more often when you are alone or in social situations? Does time of day contribute? Do you typically consume the foods that you crave?

There could be other bioactive ingredients in chocolate that make it special. For example, chocolate contains significant amounts of riboflavin (vitamin B$_2$), magnesium, and antioxidants, all of which enhance health. Perhaps deficiencies of these vitamins and minerals contribute to chocolate craving. For example, women tend to have increased cravings for chocolate when experiencing premenstrual syndrome, a time associated with reduced levels of magnesium (Bruinsma & Taren, 1999). However, many infrequently craved foods contain much higher amounts of magnesium (including barley, spinach, and pumpkin seeds). And riboflavin deficiency is an unlikely explanation for chocolate craving because riboflavin concentrations in chocolate are some 20-fold lower than they are in less preferred foods such as liver. So, despite some possible health benefits of chocolate, these are implausible as the basis for chocolate craving.

Chocolate, especially milk chocolate, has an appealing taste, smell, and creamy texture. It seems that the pleasurable orosensory (i.e., smell and mouth feel) aspects of chocolate and the innately reinforcing qualities of the macronutrients in chocolate (carbohydrate and fat), rather than any particular chemical or micronutrient, are the bases for chocolate craving. Exposure to the sight or smell of chocolate can trigger intense and difficult-to-ignore cravings, particularly among people who claim to be "chocolate lovers" or chocolate cravers. You have probably heard these people referred to as "chocoholics," and maybe you've used this term to characterize your own affection for chocolate. The idea of chocolate addiction compares the intense cravings for chocolate to the cravings drug addicts have for particular substances of abuse. In support of this, fMRI studies have revealed that exposure to the sight and/ or taste of chocolate triggers different brain activity for chocolate cravers compared with non-cravers (Rolls & McCabe, 2007). Specifically, areas associated with pleasure and reward show enhanced activity in the chocolate cravers' brains, much like drug addicts' brains show increased activity in the same brain regions upon exposure to drug paraphernalia (Kühn & Gallinat, 2011; Yokum et al., 2011).

Psychological and Sociocultural Explanations for Chocolate Craving

Despite the fact that chocolate is the most frequently craved food, it is not the most consumed food. In fact, some people, despite their reported liking of chocolate, refrain entirely from eating it or consume it infrequently and/or in small amounts. In Western society, chocolate is considered an indulgence and a treat. It is often given as a gift. Perhaps the belief that chocolate is "nice but naughty" actually makes it more desired.

In evolutionary terms, the availability of chocolate is a recent event for most of the world's population. The first record of cultivation of cacao dates from Aztec civilizations, and it was imported into Europe by the conquistadors (Poelmans & Swinnen, 2016). Cacao itself is bitter, and the word *chocolate* derives from the Nahuatl words for "bitter drink." The addition of sugar and milk enhances the orosensory and mouth feel of chocolate in our contemporary culture.

Talking Point 10.5 Is It New?

Do you think that people had food cravings before the global availability of sweet chocolate? If so, what food cravings do you think they might have had?

CAN SOMEONE ACTUALLY BE A FOOD ADDICT?

The mood–food connection is well supported by both anecdotal and empirical evidence. Perhaps, extending the idea, some people actually self-medicate using tasty food to improve mood and become dependent on certain foods to feel good. This is the cycle in which drug addicts find themselves: Intense cravings and need for the drug in order to function and feel normal or good. Addiction is also associated with uncontrolled consumption. Is it plausible that certain foods can be addictive like cocaine, heroin, and nicotine can be? One problem with this line of thinking is that we all need food to survive, but we do not need recreational drugs. Another caveat is that we are all exposed to food (we all consume food from the day that we are born), whereas not everyone ingests recreational drugs. So, if food can be problematically addictive, why doesn't everyone suffer in this way? There are two ways to think about this. The first is that only some individuals are genetically and physiologically predisposed to become food addicts. Another way is to consider that we are all predisposed, but some of us have mechanisms and strategies to resist food; this is referred to as **dietary restraint**.

People with high levels of restraint can resist the temptation to consume delicious looking and smelling foods (e.g., freshly baked cookies) despite their liking of such food. Conversely, people with low restraint are unable to resist similar temptations, regardless of a possible desire to avoid unhealthy foods, and are more likely to consume more than intended (Lawson et al., 1995). Many factors contribute to the different levels of dietary restraint that people have, including a desire to lose weight or maintain a healthy weight, gender (men generally exhibit more restraint than women [Hallam et al., 2016], religion (e.g., fasting during the days of Ramadan or giving up a favorite food for Lent), ethics (e.g., many vegans and vegetarians refrain from eating meat because of a personal conviction that animal consumption and/or poor treatment of animals is unethical), and for other health-related issues (e.g., avoiding high-sodium foods in an effort to lower blood pressure). An individual's personality also contributes; people with impulsive personalities typically have lower levels of dietary restraint. As discussed in other chapters, low dietary restraint can result in overeating and obesity, as with binge eating disorder (Van Strien & Van de Laar, 2008); however, high restraint is often associated with the eating disorder anorexia nervosa (Bulik et al., 2000).

BOX 10.1

"Junk food" is generally defined as food and beverages that are:

- Highly palatable to that individual.
- Usually low in protein and nutrients and high in refined sugar, fat, and salt.
- High in overall caloric density and can be consumed rapidly.
- Sometimes consumed within meals but often as snacks; often from fast food providers.
- Highly processed, containing added chemicals, preservatives, and artificial ingredients.
- Over time, likely to induce weight gain and metabolic disorders.
- Associated with compulsion-like consumption that has some characteristics of substance abuse.

Sources: Johnson & Kenny (2010); Smith (2006).

Our current food environment is quite different from that of our ancestors, with palatable and energy-dense foods easily available. Some evidence supports a link between our obesogenic environment and food addiction. People with low dietary restraint have a more difficult time resisting the temptation of overconsuming appealing food in today's food environment, but perhaps they would be able to resist bland food. To examine that idea using an animal study, Johnson and Kenny (2010) compared the consumption of nutritionally complete, but monotonous, rat chow with that of a palatable "junk food" diet (refer to our definition of this diet). Johnson and Kenny selected tasty, well-liked food from their school cafeteria, including bacon, sausage, pound cake, frosting, and cheesecake, as their junk food diet. Their experiment had three conditions: One group of rats was given rat chow ad libitum plus extended (nearly unlimited) access to the junk food diet; another group of rats had rat chow ad libitum with one hour of access to the junk food diet; and the control group had rat chow ad libitum only. After 40 days of the assigned diet, the rats experienced foot shock in the presence of a particular light stimulus, thus quickly developing a conditioned fear of the light. On test day, all rats had access to the junk food diet and all demonstrated interest in the food. However, the presence of the feared light stimulus, no longer paired with a foot shock, suppressed eating of the junk food in the control and one-hour-access groups but not in the extended-access group. It is interesting that, even in a sated (not hungry) state, the junk food-fed rats had such an apparent liking of highly palatable food that they were willing to risk experiencing the unpleasant foot shock. Drug-addicted rats similarly lever press for injections of particular drugs even in the presence of cues associated with punishment.

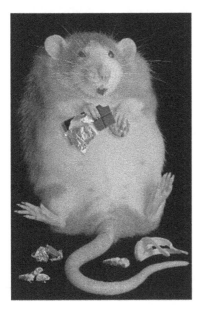

IMAGE 10.6 Rats show evidence of junk food addiction

Talking Point 10.6 What Lengths?

Have you ever gone to great lengths to obtain any of the types of foods in the junk food diet that the rats were so fond of? Perhaps a late night or early morning trip across town for pancakes and bacon? Maybe a special outing for ice cream? Do you think these behaviors support the idea that palatable foods can be addictive? Why or why not?

The rats on the junk food diet in the Johnson and Kenny (2010) study gained twice the weight of the rats in the other two conditions; they apparently enjoyed our Western diet! They also showed behavioral and biological markers that characterize drug addiction (discussed later). They were willing to risk an aversive stimulus to get the junk food and routinely ate far more calories than the control rats when given the palatable food, but not when given regular chow. These findings parallel data from human studies indicating that obese individuals (compared with lean individuals) have more intense cravings for palatable high-energy foods and demonstrate reduced restraint when exposed to these foods (Stice et al., 2008). In the Johnson and Kenny study, rats were not "addicted" to the junk food diet right from the start. It was not until they had been exposed to it for some time that these characteristics of addiction became apparent. All rats tested in the extended-access group showed signs of addiction, and, although they were all from a similar genetic background, the evidence suggests that the addiction is a result of environmental exposure more than biological predisposition. Further, the abundance of vending machines, other commercial devices, and delivery services at workplaces and certainly on college campuses enables convenient impulsive and compulsive eating of junk food.

NEUROBIOLOGY OF FOOD ADDICTION

Interest in brain reward circuitry stems from the finding in the 1950s by Olds and Milner (1954) that rats will lever press for intracranial brain stimulation in lieu of food, water, or sleep. The **mesolimbic dopamine system** (Figure 10.1), including the ventral tegmental area (VTA), nucleus accumbens, and several cortical regions, and the **endogenous opioid system** are particularly associated with reward and pleasure (see also Chapter 6). Exposure to pleasurable stimuli, such as food, water, sex, drugs, roller coaster rides, and so on, activates brain "reward" circuitry, reinforcing our experiences and leading us to want to repeat them. These mechanisms presumably evolved so that our ancestors would enjoy food, water, and sex enough that they would seek them out, despite the risks and efforts required, for survival. The pathways, though, did not evolve so that we would enjoy, and possibly become addicted to, drugs or so that we would stand in line again and again to repeat the ride on a thrilling roller coaster. Drugs of abuse, in particular, can be considered super-stimuli, activating our reward pathways more powerfully than do naturally reinforcing stimuli. Recent evidence (e.g., Avena et al., 2012; Fletcher & Kenny, 2018; Johnson & Kenny, 2010) indicates that the extremely palatable food in our environment may also be a super-stimulus. This could explain the addiction-like behaviors and neurobiological changes of the junk food-fed rats and, perhaps, the overconsumption of energy-dense food by many people in Western culture.

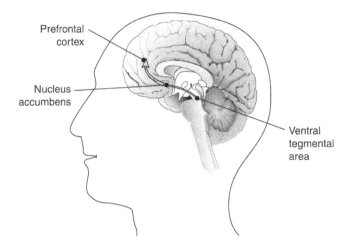

FIGURE 10.1 The mesolimbic dopamine system

Reports of people feeling unable to resist sweet snacks or people experiencing a depressed mood when they are deprived of the palatable food they are accustomed to consuming at a particular time every day are well established. These symptoms – compulsion to consume the palatable food and mood change or withdrawal when the craved food is not consumed – resemble the symptoms of drug addiction. Dr. Bart Hoebel of Princeton University and colleagues were among the first to formally propose the idea of sugar addiction, at least in rats. They found that rats intermittently fed sugar demonstrated the hallmark signs of addiction, including withdrawal, bingeing when receiving access, craving, and increased interest in other drugs (cross-sensitization; Avena et al., 2008). It has also been demonstrated that rats will lever press for saccharin over cocaine, suggesting that the sweet taste is a very powerful reinforcer (Lenoir et al., 2007). The junk food diet study by Johnson and Kenny further supports these claims. We recommend Koob and Volkow (2016) for a thorough review of research surrounding the neurobiology of obesity and drug addiction. The following is an overview of some key findings on the neural mechanisms that could underlie sugar or palatable food addiction.

Dopamine System

Dopamine release from nerve terminals in the **nucleus accumbens (NAc)** upon exposure to sugar and other palatable foods or drugs of abuse has been well documented (Kenny, 2011). Each exposure to sugar or addictive drugs triggers release of dopamine in the NAc, and, over time, this leads to changes in the availability or function of dopamine receptors. With repeated exposures, drug abusers tend to need more of their drug for it to have its initial effect; this is referred to as **tolerance**. Tolerance is explained, in part, by the down-regulation of dopamine receptors and, therefore, blunted dopamine activity. Higher doses of a drug are needed in order to activate more of the functional dopamine receptors. Perhaps this also happens with sugar or palatable food addiction, so that people need to consume increasingly more palatable food over time to experience the good, or "comforted," feeling they recall having with that food.

It would be easy to assume that sugar, because it is associated with calories, is innately reinforcing and consequently always triggers dopamine release. However, modifications to the neurobiological response can be made based on postingestive consequences. For example, dopamine activity within the NAc increases when rats ingest a sweet-tasting saccharin solution (an innately liked taste) for the first time. However, in rats with a conditioned taste aversion to saccharin produced by pairing nausea-producing lithium chloride injections with saccharin ingestion, dopamine activity is reduced when they are given oral saccharin infusions (Mark et al., 1991). (Note that they will actively avoid *drinking* saccharin; hence, the oral infusion is used to expose them to the taste for a sufficient period for the dopamine measurements. Rats with a conditioned aversion will actively reject – the rat equivalent of spitting out – saccharin during this test.) Further, dopamine release after a positive association has been made with sugar, palatable food, or addictive drug is actually higher on *anticipation* of its delivery than on the actual receipt of it (Pelchat et al., 2004; Volkow et al., 2003; Weltens et al., 2014). So, although dopamine is released initially in response to a pleasurable or rewarding stimulus, after conditioning, its release is shaped by learned expectations about the consequences of the anticipated stimulus.

The binding of dopamine to its D2 receptor subtype in the striatum, a brain region associated with pleasure and motivated behaviors, is elevated by palatable food consumption or addictive drug use. A reduction of D2 receptors in the striatum, sometimes referred to as **striatal dysfunction**, is associated with drug abuse. Some theorists believe that this indicates that drug addicts have a blunted "reward" response and thus seek drugs as a way to boost their sluggish reward systems (Stice et al., 2010). Similarly, obese humans and rats have reduced D2 receptor expression in the striatum. Johnson and Kenny (2010) discovered that striatal D2 receptor expression in the junk food diet rats was inversely related to weight gain after about 1.5 months on the palatable diet. It seems that a decrease in D2 receptors is a response to overactivation of the reward pathway. This consequently leads to increased desire for activation of the pathway through pleasurable stimuli such as palatable food or addictive drugs.

Interestingly, despite the reduction in striatal D2 receptors, the brains of obese individuals show enhanced striatal activity in response to food cues (Ferrario, 2017; Stice et al., 2010). Some researchers believe that obese people have heightened activity associated with anticipated food reward, but a decreased activity in response to the actual receipt of food. This could underlie intense food craving and wanting, but blunted satisfaction on consuming the desired food, and a continued feeling of wanting more. Although we do not yet know if changes in the human brain precede obesity or are a result of obesity, the results of the study by Johnson and Kenny, among others, suggest that it is the latter: Overconsumption, particularly of palatable food, reduces dopamine activity within the striatum eliciting an increased yearning for more palatable food.

Endogenous Opioid System

Activity of the **endogenous opioid system** is associated with pleasurable stimuli, including addictive drug ingestion. Opioid drugs, including heroin, morphine, and oxycontin, work as direct agonists of the opioid system by binding and activating endogenous opioid receptors. Other drugs of abuse activate the system indirectly, but also powerfully. For example, drugs such as alcohol, nicotine (in cigarettes), and cocaine activate other neurotransmitter systems directly, but trigger indirect activity of the opioid system. We know this because opioid antagonist drugs can effectively reduce alcohol, cigarette, and cocaine use by addicts, seemingly because the drugs are no longer as pleasurable when activity of the opioid system is blocked.

Certainly, consumption of sweet and palatable food is pleasurable, and so the opioid system is likely involved. Naloxone and naltrexone, two opioid receptor blockers used in drug addiction research and therapy, reduce the hedonic ratings of sweet and palatable tastes and smells and can reduce binge consumption associated with binge eating disorders (Drewnowski et al., 1995). Naloxone, in particular, has been shown to reduce sugar consumption in rats conditioned to receive sugar following a cue (Grimm et al., 2007). The opioid blocker seems to negate the sugar craving induced by the conditioned stimulus. Further, injections of an opioid receptor stimulant (DAMGO) into the nucleus accumbens of rats have been shown to increase consumption of palatable solutions (water with sucrose, saccharin, or salt) but not water alone (Zhang & Kelley, 1997, 2002). The endogenous opioid system seems to be involved in selective preferences for palatable tastes and, perhaps, palatable food addiction and overconsumption (Smith & Robbins, 2013).

BOX 10.2 DOES WEIGHT AFFECT BRAIN REACTIVITY TO FOOD CUES?

Stice and colleagues (2008) conducted an fMRI study to assess brain activity associated with anticipation compared with receipt of a palatable food by obese and lean adolescent girls. Particular cues preceded the delivery of a palatable chocolate milkshake, a tasteless solution, or nothing while the girls were in the MRI scanner. When anticipating and receiving the "rewarding" taste of the milkshake, obese girls (compared with lean girls) showed greater activation in areas of the cortex associated with food taste, reward, and craving, including the gustatory cortex, insular cortex, and anterior cingulate cortex. The researchers also found that BMI was inversely correlated with activity in the caudate (a part of the striatum) in response to food consumption. These findings support the theory that food "wanting" is enhanced with increased body weight, but enjoyment or satisfaction on food consumption is inversely correlated with weight. In another fMRI study, the activity in reward-associated brain regions was modulated by the *label* of the palatable food. Brain activation was higher with anticipation of the regular milkshake than with anticipation of the milkshake labeled "low fat," supporting the idea that obese individuals are more responsive to external food cues such as anticipated palatability (Ng et al., 2011). Further, this enhanced activation of the reward pathway hinders the ability to restrain and lose weight.

Orexin System

An increasing amount of evidence indicates a role of the **orexin** (a peptide also known as hypocretin) system in drug abuse and palatable food consumption (Aston-Jones et al., 2010). Orexin receptors have been found in the hypothalamus (associated with maintaining homeostasis and motivation) and mesolimbic regions (associated with reward). Orexin signaling seems to modulate dopamine activity within the mesolimbic region, enhancing the reward produced by pleasurable stimuli and increasing the motivation to seek out such stimulation. However, orexin antagonists do not block food-deprived rats' consumption of chow, indicating that orexin activity is involved in hedonic food consumption and drug use but not hunger-induced food consumption (Choi et al., 2010).

Direct administration of orexin into rat brains triggers selective eating of palatable high-fat food. Findings also indicate that, when rats are conditioned to receive palatable food, such as chocolate, at regular intervals or on particular cues, orexin signaling increases when rats "expect" the treat. Additionally, orexin antagonists have been shown to reduce impulsivity, a problem associated with drug abuse and binge eating. Orexin activity, thus, seems to facilitate eating for pleasure rather than for physiological need, which can drive overconsumption of high-fat and high-calorie palatable foods.

Cannabinoids

Marijuana smoking has, for centuries, been linked with increased food consumption, particularly of snack or junk food. Tetrahydrocannabinol (THC), the psychoactive substance in marijuana, activates the cannabinoid system, stimulating hunger for and palatability of hedonic foods. Much of the information about marijuana and increased hunger and eating has been in the form of anecdotal reports from marijuana users. However, in the 1990s, researchers discovered that THC administration in rats and mice triggered hyperphagia, and that blockage of the cannabinoid system prevented the overconsumption. This empirical evidence of the hyperphagic effects of cannabinoid stimulation led to attempts to better understand its role in eating behavior and possibilities of the use of antagonist drugs for the treatment of obesity.

THC and other cannabinoids work by binding endogenous cannabinoid receptors (primarily the CB1 receptor subtype) in the brain and periphery. Cannabinoid receptors have been found in areas of the brain associated with eating regulation and motivation (e.g., regions of the hypothalamus), areas associated with reward or pleasure (e.g., nucleus accumbens), and peripheral regions involved in digestion (e.g., intestines; Kirkham, 2009). Researchers realized that, if endogenous receptors exist, there must be some natural chemicals within the body that bind to them. This awareness led to the discovery of endocannabinoids, the brain's endogenous THC-like neurotransmitters. Endocannabinoid release is activated by pleasurable experiences, and this neural activity enhances their hedonic value. This system apparently works in conjunction with the orexin, dopamine, and opioid systems within the hypothalamic and reward pathways of the brain to additively enhance reward associated with palatable food consumption and the memories associated with such consumption. Endocannabinoids seem to play a role in appetite stimulation and motivation to seek out and consume food, particularly palatable food (Abel, 1975; Foltin et al., 1988).

Recent evidence helps explain the "munchies" (selective eating of high-energy snack foods) associated with marijuana use. Antagonists of this system effectively result in reduced eating and weight loss in humans and animals. However, cannabinoid antagonist drugs are currently not used as weight loss medication because they are associated with an increased risk for depression (Izzo & Sharkey, 2010). There is, however, current exploration of the effects of targeting cannabinoid receptors in the periphery (specifically in the intestines) to facilitate weight loss without the adverse psychological effects (Behl et al., 2021).

CONCLUDING REMARKS

The concept of "food addiction" is supported by a growing number of studies, including anecdotal human reports and empirical human and animal evidence. Many overweight people claim that their favorite foods are too irresistible, and this issue likely underlies the failure of many diet or weight loss efforts. In the documentary film *Super Size Me* (2004), Morgan Spurlock exclusively consumed food from fast-food restaurants for 30 days in an effort to explore the health risks, if any, of frequent consumption of heavily processed foods high in carbohydrate and fat (e.g., soda, cheese-burgers, French fries, and milkshakes). He gained a large amount of weight (about 25 lbs) in a very short period of time, which is perhaps not surprising considering his significant increase in daily energy consumption. More surprising to Spurlock, and of interest to us, were his reported mood swings, depression, and lethargy while on the fast-food diet. Further, his depressed mood was relieved by the consumption of his palatable and energy-dense meals. His cycle of craving, bingeing, and having associated mood swings is consistent with that described by drug addicts. Anecdotal reports such as Spurlock's support the notion that food can have profound effects on mood and can have addictive-like qualities.

Recent fMRI studies indicate that brain regions associated with taste and pleasure are more intensely activated in obese compared with lean people when they are exposed to food cues (e.g., Gearhardt et al., 2011). This is consistent with evidence showing that drug addicts have increased activity in pleasure-associated regions when exposed to cues such as pictures of drug paraphernalia. As previously discussed in this chapter, other behavioral and biological markers are similar for drug addicts and obese people or animals (perhaps "food addicts"). The neural mechanisms that underlie food liking and craving and the motivation to seek out and consume food are consistent with those that underlie drug abuse. It seems that the palatable high-energy foods so prevalent in our society overactivate reward pathways, resulting in neurophysiological and behavioral symptoms of addiction. Importantly, the addiction model of overeating is likely an insufficient explanation of the complex reasons for disordered or unhealthy eating behaviors among our diverse population; however, the parallels between addiction to drugs and overconsumption of palatable foods warrant consideration and continued investigation, particularly regarding treatment for obesity.

QUESTIONS TO ASK YOURSELF

Let's review and apply your knowledge. Take some time to answer these chapter questions:

1 How may serotonin activity impact carbohydrate craving?
2 Describe the impact that stress has on eating behaviors.
3 What is the evidence that cravings are usually not need-based?
4 What are the leading explanations for chocolate cravings?

5 Provide at least four pieces of evidence supporting the idea that palatable food can be addictive.
6 Which neurotransmitter systems seem to underlie food addiction? What is the supporting evidence for their involvement?
7 How does our current food environment impact cravings for comfort or junk foods, which can lead to binges (behaviors associated with addiction)?

GLOSSARY

Dietary restraint	The extent to which food is resisted.
Dopamine	A neurotransmitter associated with reward, motivation, and movement.
Endogenous opioid system	The brain system involved with pain relief.
Glucocorticoids	A class of steroid hormones produced in response to stress. In humans, cortisol is the principal glucocorticoid.
Hypothalamic–pituitary–adrenal (HPA) axis	The interaction between the hypothalamus, pituitary gland, and adrenal glands to regulate the body's response to stress.
Insulin	A hormone released from the pancreas that allows cells to absorb glucose from blood.
Mesolimbic dopamine system	A brain pathway extending from the ventral tegmental area in the midbrain to forebrain regions associated with pleasure and reward.
Nucleus accumbens (NAc)	A forebrain region associated with pleasure and reward.
Orexin	A neurotransmitter involved with appetite and arousal.
Serotonin (5-HT)	A neurotransmitter involved with mood, appetite, and sleep.
Striatal dysfunction	Altered activity of dopamine in the striatum.
Tolerance	The reduced effect of a drug after repeated use, so that a higher dose is needed for it to have its initial effect.
Tryptophan	The amino acid from which serotonin is synthesized.

REFERENCES

Abel, E. L. (1975). Cannabis: Effects on hunger and thirst. *Behavioral Biology, 15,* 152–281.

Aston-Jones, G., Smith, R. J., Sartor, G. C., Moorman, D. E., Massi, L., Tahsili-Fahadan, P., & Richardson, K. A. (2010). Lateral hypothalamic orexin/hypocretin neurons: A role in reward-seeking and addiction. *Brain Research, 1314,* 74–90.

Avena, N. M., Gold, J. A., Kroll, C., & Gold, M. S. (2012). Further developments in the neurobiology of food and addiction: Update on the state of the science. *Nutrition, 28* (4), 341–343.

Avena, N. M., Rada, P., & Hoebel, B. G. (2008). Evidence for sugar addiction: Behavioral and neuro-chemical effects of intermittent, excessive sugar intake. *Neuroscience & Biobehavioral Reviews, 32,* 20–39.

Barrett, B., Muller, D., Rakel, D., Rabago, D., Marchand, L., & Scheder, J. C. (2006). Placebo, meaning, and health. *Perspectives in Biology and Medicine, 49* (2), 178–198.

Behl, T., Chadha, S., Sachdeva, M., Sehgal, A., Kumar, A., Venkatachalam, T., Hafeez, A., Aleya, L., Arara, S., Batiha, G. E., Nijhawan, P. & Bungau, S. (2021). Understanding the possible role of endocannabinoid system in obesity. *Prostaglandins & Other Lipid Mediators, 152,* 106520–106534.

Bruinsma, K., & Taren, D. L. (1999). Chocolate: Food or drug? *Journal of the American Dietetic Association, 99* (10), 1249–1256.

Bulik, C. M., Sullivan, P. F., Fear, J. L., & Pickering, A. (2000). Outcome of anorexia nervosa: Eating attitudes, personality, and parental bonding. *International Journal of Eating Disorders, 28* (2), 139–147.

Cantor, M. B., Smith, S. E., & Bryan, B. R. (1982). Induced bad habits: Adjunctive ingestion and grooming in human subjects. *Appetite, 3,* 1–12.

Choi, D. L., Davis, J. F., Fitzgerald, M. E., & Benoit, S. C. (2010). The role of orexin-a in food motivation, reward-based feeding behavior and food-induced neuronal activation in rats. *Neuroscience, 167,* 11–20.

Corsica, J. A., & Spring, B. J. (2008). Carbohydrate craving: A double-blind, placebo-controlled test of the self-medication hypothesis. *Eating Behaviors, 9* (4), 447–454.

Dallman, M. F. (2010). Stress-induced obesity and the emotional nervous system. *Trends in Endocrinology and Metabolism, 21* (3), 159–165.

Dallman, M. F., Pecoraro, N. C., & la Fleur, S. E. (2005). Chronic stress and comfort foods: Self-medication and abdominal obesity. *Brain, Behavior, & Immunity, 19* (4), 275–280.

Drewnowski, A., Krahn, D. D., Demitrack, M. A., Nairn, K., & Gosnell, B. A. (1995). Naloxone, an opiate blocker, reduces the consumption of sweet high-fat foods in obese and lean female binge eaters. *American Journal of Clinical Nutrition, 61* (6), 1206–1212.

Ferrario, C. R. (2017). Food addiction and obesity. *Neuropsychopharmacology, 42* (1), 360–361.

Fletcher, P. C., & Kenny, P. J. (2018). Food addiction: A valid concept? *Neuropsychopharmacology, 43* (13), 2506–2513.

Foltin, R. W., Fischman, M. W., & Byrne, M. F. (1988). Effects of smoked marijuana on food intake and body weight of humans living in a residential laboratory. *Appetite, 11,* 1–14.

Foster, M. T., Warne, J. P., Ginsberg, A. B., Horneman, H. F., Pecoraro, N. C., Akana, S. F., & Dallman, M. F. (2009). Palatable foods, stress, and energy stores sculpt corticotropin-releasing factor, adrenocorticotropin, and corticosterone concentrations after restraint. *Endocrinology, 150* (5), 2325–2333.

Gearhardt, A. N., Yokum, S., Orr, P. T., Stice, E., Corbin, W. R., & Brownell, K. D. (2011). Neural correlates of food addiction. *Archives of General Psychiatry, 68* (8), 808–816.

Gibson, E. L. (2006). Emotional influences on food choice: Sensory, physiological and psychological pathways. *Physiology and Behavior, 89,* 53–61.

Grimm, J. W., Manaois, M., Osincup, D., Wells, B., & Buse, C. (2007). Naloxone attenuates incubated sucrose craving in rats. *Psychopharmacology, 194* (4), 537–544.

Hallam, J., Boswell, R. G., DeVito, E. E., & Kober, H. (2016). Focus: Sex and gender health: Gender-related differences in food craving and obesity. *The Yale Journal of Biology and Medicine, 89* (2), 161–173.

Izzo, A. A., & Sharkey, K. A. (2010). Cannabinoids and the gut: New developments and emerging concepts. *Pharmacology & Therapeutics, 126,* 21–38.

Johnson, P. M., & Kenny, P. J. (2010). Dopamine D2 in addiction-like reward dysfunction and compulsive eating in obese rats. *Nature Neuroscience, 13,* 635–641.

Kenny, P. (2011). Common cellular and molecular mechanisms in obesity and drug addiction. *Nature Reviews Neuroscience, 12,* 6538–6651.

Kirkham, T. C. (2009). Cannabinoids and appetite: Food craving and food pleasure. *International Review of Psychiatry, 21,* 163–171.

Koob, G. F., & Volkow, N. D. (2016). Neurobiology of addiction: A neurocircuitry analysis. *The Lancet Psychiatry, 3* (8), 760–773.

Kühn, S., & Gallinat, J. (2011). Common biology of craving across legal and illegal drugs – a quantitative meta-analysis of cue-reactivity brain response. *European Journal of Neuroscience, 33* (7), 1318–1326.

Lawson, O. J., Williamson, D. A., Champagne, C. M., DeLany, J. P., Brooks, E. R., Howat, P. M., & Ryan, D. H. (1995). The association of body weight, dietary intake, and energy expenditure with dietary restraint and disinhibition. *Obesity Research, 3* (2), 153–161.

Lenoir, M., Serre, F., Cantin, L., & Ahmed, S. H. (2007). Intense sweetness surpasses cocaine reward. *PLoS ONE, 2* (8), 1–10. doi:10.1371/journal.pone.0000698

Lieberman, H., Wurtman, J., & Chew, B. (1986). Changes in mood after carbohydrate consumption among obese individuals. *American Journal of Clinical Nutrition, 45,* 772–778.

Mark, G. P., Blander, D. S., & Hoebel, B. G. (1991). A conditioned stimulus decreases extracellular dopamine in the nucleus accumbens after the development of a learned taste aversion. *Brain Research, 551* (1), 308–310.

Michener, W., & Rozin, P. (1994). Pharmacological versus sensory factors in the satiation of chocolate craving. *Physiology & Behavior, 56* (3), 419–422.

Ng, J., Stice, E., Yokum, S., & Bohon, C. (2011). An fMRI study of obesity, food reward, and perceived caloric density. Does a low-fat label make food less appealing? *Appetite, 57* (1), 65–72. doi:10.1016/j.appet.2011.03.017

Olds, J., & Milner, P. (1954). Positive reinforcement produced by electrical stimulation of septal area and other regions of rat brain. *Journal of Comparative Physiological Psychology, 47* (6), 419–427.

Oliver, G., & Wardle, J. (1999). Perceived effects of stress on food choice. *Physiology & Behavior, 66* (3), 511–515.

Parsey, R. V., Oquendo, M. A., Ogden, R. T., Olvet, M., Simpson, N., Huang, Y. Y., & Mann, J. J. (2006). Altered serotonin 1A binding in major depression: A [carbonyl-C-11] WAY100635 positron emission tomography study. *Biological Psychiatry, 59* (2), 106–113.

Pelchat, M. L. (1997). Food cravings in young and elderly adults. *Appetite, 28* (2), 103–113.

Pelchat, M. L., Johnson, A., Chan, R., Valdez, J., & Ragland, J. D. (2004). Images of desire: Food-craving activation during fMRI. *NeuroImage, 23,* 1486–1493.

Pelchat, M. L., & Schaefer, S. (2000). Dietary monotony and food cravings in young and elderly adults. *Physiology & Behavior, 68* (3), 353–359.

Poelmans, E., & Swinnen, J. (2016). A brief economic history of chocolate. In M. P. Squiccuarini & J. Swinnen (eds.), *The economics of chocolate* (pp. 11–42). Oxford: Oxford University Press.

Rolls, E. T., & McCabe, C. (2007). Enhanced affective brain representations of chocolate in cravers vs. non-cravers. *European Journal of Neuroscience, 26* (4), 1067–1076.

Smith, A. F. (2006). *Encyclopedia of junk food and fast food.* Bloomsbury Academic.

Smith, D. G., & Robbins, T. W. (2013). The neurobiological underpinnings of obesity and binge eating: A rationale for adopting the food addiction model. *Biological Psychiatry, 73* (9), 804–810.

Stice, E., Spoor, S., Bohon, C., Veldhuizen, M., & Small, D. (2008). Relation of reward from food intake and anticipated food intake to obesity: A functional magnetic resonance imaging study. *Journal of Abnormal Psychology, 117,* 924–935. doi:10.1037/a0013600

Stice, E., Yokum, S., Blum, K., & Bohon, C. (2010). Weight gain is associated with reduced striatal response to palatable food. *The Journal of Neuroscience, 30* (39), 13105–13109.

Van Strien, T., & Van de Laar, F. A. (2008). Intake of energy is best predicted by overeating tendency and consumption of fat is best predicted by dietary restraint: A 4-year follow-up of patients with newly diagnosed Type 2 diabetes. *Appetite, 50* (2), 544–547.

Volkow, N. D., Wang, G. J., Maynard, L., Jayne, M., Fowler, J. S., Zhu, W., … Pappas, N. (2003). Brain dopamine is associated with eating behavior in humans. *International Journal of Eating Disorders, 33*, 136–142.

Weingarten, H. P., & Elston, D. (1991). Food cravings in a college population. *Appetite, 17* (3), 167–175.

Weltens, N., Zhao, D., & Van Oudenhove, L. (2014). Where is the comfort in comfort foods? Mechanisms linking fat signaling, reward, and emotion. *Neurogastroenterology & Motility, 26* (3), 303–315.

Wurtman, R., & Wurtman, J. (1995). Brain serotonin, carbohydrate craving, obesity, and depression. *Obesity Research, 3* (4), 477S–480S.

Yokum, S., Ng, J., & Stice, E. (2011). Attentional bias to food images associated with elevated weight and future weight gain: An fMRI study. *Obesity, 19* (9), 1775–1783.

Zellner, D. A., Garriga-Trillo, A., Rohm, E., Centeno, S., & Parker, S. (1999). Food liking and craving: A cross-cultural approach. *Appetite, 33*, 61–70. doi:10.1006/appe.1999.0234

Zellner, D. A., Loaiza, S., Gonzalez, Z., Pita, J., Morales, J., Pecora, D., & Wolf, A. (2006). Food selection changes under stress. *Physiology & Behavior, 87* (4), 789–793.

Zellner, D. A., Saito, S., & Gonzalez, J. (2007). The effect of stress on men's food selection. *Appetite, 49*, 696–699.

Zhang, M., & Kelley, A. E. (1997). Opiate agonists microinjected into the nucleus accumbens enhance sucrose drinking in rats. *Psychopharmacology, 132* (4), 350–360.

Zhang, M., & Kelley, A. E. (2002). Intake of saccharin, salt, and ethanol solutions is increased by infusion of a mu opioid agonist into the nucleus accumbens. *Psychopharmacology, 159* (4), 415–423.

CHAPTER 11

Eating Disorders and Treatment

After reading this chapter, you will be able to

- Understand the clinical conditions of anorexia nervosa, bulimia nervosa, and binge eating disorder.
- Recognize personality and behavioral differences and similarities associated with different eating disorders.
- Know the leading biological, psychological, and sociocultural explanations for eating disorders.
- Describe the most effective contemporary treatments for eating disorders and the issues surrounding treatment.
- Appreciate animal models of eating disorders.

Estimates indicate that between 1% and 3% of the U.S. population (roughly 8 million people) suffer with a diagnosed eating disorder, and many more suffer from subclinical (less severe) disordered eating (Galmiche et al., 2019; Watson & Bulik, 2013). In comparison with the percentage of the population that is overweight or obese (~70%), the incidence of these eating disorders may seem low; however, eating disorders are severely debilitating and have the highest death rate of any psychiatric illness (Galmiche et al., 2019; Watson & Bulik, 2013). Further, the frequency of eating disorders is much higher among certain groups of people, including college students, actors, models, and athletes participating in "appearance sports" (sports with an emphasis on appearance, weight, speed, or diet – e.g., dance, gymnastics, swimming, running, and wrestling; Prouty et al., 2002; Sundgot-Borgen & Torstveit, 2004; Zucker et al., 1999). The *Diagnostic and Statistical Manual for Mental Health Disorders* (5th ed.; DSM-5) provides criteria for the diagnosis of anorexia nervosa and bulimia nervosa (American Psychiatric Association [APA], 2013). The diagnosis of binge eating disorder was added to the most recent edition of the DSM and is the most prevalent of all eating disorders (Goode et al., 2020).

It is important to bear in mind that the distinction between disordered eating and normal eating is often unclear. We all, at times, have "peculiar" eating habits and food preferences or aversions. Dieting and being concerned about weight are considered normal in our society. So, when does "normal" behavior become "abnormal?" The important difference with clinically disordered eating is the extreme persistence regarding ritual-istic or restrained eating behaviors, and this is associated with particular personality types

DOI: 10.4324/9781032621401-11

and ways of thinking. In this chapter, we discuss the symptoms associated with anorexia nervosa, bulimia nervosa, and binge eating disorder, risk factors, leading explanations for these disorders, and best current treatments.

ANOREXIA NERVOSA

Anorexia nervosa (AN) is characterized by extreme thinness and a desire to lose weight or maintain an abnormally low weight. According to the DSM-5 criteria (see Table 11.1), a diagnosis of AN can be made if an individual is considerably underweight and fears gaining weight; thus, the diagnosis does not apply to sufferers of metabolic disorders or other illnesses that cause weight loss if those individuals hope to return to a healthy weight. The psychology and distorted body image associated with AN are significant aspects of the illness and its diagnosis (APA, 2013).

TABLE 11.1 DSM-5 diagnostic criteria for anorexia nervosa

1 Restriction of food intake leading to significantly low body weight.
2 Intense fear of gaining weight.
3 Disturbed body perception and/or denial of the seriousness of the current low weight.

Source: Adapted from APA (2013).

BOX 11.1 HOW CAN BODY PERCEPTION BE MEASURED?

Several techniques have been used by different groups of researchers to assess perceived body size. Results of these studies consistently indicate that people with AN overestimate their body size and are more dissatisfied with their body size compared with peers without eating disorders (e.g., Farrell et al., 2005). In one such study, photographed images of the participants were projected in front of them adjacent to a full-length mirror, allowing them to simultaneously see their actual reflection (Shafran & Fairburn, 2002). The participants were asked to have the experimenters adjust the projected image until it matched what they saw in the mirror. The participants with eating disorders significantly overestimated their body size compared with those without eating disorders. This study was one of the first to allow the participants to actually see their own reflection as they estimated body size; most studies require participants to recall their size from memory.

Katie

When Katie started high school, kids occasionally teased her about being "chubby," and a friend suggested that she would probably be more popular if she lost a little weight.

She decided to cut out desserts and candy from her diet in hopes of shedding a few pounds. After several months of dieting and increasing her exercise, she started receiving compliments from friends and family members. Her mom proudly took her out shopping for some cute new clothes, and the boy she had a crush on asked her out. Liking her success, Katie eliminated bread and meat from her diet. She also increased her exercise regimen from every other day to every day. Within two years, the compliments turned to looks of concern. Katie, 5′ 4″ in height, now weighed 95 lbs. (Weights between 110 and 145 lbs are considered healthy for someone of her height [Division of Nutrition, Physical Activity, and Obesity, National Center for Chronic Disease, 2011].) She was an excellent student, made straight As, and thought she looked great, although she believed she could look better if she lost a little more weight. Katie assumed the people questioning her weight and health were just jealous of her looks and ability to control her diet so well. Her parents became concerned about her shrinking appearance and her obsession with her exercise regimen, but they assumed she was going through a teenage girl "phase" and would soon return to normal eating habits. However, when she visited her family physician for an annual check-up, she was asked about her menstrual cycle. Katie happily answered that she hadn't had a period in more than a year. Her physician realized that Katie's low weight, denial of its seriousness, amenorrhea (cessation of menses), and refusal to gain weight were symptoms of anorexia nervosa. Her parents were consulted, and she spent the next three months in an inpatient facility focused on helping her restore weight and develop healthier eating habits and body image. We will return to Katie's story a little later in this chapter.

Katie's story is typical of how many eating disorders begin – with an effort to lose some weight. AN has an average age of onset between 14 and 18 years, a time of hormonal fluctuation and heightened social pressures (APA, 2000). Individuals with AN are often characterized as perfectionists and are usually competitive and high achieving. They view their weight loss as success and become fixated on losing more weight and being the "thinnest" person in their peer group. Frequently, as with Katie, their weight loss is initially met with praise and reinforcement. Thus, severe calorie restriction, meal rituals, and excessive exercise become obsessions. They hold distorted thoughts about their body size and appearance, usually estimating themselves to be much larger and less attractive than they actually are (Farrell et al., 2005).

Two patterns are associated with AN: The restricting type is characterized by severe and persistent calorie restraint, and the binge eating/purging type involves efforts to eliminate consumed food (e.g., self-induced vomiting, excessive exercise, or laxative or diuretic misuse). AN is considered the most severe psychological disorder, with 15–20% of sufferers dying within 20 years of the onset of their disorder (Arcelus et al., 2011; Birmingham et al., 2005; Fichter & Quadflieg, 2016). Suicide and cardiovascular problems are the leading causes of death among anorexics (Fichter & Quadflieg, 2016; Herzog et al., 2000). As discussed, people with AN are rarely sufficiently pleased with their weight or appearance and are severely distressed by issues surrounding food. Anorexics often isolate themselves socially: They avoid the unwanted comments or concerned looks from friends or family members. Further, people with AN are preoccupied with food (reading recipe books, planning and preparing food for others, learning how to disguise their minimal intake and food regimens, etc.). So, over time, they withdraw from others, which contributes to a sense of loneliness, despair, and self-loathing. Depression and anxiety are often co-morbid with AN (Silberg & Bulik, 2005; Swinbourne et al., 2012; Watson & Bulik, 2013).

Medical Problems Associated with AN

The medical problems associated with AN are consistent with those associated with starvation (Katzman, 2005). With energy intake below its needs, the body attempts to conserve its resources and preserve its vital functions. Medical consequences include low blood pressure, heart rate, and body temperature; amenorrhea (absence of the menstrual cycle in females of menstruation age); dry and brittle skin, hair, and nails; and lanugo (fine, downy hair normally present on third trimester fetuses) on the face and extremities. The reduced body temperature results in heightened sensitivity to cold temperatures, something anorexics often complain about (Brown et al., 2000).

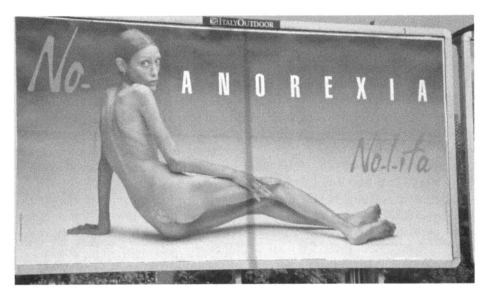

FIGURE 11.1 Isabelle Caro, a French model and actress, struggled with anorexia and died in 2010 at age 28 years as a result of medical complications associated with AN. Her picture was used as part of an anorexia awareness campaign in Italy and other countries
Source: *Los Angeles Times.*

Although not required for the diagnosis, amenorrhea is often associated with AN owing to a decrease in several hormones, including estrogen (Klibanski et al., 1995; Misra & Klibanski, 2016). Estrogen helps support bone density in females; consequently, low levels increase the likelihood of early-onset osteoporosis, a disorder associated with bone fractures and reduced height. Estrogen disturbances can also result in reproductive difficulties and infertility. People with AN have increased risks for electrolyte imbalances and cardiovascular problems, particularly if vomiting, diuretics, or laxatives are used as methods of purging. Cardiac arrest as a result of electrolyte and fluid imbalance can result in sudden death. Anorexics also commonly suffer sleep disturbances, perhaps because of an imbalance of serotonin (a neurotransmitter associated with the homeostatic regulation of eating and sleep) or a persistent desire to burn calories leading to a need to busy themselves even during nighttime hours (Haleem, 2012).

Let's return to Katie: In the years that followed inpatient treatment, Katie remained underweight and continued to use excessive exercise as a means of purging the food she ate. She became increasingly rigid with her eating and exercise routines, isolating herself from close relationships with others. Now at age 35, Katie's thin hair and hunched posture (a result of early-onset osteoporosis) make her appear much older than she actually is. Katie has realized the unfortunate consequences of her years of starving herself, but much of the damage is irreversible.

Generally, the more chronic the symptoms of AN, the more resistant people are to treatment. The rigid personality, fear of weight gain, and long-term medical consequences associated with AN contribute to the difficulties in treating and preventing relapse in this population, as with Katie. Thus, early identification and treatment of AN symptoms are critical for recovery.

BULIMIA NERVOSA

Bulimia nervosa (BN) is more prevalent than AN, affecting between 1% and 3% of the population (AN affects less than 1% of the population; Castillo & Weiselberg, 2017). BN is characterized by cycles of food binges and purges (getting rid of the excessive food consumed during a binge).

A *binge* is an excessive amount of food eaten within a limited amount of time (less than about two hours; APA, 2013). Binges cause uncomfortable fullness and feelings of shame and guilt; thus, purges serve as compensatory behavior. Commonly used purging methods include: Self-induced vomiting; misusing laxatives, diuretics, or enemas; and excessive exercising. The term *excessive exercise* refers to exercise performed not for enjoyment, and not because of participation on a sports team or training for an athletic event, or even for health, but rather as a means of burning off calories recently consumed. This type of exercise involves a psychology that differs in key ways from exercise performed for enjoyment, health, or sport.

Binges usually occur when the individual is alone and are done secretly. The eating is beyond physiological needs, and hunger is not a necessary prerequisite for a binge – psychological factors such as stress, loneliness, or depressed mood can prompt binge eating (Mathes et al., 2009). Foods consumed during binges are normally soft textured and require little or no chewing (e.g., cookie dough, ice cream, breads and sandwiches, milkshakes, juices and sodas, cookies, and cake), are frequently sweet tasting, high in calories and fat (Latner & Wilson, 2000), and are considered "forbidden." Binges usually contain more than 1,000 calories (often more than 4,000; Heaner & Walsh, 2013; Kaye et al., 1992). In other words, in a single "sitting" or bout, one may consume more than the recommended caloric intake for an entire day. People with BN describe their binges as numbing, pleasurable, and even euphoric. However, the "high" is quickly followed by a "low." After bingeing, bulimics feel guilty, ashamed, and worried about weight gain and often experience self-hatred and depression (Hayaki et al., 2002). Bulimics are concerned about their appearance and are fearful of gaining weight. Purging helps alleviate the guilt and discomfort associated with the out-of-control bingeing and eliminates some of the food consumed, but it also causes guilt and shame. Further, because purging empties the stomach, hunger follows, and the cycle of binge eating and purging continues (Figure 11.2).

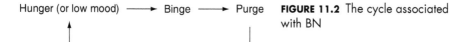

FIGURE 11.2 The cycle associated with BN

TABLE 11.2 DSM-5 diagnostic criteria for bulimia nervosa

1	Recurrent episodes of binge eating
2	Recurrent inappropriate purging behavior to prevent weight gain
3	The symptoms occur, on average, at least once a week for three months
4	Inappropriate focus on shape and weight

Source: Adapted from APA (2013).

People with BN are typically within 10 lbs of the expected or healthy weight for their height. It is often assumed that they should be underweight because purging "undoes" the binge; however, purging methods do not allow 100% compensation. Vomiting, for example, results in the elimination of only about half of the calories consumed in a binge (Latner & Wilson, 2000). Further, recurrent purging disrupts the body's ability to regulate hunger and satiety, leads to more frequent feelings of hunger, and alters the digestion and metabolism of food consumed. The diagnosis of BN requires that bingeing and purging behaviors occur at least once a week (see Table 11.2), but these behaviors are usually far more frequent; for some sufferers, episodes occur more than 30 times per week (Kaye et al., 1992).

Medical Problems Associated with BN

The medical problems associated with BN are generally related to the means of purging. People who use forced vomiting as a frequent purging method risk damage to their teeth, gums, and esophagus. Gastric acids cause erosion of tooth enamel, making teeth prone to cavities and decay. It is not uncommon for a dentist or dental hygienist to be among the first to identify symptoms of BN (DeBate et al., 2005). Acids can also cause ulceration of the esophagus and swallowing difficulty. Frequent forced vomiting can result in reflexive, unwanted vomiting (this is called *reverse peristalsis*). Misuse of laxatives and diuretics can cause kidney damage, bowel control problems, and electrolyte imbalances that can be fatal.

Andrea

Andrea, a bright and ambitious college student, had interests in opera, foreign languages, and human rights and a desire to "save the world." She was fluent in Spanish, was studying German, and planned to tackle the Japanese language next. She was an ardent supporter of human rights and planned to use her degree in international business and politics to improve the lives of others around the world. Andrea was a loving daughter, sister, and friend. Unfortunately, she suffered with bulimia nervosa. Her mother beautifully describes her and shares entries from her journals written during high school and college in the book *Andrea's Voice* (Smeltzer et al., 2006). Andrea's mood swings, self-hatred, and frustration elevated during the months she battled bulimia. She wrote in her journal about her desire to "win" the battle and described her disappointment and resentment when she had setbacks. In one entry, she wrote that she feared she needed to cut back on her purging (vomiting) because she was starting to experience reflexive vomiting and was unable to keep food down (reverse peristalsis). Despite her tremendous accomplishments in life and promising future, Andrea felt imprisoned by her illness, angry at her captor, and alone. Tragically, after a 13-month battle with bulimia, an electrolyte imbalance caused her heart to fail, and she died in her sleep at age 19 years.

BINGE EATING DISORDER

Binge eating disorder (BED) is associated with large, uncontrolled, recurrent bouts of food consumption within two hours. BED affects about 3% of the population; women are diagnosed at slightly higher rates than men (Reslan & Saules, 2011). Binges are followed by distress and feelings of disgust and disappointment. People with BED feel that they cannot control their food consumption. As with BN, the foods consumed during a binge are often soft and can be quickly chewed and swallowed, such as breads and snack foods, and consumed secretly. Unlike BN, the binge is not followed by a purge; consequently, high weights and obesity are often co-morbid with BED (Leehr et al., 2015; Wilfley et al., 2016). BED also differs from BN in having a later age of onset, typically in early adulthood rather than adolescence.

About 33% of our adult population meets the criteria for obesity based on body mass index (BMI), and only about 3% of our population is diagnosed with BED. So, the majority of obesity is not associated with BED. And not all people with BED are obese (Wilfley et al., 2016). Further, obese individuals with BED have higher rates of depression and lower self-esteem than those without BED.

Medical Problems Associated with BED

Elevated body weights are often associated with BED and related health problems, which include type 2 diabetes, metabolic syndrome, hypertension, and sleep disturbances/sleep apnea. People with BED have both reduced quality of life and activity level and increased likelihood of earlier death compared with those without BED (Giel et al., 2022).

TABLE 11.3 DSM-5 diagnostic criteria for binge eating disorder

1	Recurrent episodes of binge eating
2	Marked distress regarding binge eating
3	The symptoms occur, on average, at least once a week for three months
4	The absence of compensatory behaviors (e.g., purging)

Source: Adapted from APA (2013).

TABLE 11.4 Other eating disorders included in DSM-5

In addition to anorexia nervosa, bulimia nervosa, and binge eating disorder, the DSM-5 also includes the following disorders:

1	Avoidant restrictive food intake disorder – a disorder associated with reduced food intake and inability to meet nutritional needs
2	Other specified feeding and eating disorder – a diagnosis given when symptoms of AN, BN, or BED are subclinical and do not meet the criteria for those disorders
3	Pica – characterized by the consumption of non-foods, such as paper or dirt
4	Rumination disorder – a condition in which people repeatedly and unintentionally spit up undigested food

Source: APA (2013).

Risk Factors for AN and BN

About 80% of people with AN or BN are females, often between ages 14 and 35 years. Until recently, eating disorders were only considered problems in Western countries, reported primarily among people in North America and Western Europe. However, rates of eating disorders are now rising in industrialized countries around the world. In Japan, for example, a culture that values thinness particularly among women, eating disorders are among the fastest-growing psychiatric problems for females in adolescence and early adulthood (Nakai et al., 2021; Thomas et al., 2016). Rates of eating disorders have likewise risen among Hispanic and African American females and among young males, groups of people in our culture that, until recently, did not emphasize extreme thinness (Pike et al., 2014; Smink et al., 2012; Wood et al., 2010).

The average age of onset of AN and BN is during adolescence or early adulthood, most often between ages 15 and 21 years, with AN usually occurring at younger ages than BN (Hoek & Van Hoeken, 2003; Hudson et al., 2007). Depression, anxiety, and substance abuse are frequently co-morbid with AN and BN (Hudson et al., 2007; Kaye, 2008; Swinbourne et al., 2012). These may contribute to the onset of eating disorders or they could be consequences of them; however, evidence indicates that other factors underlie eating disorders and the co-morbid disorders (e.g., personality, serotonin imbalance, genetics; Kaye et al., 2009; Stice et al., 2004). Stimulants (e.g., cocaine, methamphetamine, nicotine), which speed up metabolism and reduce feelings of hunger, are often abused by people with eating disorders. People with BN are more likely than people with AN to additionally abuse alcohol and marijuana, as these can contribute to weight gain (Root et al., 2010).

Different personality characteristics are associated with AN and BN. As discussed previously, anorexics are typically perfectionists, exercising high levels of self-control and harm avoidance, and hold themselves to idealistic standards (Kaye, 2008). Consequently, they tend to be very self-critical. They are paradoxically obsessed with food and eating rituals, yet steadfast in their restraint from eating in their pursuit of weight loss. Many have symptoms of obsessive-compulsive personality disorder. Because they tend to isolate themselves so that they can pursue their eating and exercise rituals without receiving negative attention, they can exhibit symptoms of avoidant personality disorder (Diaz-Marsá et al., 2000; Waller et al., 2013).

Bulimics are less controlling and restrained than anorexics. Rather, bulimics tend to be more impulsive and have more erratic mood swings. Some people with BN have symptoms of borderline personality disorder, which is characterized by emotional instability and impulsiveness. Bulimics tend to be highly concerned with pleasing and being attractive to others, whereas anorexics are more focused on meeting their own goals and adhering to their stringent standards. These personality traits seem to differentially increase an individual's risk of either AN or BN (Tyrka et al., 2002; Waller et al., 2013).

Risk Factors for BED

The majority of people with BED have a mental health problem in their lives. Many have co-morbid depression, anxiety, substance use disorder, or post-traumatic stress disorder (PTSD) and are at increased risk for self-harm and suicide attempts (Keski-Rahkonen, 2021; Wilfley et al., 2016). Rates of BED are higher among non-heterosexuals than heterosexuals. War veterans are a high-risk population for the BED diagnosis, likely because of their increased risk for PTSD. Childhood abuse, neglect, violence, and restricted access to food during childhood are risk factors for the later development of BED-related symptoms. Further, the frequent co-morbidity with trauma and PTSD indicates that the binge behavior with BED may be an attempt to cope with the trauma (Keski-Rahkonen, 2021). As with AN, BED is often co-morbid with obsessive-convulsive and/or avoidant personality disorders (Farstad et al., 2016).

BIOPSYCHOSOCIAL EXPLANATIONS OF AN AND BN

Eating disorders are found primarily in industrialized societies that emphasize a thin appearance. Media and marketing contribute to the pervasiveness of particular attractiveness ideals. In the 1960s, super-thin models, such as Twiggy, were glamorized. Some theorists postulate that this idealization of a thin body type led people (women, in particular) to hold themselves to this standard and judge themselves harshly, resulting in restrained and disordered eating for some. Another poignant example of the influence of media occurred in Fiji. Eating disorders and body image issues were minimal among the Fijian population (with only one reported case of AN) prior to the 1995 introduction of television. Rates of body dissatisfaction and disordered eating increased significantly within just a few years of media exposure and had a particularly negative impact among adolescent girls (Becker et al., 2002).

However, it is important to consider this: Media messages idealizing the thin body image are pervasive; yet only between 1% and 3% of our population has a diagnosable eating disorder. If media or other social influences bear full responsibility for disordered eating, then, theoretically, everyone within that culture would suffer, and clearly that is not the case. Historical investigation reveals that disordered eating occurred among early Christians and during the Renaissance, usually for ritualistic or religious reasons (Miller & Pumariega, 2001). Early Christians are known to have refrained from food consumption as a demonstration of selflessness and purity (the psychology behind their restraint is clearly different from that associated with AN, but the behaviors can appear alike). And, similar self-imposed food restriction occurs today in non-Western cultures (e.g., fasting among Buddhists as a practice of self-control).

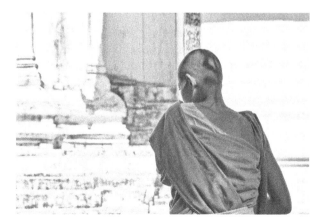

IMAGE 11.1 Buddhist monk at a place of worship

Whereas it is quite clear that sociocultural influences contribute to distorted body image and eating behaviors, other factors must additionally contribute. In this section, we explore the **biopsychosocial model** to explain AN and BN. According to this model, biological, psychological, and sociocultural factors are separate but have additive or synergistic effects, increasing an individual's risk for developing an eating disorder.

Biological Factors

Eating disorders occur at much higher rates within families than among the general population, and the closer someone is related to an individual with an eating disorder, the greater the risk that person has of developing an eating disorder as well, even when raised in a different environment (Klump et al., 2009). Studies of identical (monozygotic) and fraternal (dizygotic) twins indicate a 50–80% genetic contribution to the vulnerability for AN or BN (Bulick et al., 2006; Kaye, 2008; Kendler et al., 1991, 1995; Klump et al., 2001). It seems that some people may have shared genetic liability for the development of eating disorders. Of particular interest to researchers are genes, neurotransmitters, and brain pathways associated with appetite, impulse control, motivation, and reward.

Serotonin

Several groups of researchers have found evidence implicating a role of the genes involved in the synthesis of the neurotransmitter **serotonin** and its receptors in eating disorders (Haleem, 2012; Kaye, 2008). Serotonin activity is associated with satiety, mood, and inhibition. People with AN or BN are at increased risk for co-morbid depression, which is also associated with irregular serotonin activity (Haleem, 2012). However, it seems that serotonin activity associated with AN differs from that associated with BN. For example, people with AN exercise high levels of dietary restraint and inhibition, whereas people with BN have impulse control difficulties, indicating that serotonin activity may be high in the brains of people with AN and low in those with BN. Further, symptoms of BN are typically reduced by antidepressant medications that increase serotonin activity, but these medications are unreliable in the treatment of AN (Ferguson et al., 1999; Kaye, 2008). This further supports the theory that serotonin activity is lower than normal for bulimics, but higher for people with anorexia.

People with AN have reduced brain volume, particularly in chronic cases. Thus, in studies of brain irregularity, it is difficult, and often impossible, to determine which factors are *causal* versus *consequential* of the disorder (Kaye et al., 2009). With AN, a cycle of below normal consumption of food and weight loss drives a continued effort to restrict calories and lose more weight. Some evidence supports the theory that anorexics have higher than normal levels of serotonin activity *prior* to the onset of their symptoms, which contribute to their feelings of satiety, nervousness about food consumption, and drive for thinness and perfection. Further, food consumption elevates the already high levels of serotonin, whereas starvation serves to reduce levels and stabilize mood. So, people with AN may actually avoid food as an attempt reduce their anxiety. (We recommend Kaye et al. [2009] and Frank et al. [2019] for reviews of the neurobiology of AN.)

Dopamine and the Endogenous Opioid System

Individuals with AN have blunted enjoyment of palatable food (along with decreased enjoyment of other typically rewarding or enjoyable stimuli; Kaye et al., 2009), whereas people with BN frequently report euphoric-like feelings associated with binge episodes. These dissimilar emotional states associated with these two eating disorders indicate that the brain's reward pathways may respond in different ways to food-related stimuli.

The use of fMRI technology has provided evidence of differences in brain activity in people with AN and BN compared with those without an eating disorder. Non-eating disordered people usually have elevated neural activity on seeing or consuming appetizing food (e.g., brownies, pizza, candy) in areas of the brain associated with pleasure and reward. However, these stimuli have the converse effect on the brain activity of people with AN, indicating disturbances within the **dopamine** system, which persists after recovery from symptoms (Kaye et al., 1999). Dopamine dysfunction could contribute to the diminished reward response associated with food-related stimuli in the brains of people with AN and their reduced motivation to consume food (Kaye et al., 2009). Interestingly, people with AN have increased activity in areas of the brain associated with pleasure and reward in response to images of thin bodies (Frank, 2013).

Conversely, the brain activity in regions associated with reward and pleasure of people with BN is greater than that of non-BN people when exposed to food-related stimuli. This provides a biological explanation for the intense craving for food and the blunted ability to control the amount of food consumed in a binge. In addition to dopamine within the reward regions of the brain, endogenous opioids (endorphins) are also involved in eating behavior. One group of researchers found that naloxone, a drug that blocks opioid receptors in the brain, reduced palatable food consumption among people with BN (or with binge eating disorder) but not among normal-weight or obese non-bingeing individuals (Drewnowski et al., 1995). Along with the reduced activity of serotonin, the neurobiological alterations of reward circuitry may help explain the impulse-control problems and overconsumption associated with binge eating.

Psychological Factors

People with AN and BN have distorted attitudes about eating and body weight. They have frequent negative thoughts about their appearance and their eating behaviors. From the **cognitive perspective** in the field of psychology, their maladaptive and negative thoughts lead to attempts to restrain eating and lose weight. In other words, the thoughts precede the behaviors. Further, the cycle of negative thinking coupled with unhealthy eating behaviors is reinforcing, and the person becomes more convinced of his or her distorted thoughts about weight and eating and is increasingly compulsive about his or her eating behaviors (more restraining with AN or more frequent bingeing and purging with BN). Body dissatisfaction and perceived pressure to be thin are among the leading psychological risk factors for eating disorders (Rohde et al., 2015).

Theorists from the **psychodynamic perspective** in psychology posit that disordered eating behaviors stem from misuse of food by parents during an individual's childhood (Bruch, 1973; Zerbe, 2008). Parents sometimes use food as a means of soothing children. This can lead to a lifelong emotional association with food. Children parented in this way learn to seek food for comfort, rather than nutrition, which can result in binge eating (BN) or to food restriction as a means of self-punishment (AN) later in life. **Behavioral**

theorists also believe that this early experience with food is influential because children learn to model their parents' eating behaviors. So, parents who eat food as a means of comforting themselves are likely to unintentionally teach the same behavior to their children.

Sociocultural Factors

Historically, societies struggled with food scarcity, and low weight was due to inability to obtain sufficient amounts of food. In such societies, people of heavier weights were considered healthier, more attractive, and of higher social status than people of low weights. In our current society, the opposite is true. Exposure to media perpetuating this thin-ideal image is correlated with body dissatisfaction and disordered eating (Stice et al., 1994; Thompson & Stice, 2001). Sociocultural influences, including media, family, and peers, may have a negative impact on body satisfaction, putting genetically vulnerable individuals at greater risk of developing an eating disorder. Children of parents who exercise high levels of dietary restraint and emphasize weight loss are at increased risk of disordered eating (Baker et al., 2000; Birch & Fisher, 2000). Further, children of *authoritarian* parents (parents who are controlling, set strict rules, and expect obedience) have a reduced ability to regulate calorie needs (Johnson & Birch, 1994) and are more likely to eat in the absence of hunger (Birch & Fisher, 2000). Girls are apparently more affected than boys by parental behaviors, especially by the mother's behaviors and attitudes. Daughters of mothers who are preoccupied with weight, restrict or limit foods, and/or encourage their daughters to lose weight are at a particularly increased risk for disordered eating (Francis & Birch, 2005). Parents who encourage healthy eating and explain the benefits of a healthy lifestyle, offer healthy options from which children can select their food, and eat together as a family have children with healthier lifelong eating habits (Patrick et al., 2005). It is important to note, though, that the shared disordered eating between mothers and daughters or within families may be attributed to environment and learning, but it also may be due to shared genetics responsible for perfectionistic or obsessive personality types.

Biopsychosocial Explanations for BED

As with BN, people with BED have blunted impulse control. Binge eating behavior is linked to stress and difficulty with emotional regulation (Kessler et al., 2016).

Biological Factors

Neuroimaging studies have revealed that people with BED have greater activity in regions of the brain associated with reward and craving (e.g., the striatum) when exposed to pictures of high-calorie food than people without BED. There is also increased brain activity in the cortex of people with BED when exposed to food-related stimuli (Kessler et al., 2016). Taken together, these neurobiological differences provide insight into the difficulty people with BED have with impulsivity and portion control. They have a greater desire for food and they think about food more often than people without BED. Some researchers compare the compulsive binge eating and brain reactivity to food stimuli to similar patterns seen with drug addiction. Altered dopamine activity within the reward pathway of the brain is the major chemical contributor to binge eating behavior.

Psychological Factors

As discussed, BED is often associated with childhood maltreatment and/or a traumatic event. Binges are used to cope with the distress of the trauma. People with BED have a reduced ability to regulate emotions and are at increased risk for depression and self-harm. Binge eating provides temporary improvement in mood (Leehr et al., 2015).

From the behavioral perspective, binge eating behavior can stem from parents' misuse of food as a form of comforting and soothing. An adult with BED may continue to associate food with comfort, and this can further contribute to improved mood.

Sociocultural Factors

Commensal eating (eating in groups) facilitates healthful food consumption and helps us learn how to eat foods that may be new (e.g., with fingers, fork, condiments, etc.). In recent decades, it has become increasingly normal for us to eat alone, perhaps in our car on the way to school or work or while watching our favorite shows in the comfort of our bed. Because binge eating is usually done secretly, the problematic behavior may go unnoticed for a long time, because food consumption in isolation raises little to no concern among loved ones or roommates.

Abuse or neglect by parents during childhood is often associated with BED. Children may find comfort from food and continue this association into adulthood. And, with such convenient access to highly palatable food in developed countries, people with BED can easily obtain their source of comfort.

TREATMENTS

Only a small percentage of people with eating disorders receive treatment, and an even smaller percentage complete the recommended therapeutic phases (Halmi et al., 2005; Hudson et al., 2007; Noordenbos et al., 2002). People with AN are particularly resistant to treatment and unlikely to initiate a search for help for several reasons – an individual's denial of the seriousness of the disorder, refusal to make changes in eating behaviors or gain weight, the expense of treatment, and under-diagnosing of disordered eating by physicians (Walsh et al., 2000). However, recognition of symptoms, support, and treatment are critically important for recovery from eating disorders. Leading contemporary treatments involve individual, group, and family therapy; nutrition counseling; and often medication, especially when other psychological disorders are co-morbid with the eating disorder.

The first step in treating AN is helping the individual restore weight. This process is more challenging than it sounds, particularly in chronic cases. Digestion is slowed for these individuals, resulting in discomfort when they consume meals larger than what they have become accustomed to eating. Further, weight gain causes distress for people with AN, as this has been their fear. Behavioral tactics are usually the most effective methods for helping people with AN gain weight (Kaye et al., 2000). Rewards, such as praise and computer or television time, are given when a person eats appropriately. This process can take place in an inpatient treatment center or at an individual's home, which often involves family supervision and support. Typically, a nutritionist or other trained professional creates a daily meal plan with gradual caloric increases over the span of several weeks (usually about 100 additional calories per week until weight is restored). This method, in contrast with force-feeding of a high-calorie diet in the first few days of treatment, is more tolerable to the person with AN, both physiologically and psychologically. People with BN are able to begin psychological therapy and medication immediately on diagnosis as they are usually within a healthy weight range (Kaye et al., 2000). For BED, treatment is focused on the binge eating behavior, restraint, and weight loss. The most frequently prescribed medications for eating disorders are selective serotonin reuptake inhibitors (SSRIs), which are also antidepressants and work by elevating serotonin neurotransmission (Kaye, 2008; Sim et al., 2010).

Cognitive-behavioral therapy (CBT) is the leading type of psychological therapy for eating disorders (Bulik et al., 2007; Iacovino et al., 2012; Yager & Powers, 2007). CBT addresses an individual's maladaptive thoughts about food and body weight and also reinforces healthy eating behavior. For BED and BN, major goals of CBT are improved restraint and healthier coping techniques. Exposure and response prevention therapy can be used to help people with BN or the binge eating–purge type of AN. With this, the therapist may sit with the client as they eat a meal and wait with them as food moves through their digestive system, while preventing compensatory behavior. It may take multiple exposures of eating without purging for this behavior to feel normal and to not cause distress. **Dialectical behavior therapy**, a newer form of CBT, is used to train people to better regulate their emotions and be more mindful of their behaviors and feelings. This is particularly helpful for people who are prone to binge eating for emotional reasons (Bankoff et al., 2012; Telch et al., 2001).

Individual therapy is usually coupled with **family and group therapy**. Because family dynamics frequently contribute to the onset of disordered eating, it is important that the family members address their issues so that they can provide a supportive environment for the individual recovering from an eating disorder (Wilson et al., 2007). Group therapy can help sufferers realize that they are not alone. Because people with AN tend to isolate themselves, and binges with BN and BED are done secretly, sufferers are usually comforted by the realization that other people also suffer in similar ways. Additionally, in group therapy, people can share tactics that they have found helpful and can support one another through the recovery process. Unfortunately, there are two main reasons for concern with group therapy – the sharing of unhealthy weight loss tactics and competition among group members to be the thinnest (this is particularly problematic among people with AN). Therapists work to ensure that the group therapy is beneficial and not harmful, as effective social and family support is important for long-term recovery.

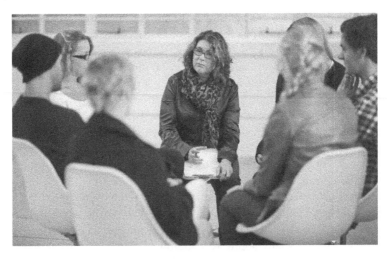

IMAGE 11.2 This is an example of a group therapy session

Is Treatment Effective?

Simply stated, improvement from eating disorder symptoms is more likely with treatment than without it (Bulik et al., 2007; Shapiro et al., 2007). Unfortunately, people with eating disorders often drop out of therapy or relapse after remission of symptoms, particularly in cases of chronic AN. However, the research on the effectiveness of therapy and specific forms of treatment is limited because of the small sample sizes and high dropout rates in most of the studies (Bulik et al., 2007). And, as discussed previously, people with eating disorders often have co-morbid psychological disorders and issues, which complicate the effectiveness of therapy. Other problematic issues surrounding treatment are expense and accessibility. Recall Katie, discussed earlier in this chapter. She was in a treatment facility for three months – the length of time recommended by most therapists and psychiatrists. The average cost of inpatient treatment for eating disorders is $30,000 per month, and insurance companies usually do not cover it. Most people cannot afford to pay nearly $100,000 for the recommended three months of treatment. Taking such a long period of time away from work or school creates an additional challenge for people suffering with eating disorders.

ANIMAL MODELS OF EATING DISORDERS

Given the obstacles to therapy and high rates of relapse, there is hope that drug treatment will be possible in the treatment of eating disorders. To test potential therapeutic agents, animal models have been examined. You may wonder if animals could be feasible models of eating disorders. With the possible exception of nonhuman primates (in whom this type of research is essentially impossible for well-justified animal welfare considerations), animals are not thought to have a developed sense of self-awareness and, in particular, of body image. So, the essential aspect of distorted body image, especially in AN, probably cannot be modeled. But other animal models have one key attribute of AN as it relates to eating: Forgoing food when it is available despite substantial weight loss. These models fall into two categories: Those that occur in nature, and those that are induced by a laboratory procedure.

Let's look first at the natural models. One of the most widely known is incubation anorexia, which refers to the loss of appetite and weight loss (often 10–15%) observed in many species of birds while they have eggs in their nest (Mrosovsky, 1990), especially when only one sex does all the incubating. You might rightly point out that the bird is put into a conflict between keeping the eggs warm and protected and leaving the nest to forage for food. However, this anorexia occurs in these birds even in a domesticated environment when abundant food is placed next to the nest. This observation leads to the conclusion that there are physiological changes (probably hormonal) during incubation that suppress appetite and, in a natural environment, will suppress hunger and keep the incubating bird "on task."

This model is not only task-related but, because birds are seasonal breeders, will be associated with specific day length (photoperiod) indicative of the season. If animals show physiological and behavioral changes in different seasons, they are said to be photoperiodic. There are other photoperiod-related changes in food intake. Many species eat less in the winter when days are short and lose substantial body weight (e.g., 20%; Iverson & Turner, 1974), and, like the incubating birds, this occurs even in captivity when food is readily available. In the natural environment, food tends to be less abundant during the winter, and expending large amounts of energy in unsuccessful foraging is a poor survival strategy. The physiological suppression of hunger then has an adaptive function. Another example is in rutting deer (Yoccoz et al., 2002): The males lose 10–15% of their body weight during rutting season, even though there is plenty of grass around; in contrast, females do not lose weight.

Unfortunately for the animal model perspective, humans are not photoperiodic with regard to mating or breeding behavior, but one could argue that some individuals, such as those prone to seasonal affective disorder, may exhibit some elements of photoperiodism. One established laboratory model that does not involve photoperiodism is called **activity-based anorexia** (ABA; Epling et al., 1983). In this protocol, animals (usually rats or mice) are given food for a restricted time each day – often two to four hours. Most species are able to adapt to this type of schedule quite well; although they don't eat as much as they would with 24-hour access, they do eat more than enough to maintain a healthy body weight. In fact, this type of time-restricted feeding regimen is common in zoos and for domestic pets. In ABA, the animals are additionally provided with a running wheel. As they lose weight, they tend to run more and so expend more energy, but their food intake does not rise commensurately (and may in fact be suppressed a bit). As a result, they are trapped in a spiral of a progressively more negative energy balance and usually have to be removed from the experiment for humane reasons when weight loss exceeds a threshold (e.g., 15%).

Another model that does not involve ABA has been found using mice in one of the authors' labs (Atalayer & Rowland, 2012). In this case, food was also restricted to 160 minutes per day but spread out across the night in several meals or feeding opportunities (we used 4, 8, or 16 opportunities of 40, 20, or 10 minutes each). Additionally, the food was available as small pellets (20 mg) for which the mice had to work by emitting a fixed number of responses. After several days, the number of responses required (the price) was increased. Food intake was highly influenced by the condition: At 25 responses per pellet, the intake was <50% that at the lowest cost (2 responses), and the mice lost weight rapidly. You might question whether, at 25 responses per pellet and only 160 minutes of total access to food, the animals were simply running out of time to acquire more food. But analysis of when pellets were taken within an opportunity showed that, even when weight was dropping, the mice ate progressively less within each window of opportunity and overall ate less than half what they could have consumed if they had used the time fully. One key feature of this procedure might be that the local rate of feeding is limited because responses need to be performed between each mouthful or pellet. (Slowing of eating by more chewing has been advocated as an appetite control device in humans and is discussed in other chapters.) This, or some other aspect of this situation, is leading to a "voluntary" failure to increase feeding duration within an opportunity.

In the case of bulimia nervosa, many animals (rats and mice in particular) are unable to vomit, and so that essential aspect (along with body image) of BN is not modeled. However, several protocols have been developed in which animals eat a large amount in a short time (i.e., binge eating). In most of these protocols, using rats or mice, the relatively bland maintenance diet (chow) is available all the time, and preferred or palatable food (e.g., cakes, hotdogs, cookies) is given occasionally. When the palatable food is given every day, intake tends to be quite high and constant from day to day, and it is compensated by a reduction in chow intake over the rest of the day, so that total caloric intake is not increased, and no weight gain occurs. However, if the palatable food is given every other day (or, in general, less predictably), the intake increases as the number of exposures increases and eventually greatly exceeds the intake of the palatable food by the daily group (Corwin, 2004; Gearhardt et al., 2011). The behavior resembles that seen with binge eating disorder. We discuss this model in greater detail in Chapter 10 in our section on junk food addiction.

Are these useful models of eating disorders? We'll leave you to debate and think about this. Regardless, the relative absence of eating disorders among animals, infants, and young children supports that we are biologically driven to eat and survive, and eating disorders defy these innate motivations.

CONCLUDING REMARKS

Eating disorders are serious, life-endangering psychiatric conditions. Biological, psychological, and sociocultural factors contribute to an individual's risk for the development and maintenance of disordered eating. Cognitive-behavioral therapy is the most effective and frequently used type of psychotherapy; however, access and affordability are hindrances to treatment for many sufferers. Early diagnosis and treatment yield the most optimistic outcomes, particularly when coupled with family and social support.

QUESTIONS TO ASK YOURSELF

Let's review and apply your knowledge. Take some time to answer these chapter questions:

- What are the criteria for the diagnosis of AN? For BN? For BED?
- Describe the personality types and behaviors most associated with AN, BN, and BED.
- What are the medical complications or problems associated with each eating disorder?
- Provide several pieces of support for a biopsychosocial explanation for eating disorders.
- What are the leading types of treatment? What are some of the issues surrounding treatment?
- Discuss research involving animal models of eating disorders. What are the advantages and limitations of animal models when studying eating disorders?

Talking Point 11.1

Could there be alternative explanations for the higher rates of eating disorders within families? Explain.

GLOSSARY

Activity-based anorexia (ABA)	A laboratory model of weight loss involving exercise and reduced food intake.
Behavioral theorists	Researchers and practitioners focused on the effects of learning on behavior.
Biopsychosocial model	The theory that psychological problems are due to interactions of biological, psychological, and sociocultural factors.
Cognitive-behavioral therapy (CBT)	Psychological therapy that addresses maladaptive thoughts and dysfunctional behaviors.
Cognitive perspective	A psychological model focused on the content and process of human thinking.
Dialectical behavior therapy (DBT)	A form of cognitive-behavioral therapy that emphasizes emotion regulation, mindful awareness, and acceptance.
Dopamine (DA)	A neurotransmitter associated with reward, motivation, and movement.
Family and group therapy	Formats in which the therapist meets with family members or groups of individuals with similar psychological issues.
Psychodynamic perspective	A theoretical model that attributes human functioning to interactions of forces and drives within the person, particularly in the unconscious mind. Childhood experiences are emphasized within this perspective.
Serotonin (5-HT)	A neurotransmitter involved with eating, sleeping, and mood.

REFERENCES

American Psychiatric Association (APA). (2000). *Diagnostic and statistical manual of mental disorders,* 4th ed., text revision. Washington, DC: Author.

American Psychiatric Association (APA). (2013). *Diagnostic and statistical manual of mental disorders,* 5th ed. Washington, DC: Author.

Arcelus, J., Mitchell, A. J., Wales, J., & Nielsen, S. (2011). Mortality rates in patients with anorexia nervosa and other eating disorders: A meta-analysis of 36 studies. *Archives of General Psychiatry, 68* (7), 172–731.

Atalayer, D., & Rowland, N. E. (2012). Effects of meal frequency and snacking on food demand in mice. *Appetite, 58,* 117–123.

Baker, C. W., Whisman, M. A., & Brownell, K. D. (2000). Studying intergenerational transmission of eating attitudes and behaviors: Methodological and conceptual questions. *Health Psychology, 19,* 376–381.

Bankoff, S. M., Karpel, M. G., Forbes, H. E., & Pantalone, D. W. (2012). A systematic review of dialectical behavior therapy for the treatment of eating disorders. *Eating Disorders, 20* (3), 196–215.

Becker, A. E., Burwell, R. A., Gilman, S. E., Herzog, D. B., & Hamburg, P. (2002). Eating behaviours and attitudes following prolonged television exposure among ethnic Fijian adolescent girls. *British Journal of Psychiatry, 180,* 509–514.

Birch, L. L., & Fisher, J. O. (2000). Mothers' child-feeding practices influence daughters' eating and weight. *American Journal of Youth and Adolescence, 27,* 43–57.

Birmingham, C. L., Su, J., Hlynsky, J. A., Goldner, E. M., & Gao, M. (2005). The mortality rate from anorexia nervosa. *International Journal of Eating Disorders, 38* (2), 143–146.

Brown, J. M., Mehler, P. S., & Harris, R. H. (2000). Topics in review: Medical complications occurring in adolescents with anorexia nervosa. *Western Journal of Medicine, 172* (3), 189–193.

Bruch, H. (1973). *Eating disorders: Obesity, anorexia nervosa and the person within.* New York: Basic Books.

Bulik, C. M., Berkman, N. D., Brownley, K. A., Sedway, J. A., & Lohr, K. N. (2007). Anorexia nervosa treatment: A systematic review of randomized controlled trials. *International Journal of Eating Disorders, 40* (4), 310–320.

Bulick, C. M, Sullivan, P. F., Tozzi, F., Furberg, H., Lichtenstein, P., & Pedersen, N. L. (2006). Prevalence, heritability, and prospective risk factors for anorexia nervosa. *Archives of General Psychiatry, 63* (3), 305–312.

Castillo, M., & Weiselberg, E. (2017). Bulimia nervosa/purging disorder. *Current Problems in Pediatric and Adolescent Health Care, 47* (–), 85–94.

Corwin, R. L. (2004). Binge-type eating induced by limited access in rats does not require energy restriction on the previous day. *Appetite, 42,* 139–142.

DeBate, R. D., Tedesco, L. A., & Kerschbaum, W. E. (2005). Knowledge of oral and physical manifestations of anorexia and bulimia nervosa among dentists and dental hygienists. *Journal of Dental Education, 69* (3), 346–354.

Diaz-Marsá, M., Luis, J., & Sáiz, J. (2000). A study of temperament and personality in anorexia and bulimia nervosa. *Journal of Personality Disorders, 14* (4), 352–359.

Division of Nutrition, Physical Activity, and Obesity, National Center for Chronic Disease. (2011). Prevention and health promotion healthy weight – it's not a diet, it's a lifestyle. Retrieved from www.cdc.gov/healthyweight/assessing/bmi/adult_bmi/english_bmi_calculator

Drewnowski, A., Krahn, D. D., Demitrack, M. A., Nairn, K., & Gosnell, B. A. (1995). Naloxone, an opiate blocker, reduces the consumption of sweet high-fat foods in obese and lean female binge eaters. *American Journal of Clinical Nutrition, 61* (6), 1206–1212.

Epling, W. F., Pierce, W. D., & Stefan, L. (1983). A theory of activity-based anorexia. *International Journal of Eating Disorders, 3* (1), 27–46.

Farrell, C., Lee, M., & Shafran, R. (2005). Assessment of body size estimation: A review. *European Eating Disorders Review, 13,* 75–88.

Farstad, S. M., McGeown, L. M., & von Ranson, K. M. (2016). Eating disorders and personality, 2004–2016: A systematic review and meta-analysis. *Clinical Psychology Review, 46,* 91–105.

Ferguson, C. P., La Via, M. C., Crossan, P. J., & Kaye, W. H. (1999). Are serotonin selective reuptake inhibitors effective in underweight anorexia nervosa? *International Journal of Eating Disorders, 25* (1), 11–17.

Fichter, M. M., & Quadflieg, N. (2016). Mortality in eating disorders – results of a large prospective clinical longitudinal study. *International Journal of Eating Disorders, 49* (4), 391–401.

Francis, L. A., & Birch, L. L. (2005). Maternal influences on daughters' restrained eating behavior. *Health Psychology, 24,* 548–554.

Frank, G. K. (2013). Altered brain reward circuits in eating disorders: Chicken or egg? *Current Psychiatry Reports, 15* (10), 396–402.

Frank, G. K., Shott, M. E., & DeGuzman, M. C. (2019). Recent advances in understanding anorexia nervosa. *F1000Research, 8,* 1–7.

Galmiche, M., Dechelotte, P., Lambert, G., & Tavolacci, M. P. (2019). Prevalence of eating disorders over the 2000–2018 period: A systematic literature review. *The American Journal of Clinical Nutrition, 109* (5), 1402–1413.

Gearhardt, A. N., White, M. A., & Potenza, M. N. (2011). Binge eating disorder and food addiction. *Current Drug Abuse Reviews, 4* (–), 201–207.

Giel, K. E., Bulik, C. M., Fernandez-Aranda, F., Hay, P., Keski-Rahkonen, A., Schag, K., Schmidt, U., & Zipfel, S. (2022). Binge eating disorder. *Nature Reviews Disease Primers, 8* (1), 16–63.

Goode, R. W., Cowell, M. M., Mazzeo, S. E., Cooper-Lewter, C., Forte, A., Olayia, O. I., & Bulik, C. M. (2020). Binge eating and binge-eating disorder in Black women: A systematic review. *International Journal of Eating Disorders, 53* (4), 491–507.

Haleem, D. J. (2012). Serotonin neurotransmission in anorexia nervosa. *Behavioural Pharmacology, 23* (5,6), 478–495.

Halmi, K. A., Argas, W. S., Crow, S., Mitchell, J., Wilson, G. T., Bryson, S. W., & Kraemer, H. C. (2005). Predictors of treatment acceptance and completion in anorexia nervosa: Implications for future study designs. *Archives of General Psychiatry, 62* (7), 776–781.

Hayaki, J., Friedman, M. A., & Brownell, K. D. (2002). Shame and severity of bulimic symptoms. *Eating Behaviors, 3* (1), 73–83.

Heaner, M. K., & Walsh, B. T. (2013). A history of the identification of the characteristic eating disturbances of Bulimia Nervosa, Binge Eating Disorder and Anorexia Nervosa. *Appetite, 71*, 445–448.

Herzog, D. B., Greenwood, D. N., Dorer, D. J., et al. (2000). Mortality in eating disorders: A descriptive study. *International Journal of Eating Disorders, 28* (1), 20–26.

Hoek, H. W., & Van Hoeken, D. (2003). Review of the prevalence and incidence of eating disorders. *International Journal of Eating Disorders, 34* (4), 383–396.

Hudson, J. I., Hiripi, E., Pope, H. G., & Kessler, R. C. (2007). The prevalence and correlates of eating disorders in the National Comorbidity Survey Replication. *Biological Psychiatry, 61* (3), 348–358.

Iacovino, J. M., Gredysa, D. M., Altman, M., & Wilfley, D. E. (2012). Psychological treatments for binge eating disorder. *Current Psychiatry Reports, 14*, 432–446.

Iverson, S. L., & Turner, B. N. (1974). Winter weight dynamics in Microtus Pennsylvanicus. *Ecology, 55*, 1030–1041.

Johnson, S. L., & Birch, L. L. (1994). Parents' and children's adiposity and eating style. *Pediatrics, 94* (5), 653–661.

Katzman, D. K. (2005). Medical complications in adolescents with anorexia nervosa: A review of the literature. *International Journal of Eating Disorders, 37* (S1), S52–S59.

Kaye, W. (2008). Neurobiology of anorexia and bulimia nervosa Purdue ingestive behavior research center symposium influences on eating and body weight over the lifespan: Children and adolescents. *Physiology and Behavior, 94*, 121–135.

Kaye, W. H., Frank, G. K., & McConaha, C. (1999). Altered dopamine activity after recovery from restricting-type anorexia nervosa. *Neuropsychopharmacology, 21*, 503–506.

Kaye, W. H., Fudge, J. L., & Paulus, M. (2009). New insights into symptoms and neurocircuit function of anorexia nervosa. *Nature Reviews Neuroscience, 10*, 573–584.

Kaye, W. H., Klump, K. L., Frank, G. K. W., & Strober, M. (2000). Anorexia and bulimia nervosa. *Annual Review of Medicine, 51* (1), 299–313.

Kaye, W. H., Weltzin, T. E., McKee, M., McConaha, C., Hansen, D., & Hsu, L. K. (1992). Laboratory assessment of feeding behavior in bulimia nervosa and healthy women: Methods for developing a human-feeding laboratory. *American Journal of Clinical Nutrition, 55* (2), 372–380.

Kendler, K. S., MacLean, C., Neale, M., Kesler, R., Heath, A., & Eaves, L. (1991). The genetic epidemiology of bulimia nervosa. *American Journal of Psychiatry, 148* (12), 1627–1637.

Kendler, K. S., Walters, E. E., Neale, M. C., Kessler, R., Heath, A., & Eaves, L. (1995). The structure of genetic and environmental risk factors for six major psychiatric disorders in women. *Archives of General Psychiatry, 52*, 374–383.

Keski-Rahkonen, A. (2021). Epidemiology of binge eating disorder: prevalence, course, comorbidity, and risk factors. *Current Opinion in Psychiatry, 34* (6), 525–531.

Kessler, R. M., Hutson, P. H., Herman, B. K., & Potenza, M. N. (2016). The neurobiological basis of binge-eating disorder. *Neuroscience & Biobehavioral Reviews, 63*, 223–238.

Klibanski, A., Biller, B. M., Schoenfeld, D. A., Herzog, D. B., & Saxe, V. C. (1995). The effects of estrogen administration on trabecular bone loss in young women with anorexia nervosa. *Journal of Clinical Endocrinology & Metabolism, 80* (3), 898–904.

Klump, K. L., Miller, K. B., Keel, P. K., McGue, M., & Iacono, W. G. (2001). Genetic and environmental influences on anorexia nervosa syndromes in a population-based sample of twins. *Psychological Medicine, 31* (4), 737–740.

Klump, K. L., Suisman, J. L., Burt, S., McGue, M., & Iacono, W. G. (2009). Genetic and environmental influences on disordered eating: An adoption study. *Journal of Abnormal Psychology, 118* (4), 797–805. doi:10.1037/a0017204

Latner, J. D., & Wilson, G. T. (2000). Cognitive-behavioral therapy and nutritional counseling in the treatment of bulimia nervosa and binge eating. *Eating Behaviors, 1* (1), 3–21.

Leehr, E. J., Krohmer, K., Schag, K., Dresler, T., Zipfel, S., & Giel, K. E. (2015). Emotion regulation model in binge eating disorder and obesity-a systematic review. *Neuroscience & Biobehavioral Reviews, 49,* 125–134.

Mathes, W. F., Brownley, K. A., Mo, X., & Bulik, C. M. (2009). The biology of binge eating. *Appetite, 52* (3), 545–553.

Miller, M. N., & Pumariega, A. J. (2001). Culture and eating disorders: A historical and cross-cultural review. *Psychiatry, 64* (2), 93–110.

Misra, M., & Klibanski, A. (2016). Anorexia nervosa and its associated endocrinopathy in young people. *Hormone Research in Paediatrics, 85* (3), 147–157.

Mrosovsky, N. (1990). *Rheostasis: The physiology of change.* New York: Oxford University Press.

Nakai, Y., Nin, K., & Goel, N. J. (2021). The changing profile of eating disorders and related sociocultural factors in Japan between 1700 and 2020: a systematic scoping review. *International Journal of Eating Disorders, 54* (1), 40–53.

Noordenbos, G., Oldenhave, A., Muschter, J., & Terpstra, N. (2002). Characteristics and treatment of patients with chronic eating disorders. *Eating Disorders, 10* (1), 15–29.

Patrick, H., Nicklas, T. A., Hughes, S. O., & Morales, M. (2005). The benefits of authoritative feeding style: Caregiver feeding styles and children's food consumption patterns. *Appetite, 44,* 243–249.

Pike, K. M., Hoek, H. W., & Dunne, P. E. (2014). Cultural trends and eating disorders. *Current Opinion in Psychiatry, 27* (6), 436–442.

Prouty, A. M., Protinsky, H. O., & Canady, D. (2002). College women: Eating behaviors and help-seeking preferences. *Adolescence, 37,* 353–363.

Reslan, S., & Saules, K. K. (2011). College students' definitions of an eating "binge" differ as a function of gender and binge eating disorder status. *Eating Behaviors, 12* (3), 225–227.

Rohde, P., Stice, E., & Marti, C. N. (2015). Development and predictive effects of eating disorder risk factors during adolescence: Implications for prevention efforts. *International Journal of Eating Disorders, 48* (2), 187–198.

Root, T. L., Pinheiro, A. P., Thornton, L., et al. (2010). Substance use disorders in women with anorexia nervosa. *International Journal of Eating Disorders, 43* (1), 14–21.

Shafran, R., & Fairburn, C. G. (2002). A new ecologically valid method to assess body size estimation and body size dissatisfaction. *International Journal of Eating Disorders, 32* (4), 458–465.

Shapiro, J. R., Berkman, N. D., Brownley, K. A., Sedway, J. A., Lohr, K. N., & Bulik, C. M. (2007). Bulimia nervosa treatment: A systematic review of randomized controlled trials. *International Journal of Eating Disorders, 40* (4), 321–336.

Silberg, J. L., & Bulik, C. M. (2005). The developmental association between eating disorders symptoms and symptoms of depression and anxiety in juvenile twin girls. *Journal of Child Psychology and Psychiatry, 46* (12), 1317–1326.

Sim, L. A., McAlpine, D. E., Grothe, K. B., Himes, S. M., Cockerill, R. G., & Clark, M. M. (2010, August). Identification and treatment of eating disorders in the primary care setting. *Mayo Clinic Proceedings, 85* (8), 746–751.

Smeltzer, D., Smeltzer, A., & Costin, C. (2006). *Andrea's voice – silenced by bulimia: Her story and her mother's journey through grief toward understanding.* Carlsbad, CA: Gürze Books.

Smink, F. R., Van Hoeken, D., & Hoek, H. W. (2012). Epidemiology of eating disorders: Incidence, prevalence and mortality rates. *Current Psychiatry Reports, 14* (4), 406–414.

Stice, E., Burton, E., & Shaw, H. (2004). Prospective relations between bulimic pathology, depression, and substance abuse: Unpacking comorbidity in adolescent girls. *Journal of Consulting and Clinical Psychology, 72* (1), 62.

Stice, E., Schupak-Neuberg, E., Shaw, H. E., & Stein, R. I. (1994). Relation of media exposure to eating disorder symptomatology: An examination of mediating mechanisms. *Journal of Abnormal Psychology, 103* (4), 836–840.

Sundgot-Borgen, J., & Torstveit, M. K. (2004). Prevalence of eating disorders in elite athletes is higher than in the general population. *Clinical Journal of Sport Medicine, 14* (1), 25–32.

Swinbourne, J., Hunt, C., Abbott, M., Russell, J., St Clare, T., & Touyz, S. (2012). The comorbidity between eating disorders and anxiety disorders: Prevalence in an eating disorder sample and anxiety disorder sample. *Australian & New Zealand Journal of Psychiatry, 46* (2), 118–131.

Telch, C. F., Argas, W. S., & Linehan, M. M. (2001). Dialectical behavior therapy for binge eating disorder. *Journal of Consulting and Clinical Psychology, 69*, 1061–1065.

Thomas, J. J., Lee, S., & Becker, A. E. (2016). Updates in the epidemiology of eating disorders in Asia and the Pacific. *Current Opinion in Psychiatry, 29* (6), 354–362.

Thompson, J. K., & Stice, E. (2001). Thin-ideal internalization: Mounting evidence for a new risk factor for body-image disturbance and eating pathology. *Current Directions in Psychological Science, 10* (5), 181–183.

Turner, H., Bryant-Waugh, R., & Peveler, R. (2010). The clinical features of EDNOS: Relationship to mood, health status and general functioning. *Eating Behaviors, 11* (2), 127–130.

Tyrka, A. R., Waldron, I., Graber, J. A., & Brooks-Gunn, J. (2002). Prospective predictors of the onset of anorexic and bulimic syndromes. *International Journal of Eating Disorders, 32* (3), 282–290.

Waller, G., Ormonde, L., & Kuteyi, Y. (2013). Clusters of personality disorder cognitions in the eating disorders. *European Eating Disorders Review, 21* (1), 28–31.

Walsh, J. M. E., Wheat, M. E., & Freund, K. (2000). Detection, evaluation, and treatment of eating disorders: The role of the primary care physician. *Journal of General Internal Medicine, 15*, 577–590.

Watson, H. J., & Bulik, C. M. (2013). Update on the treatment of anorexia nervosa: Review of clinical trials, practice guidelines and emerging interventions. *Psychological Medicine, 43* (12), 2477–2500.

Wilfley, D. E., Citrome, L., & Herman, B. K. (2016). Characteristics of binge eating disorder in relation to diagnostic criteria. *Neuropsychiatric Disease and Treatment*, 2213–2223.

Wilson, G. T., Grilo, C. M., & Vitousek, K. M. (2007). Psychological treatment of eating disorders. *American Psychologist, 62* (3), 199–216.

Wood, R., Nikel, A., & Petrie, T. A. (2010). Body dissatisfaction, ethnic identity, and disordered eating among African American women. *Journal of Counseling Psychology, 57* (2), 141–153.

Yager, J., & Powers, P. S. (eds.). (2007). *Clinical manual of eating disorders.* Washington, DC: American Psychiatric Publishing.

Yoccoz, N. G., Mysterud, A., Langvatn, R., & Stenseth, N. C. (2002). Age- and density-dependent reproductive effort in male red deer. *Proceedings of the Royal Society – Biological Sciences, 269*, 1523–1528.

Zerbe, K. J. (2008). *Integrated treatment of eating disorders beyond the body betrayed.* New York: W. W. Norton.

Zucker, N. L., Womble, L. G., Williamson, D. A., & Perrin, L. A. (1999). Protective factors for eating disorders in female college athletes. *Eating Disorders, 7*, 207–218.

CHAPTER 12

Personal Weight Loss Strategies in Obesity

After reading this chapter, you will be able to

- Discuss the effectiveness of diet and exercise for weight loss and weightmanagement.
- Appreciate the benefits of exercise for overall health (beyond weight management).
- Understand what intermittent fasting is and why your meal times are important.
- Evaluate different types of therapies involved in weight management.

The obesity epidemic has been discussed throughout this book. Obesity is not simply a cosmetic problem; it is associated with decreased quality of life, psychological distress, and numerous health problems, including cardiovascular disease and stroke, type 2 diabetes, cancer, and premature death. According to Our World in Data (2019), approximately 5 million people died prematurely in 2019 as a result of being obese – this is about 9% of the world's population.

Further, overweight and obesity have a devastating economic impact through direct (e.g., health care) and indirect (e.g., lost workdays) costs. The global economic impact of obesity was estimated to be approximately $2 trillion in 2014 (Dobbs et al., 2014). If current obesity trends continue, the World Obesity Federation (2024) predicts the global economic impact will surpass $4 trillion by 2035, which is nearly 3% of global GDP (gross domestic product); this number is estimated to be comparable to the economic impact of the COVID-19 pandemic that began in 2020.

In this chapter, we discuss preventative and treatment options for obesity, including the most common behavioral interventions to shed excess weight: Diet and exercise. We discuss the effects of intermittent fasting on weight loss and the effect of the time at which we eat. Following this is a discussion of counseling, prospective pharmacotherapies, and bariatric surgery as the next level of treatment options. We then discuss circadian clocks and their effect on body weight and food intake and conclude with a brief introduction to the emerging field of chrononutrition.

DOI: 10.4324/9781032621401-12

ENERGY BALANCE AND WEIGHT LOSS

At any given time, millions of Americans say that they want to lose weight, and millions of Americans are actively dieting. However, weight loss is difficult because it requires tremendous mental energy to perpetually override our natural programming to conserve energy, to seek high-calorie foods, and to store extra food as body fat. In this section, we will first discuss the effects of increasing energy expenditure and then contrast it with the impact of limiting energy intake on body weight regulation.

While the biological basis of overnutrition is complex enough to warrant this entire textbook, the thermodynamic basis of weight loss is simple and intuitive: Weight loss will occur when energy expenditure exceeds energy intake; that is, an individual must be in a state of negative energy balance. Energy expenditure can be divided into the following four categories: Resting metabolic rate (RMR), thermic effect of food (TEF), spontaneous physical activity (SPA), and exercise. Some of these components have been discussed in detail in Chapter 3. SPA is generally considered non-goal-oriented physical activity (e.g., fidgeting, standing, general movement that is not goal-directed), while exercise (or volitional exercise) is activity pertaining to sports and fitness (Garland et al., 2010).

On the face of it, achieving a state of negative energy balance would appear to be quite straightforward: One can either decrease one's energy intake (limit one's eating and drinking), increase one's energy expenditure (exercise), or do a combination of both. However, this idea assumes that the components of our energy balance are static, which is not the case. Upon engaging in exercise, people often compensate behaviorally by increasing their food intake or possibly reducing their SPA owing to fatigue; additionally, RMR is shown to decrease when people restrict their food intake (Donnelly & Smith, 2005). The result is that these compensatory mechanisms conserve energy, thereby making it harder for an individual to lose weight. Other variables such as age, sex, body composition, and genetic factors further complicate the energy equation.

Before we discuss whether exercise and dieting are successful tools with which to bring about successful weight loss, it is valuable to discuss what is meant by "successful weight loss." Does this mean weight loss for the duration of the diet or exercise regimen? For most people, successful weight loss requires lasting results where once, weight is lost, it is not gained back, and a healthy weight is maintained for the remainder of their lives.

EFFICACY OF EXERCISE FOR WEIGHT LOSS

Exercise by itself has numerous benefits, including improved cardiovascular functioning, improved insulin sensitivity, possible improvement in cognitive functioning, improved sense of mental well-being, lower risk of certain cancers, lower risk of falling, and improved bone health, and research continues to discover new benefits of exercise. The effect of exercise on weight loss, however, is modest at best (Donnelly & Smith, 2005, Slentz et al., 2004, Westerterp et al., 1992).

Slentz and colleagues (2004) reported significant, dose-dependent decreases in body weight in a group of sedentary and overweight or mildly obese participants (average body mass index, or BMI, was 29.7 +/− 3.2), following eight months on three different levels of exercise (high amount of vigorous exercise, low amount of vigorous exercise, low amount of moderate exercise, and no exercise). It is important to note that the participants in the study were counseled not to make any changes in their diet. Even with the highest level of exercise (20 miles jogging per week at approximately 75% peak oxygen consumption), the weight lost was only 3.5 kg (7.7 lbs) over the course of eight months, which is roughly equivalent to running 83 miles to lose 1 lb. This is more than the typical overweight person would be willing or able to do in order to lose weight.

Most people have heard of *The Biggest Loser*, a reality weight loss television show where participants often achieve dramatic weight loss through diet and exercise. One study followed 14 participants in this show for six years. Predictably, after six years, all but one participant had regained weight, and collectively they had regained a substantial portion of the lost weight. Still, participants experienced less weight gain than most dieters, an outcome that the authors speculatively attribute to the "external accountability" resulting from the extremely public nature of their weight loss. The study compared blood work drawn immediately after the 30-week competition to blood work taken six years later and found that metabolic adaptation effects from the competition were still present six years later. Participants with greater weight loss experienced greater metabolic slowing (Fothergill et al., 2016).

The second edition of the Physical Activity Guidelines for Americans (U.S. Department of Health and Human Services, 2018) emphasizes the value of any physical activity; physically active people, regardless of their body weight (normal weight, overweight, or obese), have lower risks of **all-cause mortality** compared with inactive people and, correspondingly, have a longer life expectancy (see Figure 12.1). Few behavioral choices we make can claim to be as beneficial.

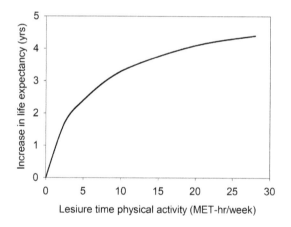

FIGURE 12.1 Estimated years of life gained as a function of average weekly level of exercise after age 40. Data redrawn from a longitudinal study of a large cohort of individuals in the National Cancer Institute database (Moore et al., 2012)

Despite the fact that research does not support the notion that exercise is an effective treatment option to combat obesity, many people are given the erroneous advice that they can exercise their way out of obesity – that, if they work out hard enough, they will lose the weight. A survey administered to a representative sample of Americans found that 71% of respondents believed that exercise was a very effective way to lose weight (Thomas et al., 2015). Furthermore, those respondents who both reported their weight status as being either overweight, very overweight, or obese and reported believing that exercise would result in meaningful weight loss were more likely to get discouraged when their weight loss was not as substantial as they had originally hoped. These results have implications for creating realistic expectations in people when they adopt an exercise program to lose weight.

EFFICACY OF DIETING AND ENERGY RESTRICTION FOR WEIGHT LOSS

In 2013, high school science teacher John Cisna ate only McDonald's food for 180 days and lost 60 lbs; however, he limited his intake to 2,000 calories per day. John's highly publicized experiment is perhaps the best example of how any diet that reduces caloric intake can provide short-term weight loss. But is this "success"? Certainly, the diet was a success for John who became famous, published a book, and became a compensated "brand ambassador" for McDonald's. Five years later, he has kept the weight off and released a second book. Is it possible that John (and countless celebrities) are able to keep the weight off because they have a significant financial motivation to do so? Can we expect the same results? No. Rarely does science provide such certain answers.

For many people, the word diet implies a temporary behavior modification that can reverse a non-temporary behavior. Implicit in the phrase "going on a diet" is the expectation that the diet will someday end; however, not being "on the diet" is what necessitated the diet (i.e., need for weight loss) in the first place. So, when the diet ends, the result is weight gain. Thus, for a diet to have a chance of working, one should instead say, "I'm changing what I eat for the rest of my life."

We now have decades of evidence demonstrating that diets are ineffective in helping us lose weight long term; in fact, some studies paradoxically suggest that dieting may also cause people to become more overweight! A study which followed both identical and fraternal twins over 25 years found that the twin who dieted more frequently was more likely to gain weight than the non-dieting twin (Pietiläinen et al., 2012). The authors concluded that intentional weight loss episodes (dieting) may cause weight gain, independent of genetic factors. Several studies have found that attempting to lose weight through dieting is highly predictive of future weight gain (Kroke et al., 2002).

EXERCISE AND DIET FADS

As previously discussed, lasting weight loss requires caloric restriction. This means a combination of eating less food and, probably, eating food that is less preferred. Ideally, this difficult dietary change should be combined with regular exercise and must be continued for the rest of one's life! The severity of the overnutrition problem, combined with the unpalatable nature of the solution, creates an environment of hopelessness, delusion, and desperation – an environment where the promise of the next new diet or exercise intervention thrives.

Despite it being a well-known secret that diet interventions and exercise interventions have both moderate and transient effects on weight loss, the fad diet and fad exercise industries are booming, with the U.S. weight loss market set to surpass $305.3 billion by 2030 (Wankhade, 2023).

The diet and exercise segments of the weight loss industry create a false sense of hope that people can attain lasting weight loss without difficult and permanent lifestyle changes. These fads (be they diet or exercise) seduce by offering a shortcut to a healthy weight. They promise us that, if we follow instructions, join a club, drink a shake, or buy a gadget, then we will lose weight without having to adjust the behaviors that caused the condition.

Exercise fads range from expensive equipment (e.g., Peloton stationary bicycles and Nordic Track treadmills) to popular exercise trends (e.g., high impact interval training or HIIT, CrossFit, and rucking). Advertisements accompanying exercise equipment make promises of weight loss following minimal effort (e.g., 8 Minute Abs or toning shoes). For those of you too young to remember these ads, search for them on YouTube! Fad diets come in many forms; some don the trappings of modern science (e.g., paleodiet, ketogenic diet), while others are cloaked in exotic mysticism (e.g., macrobiotic diets). Some fad diets are peddled by charlatans and feature dramatic before-and-after photographs and celebrity endorsements, while other fad diets are sincerely offered and may provide some people with genuine help.

INTERMITTENT FASTING AND THE TIMING OF MEALS

The practice of fasting is the voluntary abstinence from consuming food (and, in some cases, even beverages) for an extended period of time. Many religious traditions, including Buddhism, Christianity, Hinduism, Islam, and Judaism, have cultural practices which involve fasting. Fasting or hunger strike has also been used as a form of civil disobedience in which people fast as a form of political protest (e.g., Mahatma Gandhi, Indian activist and leader of the Indian Independence Movement).

While the cultural/religious practice of fasting has been around for centuries, the popularity of **intermittent fasting (IF)** in the diet world is relatively recent, thus permitting us to refer to IF as a fad diet. Intermittent fasting can be broadly divided into two categories: All-day fasts and time-restricted intake.

All-day fasts, as the name implies, involve fasting for the entire day, but there are modifications that involve significantly reduced caloric intake on the "fasting days" rather than absolute fasting. A popular version of the IF diet is referred to as the 5:2 diet, which involves five days of "regular" food intake and two days of caloric restriction during which dieters only consume between 500 and 600 calories per day. Time-restricted eating refers to limiting food consumption to specific hours of the day and then not eating (i.e., fasting) for the remainder of that day.

One of the major challenges of losing weight is constantly having to make the healthy or responsible choice when it comes to choosing what to eat. There is an extensive body of research which demonstrates that neurocircuitry involved with food choice will usually discount long-term consequences and prioritize immediate satiation. This is why dieting is difficult, and why most diets fail (Rangel, 2013). Corresponding to this challenge, the purported advantage of IF is that it reduces the decision-making challenges that are typically associated with dieting and weight loss. People are either allowed to eat ad libitum during some portion of an IF diet or they are fasting.

There are several studies documenting the effectiveness of IF for weight loss and improving cardiovascular health. However, there are also numerous studies which assert that, while IF in its various forms may be a viable weight loss option, it does not appear to be superior or more effective than traditional caloric restriction approaches (Catenacci et al., 2016; Sundfør et al., 2018).

CHRONONUTRITION AND THE TIMING OF MEALS

Implicit in IF is that the timing of food intake will be altered. It is becoming increasingly clear that *when* we eat (**chrononutrition**) may be as important as *what* we eat in relation to energy balance. Recent studies seem to support the hypothesis that the timing of food intake may have an important effect on weight gain. While it is well established that maintaining rats or mice on a high-fat diet (HFD) leads to weight gain, the question of the timing of the HFD on weight gain remains less clear. Hatori and colleagues (2012) examined the combined effects of a high-fat diet and time-restricted feeding (tRF) on weight gain, caloric intake, and a variety of metabolic parameters in mice. They divided the mice into four groups, as shown in Table 12.1.

TABLE 12.1 Study design for Hatori et al. (2012)		
	Diet type	
Food access regimen	High-fat diet	Normal chow
Time-restricted access to food *	HFD, tRF	Normal chow, tRF
Ad libitum access to food	HFD, ad libitum	Normal chow, ad libitum

* The mice in the tRF condition were given access to food for 8 hours during their active–dark phase of their light–dark cycle. Remember, mice are nocturnal (unlike humans). So, they did not have access to food for 16 hours per day. All the mice in all four groups were maintained on a 12-hr-light–12-hr-dark cycle.

This study showed no overall caloric difference in the four groups over 18 weeks of the experiment. This is an important factor, because it indicates that differences in overall intake were *not* responsible for the myriad other changes observed in circadian and metabolic patterns in these mice. Despite the absence of caloric differences, the time-restricted mice gained less weight than the ad libitum-fed rats, and these differences in weight were amplified in the HFD ad libitum–fed mice. This suggests that the time-restricted feeding pattern may have protective effects against excessive weight gain (which was seen in the HFD mice that had ad libitum access to food). Other physiological and metabolic parameters such as adiposity, glucose intolerance, leptin resistance, liver pathology, and inflammation showed improvements in the time-restricted group, and motor coordination and activity levels were found to be higher in the time-restricted group. An earlier study conducted in Zucker obese rats (a spontaneous genetic model of obesity) found a similar result whereby the ad libitum-fed rats (which had access to as much food as they wanted during the dark and light phases of the light–dark cycle) gained 23% more weight than the rats that were fed only during their dark–active phase. As in the previous study, this weight gain was seen despite an absence of overall caloric intake difference between the two groups (Mistlberger et al., 1998). Consistent with these studies, Arble and colleagues (2009) also found greater weight gain in rats fed a high-fat diet during the light phase of their dark–light cycle, as compared with rats that were fed only during the dark phase; with free access to food, rats eat most of their food during the night, which is when they tend to be most active as well. Furthermore, there were no differences in food intake or physical activity between the two groups (Arble et al., 2009). Finally, time-restricted feeding was found to be effective in combating obesity and the development of metabolic disease when mice were metabolically challenged with a variety of diets, including high-fat, high-sucrose, and high-fructose diets (Chaix et al., 2014). This same study also found that the benefits of time-restricted feeding continued even if the mice were given ad libitum access to their respective diets for two days per week – an attempt to simulate a human condition where people relax their diets during the weekends.

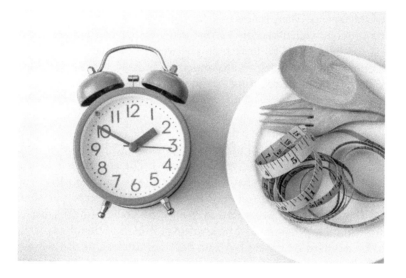

IMAGE 12.1 When we eat may have implications for our health and well-being – this is the emerging field of chrononutrition, which considers the timing of food intake in relation to one's circadian clock

These aforementioned rodent studies use protocols that model human eating behaviors, and we see the consequences as being highly similar to what we see in humans. One such study maintained two groups of overweight and obese women (with an average BMI of 32.2) on 1,400 kcal per day for 12 weeks. One group was given a high-calorie breakfast, while the second group was given a high-calorie dinner. Significantly greater weight loss was seen in the women who were given the high-calorie breakfast; this group also reported lower hunger levels and higher levels of satiety (Jakubowicz et al., 2013). Likewise, following bariatric surgery, the greatest weight loss was seen in those who had earlier meals (Ruiz-Lozano et al., 2016).

A human population at risk for altered eating times are shift workers. A clinical trial found impaired glucose tolerance in participants who engaged in nighttime eating while under a night-shift-work simulation protocol; importantly, the impaired glucose tolerance was absent in those participants who did not engage in nighttime eating despite being under the same night-shift-work simulation. These findings suggest that the impairment in glucose metabolism is associated with the atypical times when food is consumed by night-shift workers, rather than the disruption of their sleep–wake cycle itself (Chellappa et al., 2021).

Taken together, these studies make a compelling case that, in addition to the types of food we eat, the timing of food intake appears to be an important factor in maintaining a healthy body weight. The mechanism behind this phenomenon is presently unknown.

BEHAVIOR THERAPY

Weight loss is most likely to be successful when coupled with lifestyle and behavioral changes surrounding the choices we make in our diet and physical activity levels. Many people pursue behavior changes in lieu of medications, supplements, or surgery to avoid side effects and expense. Many fitness trainers, nutritionists, physicians, and other weight loss experts promote varied versions of diet and exercise plans, often depicting their own plan as the most effective. In fact, no one weight loss plan has been scientifically proven superior over others, and results are typically modest (Tsai & Wadden, 2005). Essentially, they all work by reducing calorie intake, increasing activity, and modifying behavior. Further, as with the problems surrounding accessibility of surgery for low-SES individuals, many commercial weight loss programs and fitness training sessions are not financially feasible for many obese individuals.

Weight loss is the primary goal of behavior therapy (BT), but other psychological issues may be addressed with BT (e.g., depression). The goal here is to arm subjects with a new set of eating habits that they use for the rest of their lives (i.e., relearn what and when to eat). Unfortunately, most BT programs are not tremendously effective in the long term. According to Wing and Phelan (2005), participants in behavioral weight loss programs lose an average of 7–10% of their body weight within six months of standard treatment but gain back almost 50% of the lost weight after one year. Their research indicates that approximately 20% of dieters are successful at maintaining long-term weight loss (which is defined as losing 10% of one's initial body weight and keeping it off for one year). They also report six strategies for long-term success:

> (1) engaging in high levels of physical activity; (2) eating a diet that is low in calories and fat; (3) eating breakfast; (4) self-monitoring weight on a regular basis; (5) maintaining a consistent eating pattern; and (6) catching 'slips' before they turn into larger regains.
>
> (p. 225S)

Jelalian et al. (2006) compared the effectiveness of cognitive-behavior therapy when paired with either exercise (CBT + EXER) or when paired with an Outward Bound® therapy called "peer-enhanced adventure therapy" (CBT + PEAT). Adventure therapy is designed to increase self-confidence and increase social support while also improving physical abilities. This study was done with adolescents and found that, at the end of the treatment, weight loss did not differ between the groups; however, after ten months, 35% of the CBT + PEAT group had maintained the weight loss in contrast with only 12% of the CBT + EXER group. This suggests that peer-based components of the intervention with the PEAT-treated group might be important for long-term weight management.

To examine long-term prognosis, Perri and colleagues (2001) compared two types of one-year extended BT, relapse prevention training (RPT) and problem-solving therapy (PST), with a standard BT group that did not receive any extended therapy sessions. With RPT, participants are taught methods to anticipate issues that could trigger relapse (i.e., overeating) and to plan alternative coping mechanisms or behaviors. PST involves problem-solving efforts by a health care provider to help the person manage issues on the completion of therapy. In their study, all groups received weekly two-hour group sessions for five months, including self- monitoring, goal setting, a low-calorie/low-fat diet, and a home walking program. At the end of this, all had lost (the expected) ~9% initial weight. The standard BT-only group had no additional treatment but had follow-up visits at 6 and 12 months. The RPT group had biweekly sessions for the next 12 months. Therapy included risk identification, cognitive coping, long-term planning, and so on. The PST group also had group discussions of specific problems that had arisen since the last session and guided solutions over the 12 months. The results showed that the PST group had lost significantly more weight at the end of one year compared with the BT group. Additionally, 35% of the PST participants had lost 10% or more of their body weight compared with only 6% of the BT participants. There were no significant differences between the BT and RPT groups. The elements of peer group support and discussion involved in this therapy seem particularly beneficial.

MOBILE APPS AS WEIGHT LOSS TOOLS

In recent years, there has been an explosion in the mHealth (mobile health) movement which is evidenced by (among other health-related applications) the proliferation of weight loss applications. Having so many options in the market leaves both the layperson and health care professionals bewildered as to which apps (if any) are effective. Weight loss apps typically combine fitness tracking, calorie tracking, and a motivational/reward system to keep users engaged. If designed appropriately, mobile apps have the potential to improve health and lower costs related to health care. Patel and colleagues (2015) reviewed 120 weight loss applications and found that the highest rated were Noom (Android) and Calorie Counter and Food Diary (Apple). Note that the evaluations of these apps were based on users in New Zealand, and so the usability of food tracking features was assessed based on the New Zealand markets, thus making the results of this study limited in their global application. A retrospective cohort study examining how effective mobile apps are at assisting with weight loss found that the most important factor for successful weight loss was the frequency with which users entered data on what they ate for dinner (Chin et al., 2016). This finding is particularly interesting considering the work in the field of chrononutrition which is finding that caloric intake later in the day is associated with greater weight gain. This same study also reported that another important factor for successful weight loss was the frequency with which users entered their body weight data; this finding supports the idea that the effectiveness of a mobile app lies in the engagement of the user, a principle that one can extend to all forms of diet and exercise interventions. While Chin et al. (2016) reported weight loss following the use of the mobile app, there are several studies which report that mobile app use does not result in meaningful weight loss (Laing et al., 2014; Semper et al., 2016).

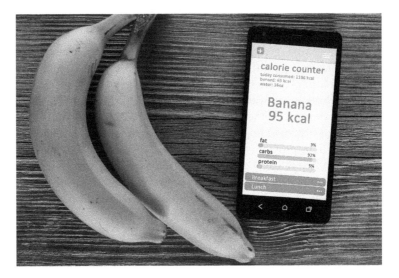

IMAGE 12.2 There are many applications now available that allow people to track their food and calorie intake

Despite their limitations, a significant advantage that apps may have over more traditional weight loss programs is the omnipresent nature of our phones and, consequently, of the apps themselves. Apps which have (1) reminders to engage in physical activity, (2) prompts to record physical activity (or automatic recording of physical activity), (3) prompts about the importance of healthy eating, (4) reminders to enter one's intake into the app, and (5) rewards/points to keep users interested may help their users adhere to the lifestyle changes required to lose weight. A comprehensive review examining the effectiveness of mobile applications with regard to weight management concluded that, while they may not be effective as the sole intervention or approach to weight management, they may have utility as a supporting tool (Ghelani et al., 2020). But, as with all weight loss endeavors, a weight loss mobile app is only effective if one commits to the program, whatever that may be.

ANTI-OBESITY DRUGS

Anti-obesity drugs generally work in one of two ways: By reducing energy intake or by increasing energy expenditure. Anti-obesity drugs work centrally (in the brain) and peripherally (e.g., in the gastrointestinal tract) and have varied mechanisms of action. In general, drugs which work by limiting energy intake do not seem to have long-term efficacy and often have serious and unpleasant side effects, including nausea, the risk of heart attack and stroke, depression, and birth defects. Owing to these risk factors and side effects, they are often only prescribed to patients who are categorized as either obese or morbidly obese.

Until recently, the most effective medications would result in weight loss of about 5–10% (usually 10–15 lbs more than placebo), which is helpful, but certainly not a "cure" for obese people, whose weight may be 50–100% over their healthy weight. Furthermore, these medications did not sustain long-term weight loss for a variety of reasons, including drug tolerance, dependance, and/or unpleasant side effects.

There have been numerous reports in the media about the relatively new class of weight loss drugs – the glucagon-like peptide-1 receptor agonists (GLP-1RAs); only time will tell if their promise of lasting weight loss will hold true or not.

Before we enter into a discussion about GLP-1RAs, we must understand more about the glucagon-like peptide-1, or GLP-1. GLP-1 is produced by specialized cells in the small intestine in response to a meal. The GLP-1 thus produced travels through the blood stream and binds to GLP-1 receptors on pancreatic β-cells, thereby stimulating them to release insulin, which then lowers blood glucose levels, thereby aiding with glucose homeostasis (Cabou & Burcelin, 2011). GLP-1 also slows down the rate of gastric emptying and reduces gut motility in humans (Shah & Vella, 2014). Furthermore, GLP-1 is synthesized in the brain, and GLP-1 receptors are found in the hypothalamus and brainstem – regions of the brain known to be associated with energy regulation (Shah & Vella, 2014). GLP-1 receptors are also found in the areas around the circumventricular organs of the brain (e.g., the area postrema); it is suggested that this may be a way peripheral GLP-1 from the intestines can access the brain (Cabou & Burcelin, 2011). The central (brain) role of GLP-1 may be to mediate satiety. Turton and colleagues (1996) found that intracerebroventricular (ICV) injections of GLP-1 inhibited feeding in fasted rats, while ICV injections of GLP-1 receptor antagonists actually doubled food intake in satiated rats.

So, with the understanding that GLP-1 inhibits food intake, slows gastric emptying, and increases feelings of satiety, it is no surprise that GLP-1 receptor agonists were considered as a target for drug therapies to help combat obesity.

The first GLP-1RA that was seen on the market was Saxenda®, which is a liraglutide. In 2014, it was approved by the U.S. Food and Drug Administration (FDA) to help adults with weight loss. In 2020, it was approved as a treatment option for children aged 12 and older. The GLP-1RAs that you have most likely heard of are the semaglutides – Ozempic® and Wegovy® – they are different doses of the same medication. Ozempic® was approved for the treatment of type 2 diabetes in 2017, while Wegovy® was approved for weight loss management in adults in 2021 (it was approved for use in children above 12 in 2022). These medications are administered via an injection. A pill form of this same medication is also available (Rybelsus®) for treatment of type 2 diabetes. A phase 3B clinical trial conducted over a period of 68 weeks demonstrated that a 2.4-mg dose of semaglutide administered weekly was more effective than a 3.0-mg dose of liraglutide administered daily, with those on the semaglutide showing an average weight change of approximately 16% from baseline, versus approximately 6% for the liraglutide group (Rubino et al., 2022).

Zepbound® – tirzepatide – was approved by the FDA in November 2023. This drug is a dual receptor agonist, engaging with both gastric inhibitory peptide (GIP) and GLP-1 receptors. Like GLP-1, GIP is produced in the intestine and stimulates insulin production (Seino et al., 2010). Azuri and colleagues (2023) examined published data to compare tirzepatide with semaglutide and found that tirzepatide resulted in approximately 18% weight loss compared with 12% weight loss in the semaglutide group. They further compared the costs of these medications and found that tirzepatide was more cost-effective, costing approximately $18,000 over 72 weeks, compared with semaglutide, which cost approximately $23,000 over 68 weeks.

As indicated above, these new drug therapies are currently very expensive, but, despite this, demand for these drugs is high, given their alluring promise of easy weight loss. An overview of some of the older anti-obesity drugs that reduce energy intake is provided in Table 12.2.

TABLE 12.2 Overview of some anti-obesity drugs that reduce energy intake

Drug	Effect	Neurotransmitter action/mechanism of action	FDA status
Contrave® (buproprion + naltrexone)	Appetite suppressant	Naltrexone: Opioid antagonist Buproprion: Dopamine reuptake inhibitor Together thought to facilitate activation of POMC neurons to produce anorectic alpha-MSH and block inhibition of this neuropeptide	Approved
Phentermine	Stimulant and appetite suppressant	Norepinephrine agonist	Approved
Qsymia® (phentermine + topiramate)	Stimulant and appetite suppressant	Norepinephrine agonist	Approved
Xenical®; low-dose OTC version called Alli® (orlistat)	Does not impact appetite; weight loss is due to reduced fat absorption in the intestines	Inhibits gastric and pancreatic enzymes necessary for the digestion of fat	Approved
Saxenda® (liraglutide); lower-dose version of this is called Victoza® – for diabetes treatment	Appetite suppressant and delayed gastric emptying	GLP-1 receptor agonist	Approved
Wegovy® (semaglutide); lower-dose version of this is called Ozempic® (injectable) and Rybelsus® (oral tablet) – both for type 2 diabetes	Appetite suppressant, delays gastric emptying, reduces cravings	GLP-1 receptor agonist	Approved
Zepbound® – for weight loss Mounjaro® – for type 2 diabetes (both are tirzepatides)	Appetite suppressant, delays gastric emptying, reduces cravings	GIP and GLP-1 receptor agonist	Approved

No FDA-approved weight loss medications work primarily by increasing energy expenditure, although drugs such as phentermine do stimulate metabolism in addition to suppressing appetite. However, many products sold as diet or herbal supplements are marketed with claims that they increase energy expenditure and result in weight loss. Substances labeled as supplements are not subject to either Drug Enforcement Administration (DEA) registration requirements of safety and proof of efficacy (which are required of controlled substances) or pre-approval by the FDA. The FDA regulates the safety of a supplement and accuracy of its marketing *after* it reaches the market. So, supplements and their constituents often change over time. For example, the over-the-counter diet supplement Dexatrim today contains different ingredients than in past formulations, because the FDA has now banned the compounds in the original formulations.

Most herbal weight loss remedies and dietary supplements have not been tested scientifically for efficacy compared with placebo, have not been tested for safety, and are not regulated for the amount or quality of the main ingredients (i.e., what it says on the label doesn't have to meet strict pharmaceutical standards of accuracy). Some dietary supplements the safety of which has not been adequately verified include white bean extract, garcinia cambogia, bitter orange, green coffee, guar gum, chitosan, forskolin, and raspberry ketone (Ríos-Hoyo & Gutiérrez-Salmeán, 2016).

CALORIE SUBSTITUTES

Calorie substitutes theoretically provide a drug- or supplement-free method of reducing energy intake without reducing the quantity of food consumed. People choose a calorie substitute to reduce overall caloric intake, either for weight management, weight loss, or diabetes management purposes. However, the research on whether calorie substitutes and low-calorie sweeteners helps with weight management or weight loss is unclear at best. There are enough studies which support their use in weight management efforts, and enough studies to refute the same claims, so that a clear picture is currently unavailable (Anderson et al., 2012). Calorie substitutes can be broadly divided into three categories: High-intensity sweeteners, sugar alcohols, and fat substitutes.

High-intensity sweeteners (or low-calorie sweeteners) are sweeteners which are many times sweeter than sugar but contain either no calories or very few calories. High-intensity sweeteners which are approved by the FDA for use as food additives include saccharin, aspartame, acesulfame potassium, sucralose, neotame, and advantame (see the FDA website for information on high-intensity sweeteners – www.fda.gov/food/food-additives-petitions/high-intensity-sweeteners). The FDA has received GRAS (generally recognized as safe) notices for steviol glycosides and luo han guo (or monk fruit) extracts and does not have additional questions regarding their GRAS status at present. This essentially means that the applications for the use of these sweeteners did not raise any red flags, but there is currently not enough data on their use to officially approve their use. See Table 12.3, which compares the sweetness of different sweeteners to table sugar (modified from U.S. Food and Drug Administration, 2018).

TABLE 12.3 High-intensity sweeteners permitted for use in food in the U.S.

Sweetener	Sweetness compared with table sugar	Examples of brand names
Acesulfame potassium (Ace-k)*	200 × sweeter	Sweet One®, Sunett®
Advantame*	20,000 × sweeter	None currently
Aspartame*	200 × sweeter	Nutrasweet®, Equal®, Sugar Twin®
Neotame*	7,000–13,000 × sweeter	Newtame®
Saccharin*	200–700 × sweeter	Sweet'NLow®, Sweet Twin®, Necta Sweet®
Luo han guo/monk fruit extracts**	100–250 × sweeter	Nectresse®, Monk Fruit in the Raw®, PureLo®

TABLE 12.3 (Continued)		
Sweetener	Sweetness compared with table sugar	Examples of brand names
Steviol glycosides (commonly called Stevia)**	200–400 × sweeter	Truvia®, PureVia®, Enliten®
Sucralose*	600 × sweeter	Splenda®

* FDA-approved; ** GRAS notice submitted; FDA has no questions

Some currently popular sweeteners include Splenda®, Truvia®, and monk fruit. Sucralose (marketed as Splenda®) is derived from sucrose and probably has the most authentic sugar flavor when compared with saccharin and aspartame (Quinlan & Jenner, 2006). As of 2008, it was believed to be the most widely used sweetener in the U.S. (Sylvetsky & Rother, 2016). Steviol glycoside sweeteners (commonly called stevia) are a class of zero-calorie sweeteners derived from the *Stevia rebaudiana* plant, which is native to parts of South America. Luo han guo, or monk fruit, sweeteners are similarly plant-derived (from the *Siraitia grosvenorii* plant, which is native to parts of China and Thailand). Both stevia and monk fruit sweeteners are relatively recent arrivals on the U.S. market (circa 2008). The largest-by-weight ingredient of Truvia® (which is sold as a stevia-based "natural" sweetener) is, in fact, not stevia but the sugar alcohol erythritol (Truvia, 2018). Sugar alcohols, also called polyols, are an example of a nutritive sweetener. While they contain some calories (ranging from 0–3 kcal/g, which is lower than table sugar, which comes in at 4 kcal/g), they are incompletely absorbed by humans, resulting in fewer calories retained following their consumption. Examples of sugar alcohols include xylitol, erythritol, and sorbitol. Sugar alcohols are frequently used in sugar-free candies and chewing gum.

Food scientists and food technologists have created a wide variety of protein, carbohydrate, and even fat-based "fat substitutes." The goal of these substitutes is to mimic the properties of fat in the food (in terms of taste, mouth feel, texture, visual appearance, etc.) while providing fewer calories per gram than fat (which is 9 kcal/g). **Olestra** is one such fat substitute. It is a fat-based fat substitute; its chemical structure is similar to the fat molecule but cannot be broken down and so is not absorbed. It gives food the satisfying "mouth feel" of fatty food and is used mainly in cooking. In a lab study of olestra, human participants were fed either a high-calorie breakfast made with real fat or an otherwise identical low-calorie breakfast made with the "fake fat" (Rolls et al., 1992). Their food intake was then monitored for the rest of the day. The people in the fake-fat group reported being hungrier in the evening and ate larger dinners, resulting in no net difference in daily caloric intake. It seems that compensation for our "norm" energy levels can blunt the effectiveness of any of the calorie substitutes. This partially explains the difficulty of maintaining weight loss through dieting or the use of calorie substitutes.

SURGERY FOR OBESITY (BARIATRIC SURGERY)

Because of the limited efficacy of everything discussed so far in this chapter, some people have looked for surgical treatments to assist them in their weight loss endeavors.

Bariatric, or weight loss surgery can be extremely beneficial for some people, particularly those who are morbidly obese and have been unable to lose weight with diet and exercise. Surgery results in average loss of about 50 kg (~100 lbs) (Higa et al., 2000) and can eliminate symptoms of type 2 diabetes and hypertension (Sugerman et al., 2003) and improve quality of life (Dymek et al., 2002). However, it is important to note that weight regain (WR) following bariatric surgery is a reality for a large number of patients who choose to undergo these types of procedures (Noria et al., 2023). This is discussed in more detail later in this chapter.

Surgery for obesity is generally allowed only for individuals who meet specific body weight and health criteria. These criteria, as outlined by the National Institutes of Health (NIH), are as follows (NIH, 2018):

(a) Individuals with a BMI ≥40.
(b) Individuals with a BMI between 35 and 39.9 who also have a serious health problem because of their obesity (such as diabetes or heart disease).
(c) Individuals with a BMI between 30 and 34.9 with a serious health problem associated with their obesity. This third category is only recommended for the adjustable gastric band procedure.

In addition to these weight and health recommendations, candidates for bariatric surgery undergo psychological and physical assessments to ensure that they are a good fit for surgery. These are discussed in some detail in the upcoming section on Factors to Consider Regarding Surgery.

These bariatric surgical procedures can be divided into three broad categories: (a) Restrictive, (b) malabsorptive, and (c) a combination of both restrictive and malabsorptive. The restrictive procedures involve limiting the amount of food the stomach can hold, while the malabsorptive procedures limit nutrient absorption thereby reducing the number of calories retained. The modifications to the stomach and intestines result in requiring changes to one's lifestyle; specifically, they necessitate the consumption of only small amounts of food at a time and the inclusion of vitamin supplements in the diet (the reduced stomach and intestinal tract interfere with the absorption of vitamins, and so higher-than-normal amounts need to be consumed).

Based on an eighth global registry report published by IFSO (International Federation for the Surgery of Obesity and Metabolic Disorders) in 2023, the most frequently performed types of weight loss surgery were sleeve gastrectomy (~60% of recorded procedures), followed by Roux-en-Y gastric bypass (~30% of recorded procedures), and one anastomosis gastric bypass (<5% of recorded procedures). The top three procedures are described in Table 12.4. The remaining ~5–6% of procedures include single-anastomosis duodeno-ileal bypass with sleeve gastrectomy (SADI-DS), biliopancreatic diversion (BPD), and adjustable gastric band (AGB) and endoscopic procedures. It is also worth noting that, as per the IFSO 2023 report, nearly 80% of the recorded operations were done on females (as defined by their chromosomes, hormones, and reproductive organs at the time of the procedures).

TABLE 12.4 Overview of the most common bariatric surgical procedures

Surgical procedure	Description	Advantages	Disadvantages
Vertical sleeve gastrectomy (VSG) or laparascopic sleeve gastrectomy (LSG)	Part of the stomach is removed, leaving a much smaller stomach; its effectiveness for weight loss is similar to RYGB	Low rates of complications and reduced surgical time	Better iron absorption occurs compared with RYGB; as it is a newer procedure, there are still fewer data available compared with RYGB
Roux-en Y gastric bypass surgery (RYGB)	Two surgical modifications are made: First, the size of the stomach is reduced and, then, it is connected to the middle part of the small intestine (the jejunum, or the Roux limb)	Most effective in terms of weight loss compared with other surgical interventions	Reduced iron and calcium absorption **Dumping syndrome**
One anastomosis gastric bypass (OAGB) or Mini-gastric bypass (MGB)	Two surgical modifications are made: The size of the stomach is reduced, and then more than half of the small intestine is bypassed	As effective as RYGB in terms of weight loss; lower rates of complications compared with RYGB	Higher rates of micronutrient deficiencies

Vertical Sleeve Gastrectomy

FIGURE 12.2 Vertical sleeve gastrectomy

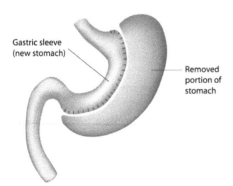

Gastric sleeve (new stomach)

Removed portion of stomach

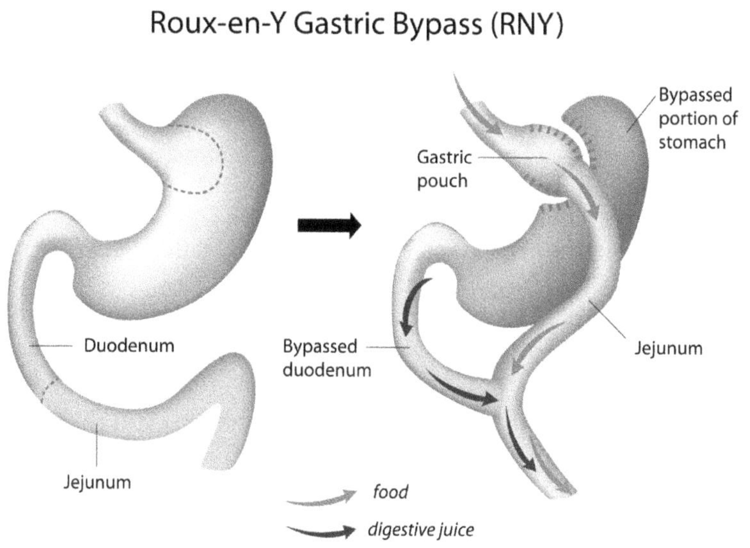

Roux-en-Y Gastric Bypass (RNY)

FIGURE 12.3 Roux-en-Y Gastric Bypass (RYGB)

ENDOSCOPIC BARIATRIC THERAPIES (EBTS)

Distinct from the metabolic and bariatric surgeries described above, there are several EBTs that have been recently approved by the FDA for use in adults with obesity. These EBTs include the use of intragastric (within stomach) balloons, a vagal stimulator, and a gastric aspiration device. These procedures are all adjustable and reversible, which may be part of their appeal. However, their utility and effectiveness remain unclear, as patients have tended to lose less weight with these procedures and also have reported higher rates of weight regain (Pratt et al., 2018).

PHYSIOLOGICAL EFFECTS OF SURGERY

As noted previously, about 70% of a patient's weight above ideal is generally lost after surgery. As expected, as most of this weight loss is in the form of fat, it is accompanied by a lowered plasma concentration of **leptin**, the satiety hormone released from fat cells (discussed in other chapters). But what about **ghrelin**, the appetite-enhancing peptide secreted by the stomach?

Studies have found reductions in plasma ghrelin levels after both LSG (Sethi et al., 2018) and RYBG (Cummings & Schwartz, 2003). Data from mouse models indicate no differences in body weight between wild-type mice and mice which have either been genetically modified to overexpress ghrelin or have had the ghrelin gene knocked out so that they have a complete absence of ghrelin (Uchida et al., 2013). Consequently, it remains unclear as to whether or not the drop in ghrelin seen in patients following bariatric surgery is of functional significance in explaining the weight loss experienced by people following these surgical procedures.

A significant health benefit associated with weight loss surgery is the remittance of symptoms of type 2 diabetes in most cases (Cummings et al., 2004). Many diabetic patients can discontinue their medication on leaving the hospital following surgery, which precedes much of the weight loss; therefore, something other than weight loss facilitates the improvement in glucose metabolism. As discussed elsewhere, obesity-related type 2 diabetes is most often due to insulin resistance. Weight loss surgery seems to restore sensitivity to insulin, quickly allowing adequate regulation of glucose. Further, the post-surgical reduction in ghrelin levels facilitates the action of insulin (Cummings et al., 2004).

Davies and colleagues (2019) conducted a review of 14 clinical studies which examined changes in gut bacteria following different types of bariatric surgery. They report an overall increase in gut bacterial species diversity following bariatric surgery, as well as meaningful changes in different species of gut bacteria. These findings are significant and warrant further examination to see whether the changes in gut microbiota are supportive of the weight loss seen following bariatric surgery.

With the recent advent of semaglutides (e.g., Wegovy, discussed earlier in this chapter) in the weight loss market, it makes sense to examine if changes in GLP-1 have been observed following bariatric surgery. In line with this, both human and animal models of VSG and RYGB bariatric surgeries have shown an increase in GLP-1 levels after surgery (Hutch & Sandoval, 2017). One thought is that, following gastric bypass surgery, the distal (ileal) gut is repositioned in such a way that it more easily comes into contact with partially digested food (chyme), which consequently stimulates specialized cells (L cells) in this region of the small intestine to secrete GLP-1 (Chambers et al., 2011). Another study found that those patients with higher levels of GLP-1 post-surgery had higher rates of weight loss (Santo et al., 2016). Weight regain (i.e., gaining back the weight lost soon after bariatric surgery) is a well-established phenomenon (Noria et al., 2023); in line with this, the elevated GLP-1 response that has been reported soon after bariatric surgical procedures was found to be absent four years after the surgery (Min et al., 2020). It is of interest to note that a study comparing the effect of weight loss following an RYGB surgical procedure with weight loss following caloric restriction found that GLP-1 levels were elevated only in those who had experienced weight loss as a result of surgery (Laferrère et al. 2008). Taken together, these studies provide a possible explanation for the role of GLP-1 in:

- Why we see successful and initially sustained weight loss following bariatric surgery.
- Why weight regain is quite common several years after bariatric procedures.
- Why weight loss following caloric restriction tends to be less successful than weight loss following bariatric surgery caloric restriction protocols.

Contrary to these findings, another study found that GLP-1 receptor-deficient mice had similar weight loss to wild-type mice, following a murine (mouse) model of RYGB and VSG surgeries (Ye et al., 2014). This would suggest that the weight loss seen following these types of bariatric surgical procedures cannot be explained by the increases in GLP-1 observed in the aforementioned studies. However, it is important to keep in mind that, when a knock-out mouse model is created, there may be compensatory mechanisms that develop of which the researchers are unaware but which could be responsible for the comparable weight loss observed in the wild-type and GLP-1 receptor-deficient mice.

FACTORS TO CONSIDER REGARDING SURGERY

One of the critical factors that is now recognized is the need for intensive medical and psychological support for surgical patients, both before and after surgery. In particular, selection of patients is important: It is unethical to do such surgery on people whose profile suggests they will not attempt to maintain the weight lost or be able to understand the limitations of their new condition. Patients must be prepared for the changes they must make to their eating behaviors and the psychological effects of body changes. Social support (family, peers, or support group) is a critical component of long-term success and increased quality of life after surgery. A standardized interview has been developed by the Medical Psychology Service of the VA Boston Healthcare System to ensure thorough assessment of patient readiness for surgery and to facilitate patient education about the procedure and behavioral changes that are needed afterward (Sogg & Mori, 2004). The focus is on seven areas:

1 Weight, diet, and nutritional history: Does the patient have a history of unsuccessful dieting?
2 Current eating behaviors: What is eaten? Is there bingeing behavior? And so on.
3 Medical history: Are there other medical conditions or recent surgeries?
4 Understanding of surgical procedures and risks: Does the patient show a "minimum understanding"?
5 Motivation and expectations: Does the patient understand realistic goals and is he/she willing to work for them?
6 Relationships and social support: Is the family willing to help/deal with weight loss?
7 Psychiatric complications: Are there any mitigating mental disorders that need treatment?

ADOLESCENTS AND SURGERY

The number of extremely overweight teenagers has risen dramatically over the past two decades, and they can have all the adverse health symptoms of adults and a reduced quality of life and self-esteem. These issues can potentially be improved with weight loss surgery. As per the NIH recommendations for teen eligibility for bariatric surgery, post-pubescent teenagers who have attained their adult height are considered eligible if they have either (a) a BMI ≥35 with a serious obesity-related health problem (e.g., diabetes or severe sleep apnea) or (b) a BMI ≥40 with a less severe health problem (e.g., high blood pressure or high cholesterol) (NIH, 2018). The question is what type of bariatric procedure should be performed on adolescents, and, if so, at what age or under what circumstances? There is a need to establish age guidelines and exclusionary factors such as drug use and the type of motivational/support factors that were discussed earlier in the Sogg and Mori (2004) checklist.

COST OF SURGERY

Weight loss surgery costs roughly $17,000–26,000 (Cremieux et al., 2008), and more if complications arise. Insurance coverage of these procedures is on the rise because, despite the high cost, analyses overwhelmingly indicate that the risks and expenses associated with obesity outweigh those associated with surgery (Salem et al., 2008). However, many employers do not purchase insurance with weight loss surgery provisions, and most insurance companies, including Medicaid/Medicare, provide coverage only at certain facilities, typically in urban settings, and often do not cover all the medications and follow-up care.

Although obesity is found among all socioeconomic status (SES) groups in Western society, morbidly obese people are overrepresented in low-SES populations and in rural communities (Livingston & Ko, 2004). The expense of surgery and the scarcity of surgical hospitals in rural compared with urban areas make weight loss surgery inaccessible for many people at the highest risk for health problems associated with obesity.

A 2016 review of the number of bariatric surgeries conducted across different states revealed that most bariatric surgeries are conducted in the northeastern part of the U.S. (Delaware, New Jersey, New York, and Massachusetts), and the fewest were conducted in the southern part of the U.S. (which typically has the highest rates of obesity). These states included West Virginia, Mississippi, Alabama, Arkansas, and Louisiana. This study concluded that insurance coverage and the economic ranking of the state were more impactful in determining whether bariatric surgery might be a treatment option than the prevalence of obesity itself (DeMaria et al., 2018).

WEIGHT REGAIN AFTER SURGERY

Whether bariatric surgery is an effective treatment option in the long term for weight loss and weight management is presently unclear. Most weight loss occurs within 18 months following the bariatric surgery (Buchwald et al., 2007; Magro et al., 2008). However, some weight gain after that is quite common. Patients with extremely high BMIs (>40), binge-eating disorder, and/or a lack of social support seem to be at the highest risk for weight regain after surgery, particularly if they do not attend enough follow-up visits and support group meetings (Magro et al., 2008). One follow-up study found that, despite losing weight initially, morbidly obese (BMI <50) and super-obese (BMI ≥50) patients who underwent RYGB surgery continued to gain weight when assessed at five and ten years after they had reached their lowest weight following the surgery (Christou et al., 2006).

CONCLUDING REMARKS

Obesity carries many risks to physical and psychological well-being. At present, the leading treatments also carry risks and are quite costly. Because losing weight once it has been gained in excess is challenging and often unsuccessful in the long term, the best course is prevention. The concept of preventive care has received increased attention among health care professionals and insurance companies and in the political arena (as it relates to health care expenses). Despite the growing obesity problem in many countries around the world, there is no established evidence-based national obesity prevention or weight loss program (Swinburn et al., 2005). Does this matter? Is obesity treatment or prevention an issue of national or global concern? Evidence overwhelmingly supports that there is a need to address the problem; the health benefits (e.g., better quality of life, increased work productivity, reduced health expenses) outweigh the expenses of preventive or weight loss programs. However, remaining questions around such a program include who should fund it, who should be targeted, and what should be done. Several studies targeting school-age children and adolescents have found prevention programs successful at reducing obesity rates and cost-effective in the long term (Taylor et al., 2007; Wang et al., 2015, 2018). We remain optimistic that heightened awareness and concern about obesity, coupled with empirical data supporting the effectiveness of prevention programs, will yield increased proactive efforts to improve the health of current and future generations.

GLOSSARY

All-cause mortality	All possible causes of death, some of which include heart disease and certain cancers.
Aspartame	Non-caloric artificial sweetener.
Behavioral therapy	A form of psychological therapy in which problematic behaviors are identified and improvements are learned.
Cannabinoid receptor blockers	Drugs that are antagonists or blockers of action of cannabinoid transmitters.
Chrononutrition	An emerging field of study which examines how circadian rhythms and timing of food intake might affect health and propensity for weight gain. The research in this field aims to answer the question: Is *when* you eat an important factor in battling weight gain?
Dopamine	Monoamine neurotransmitter located mainly in nigrostriatal (movement) and mesolimbic (reward) pathways in the brain.
Dumping syndrome	This is a complication of bariatric surgery, following reduction in stomach size. When food (especially high-sugar foods) moves too quickly from the stomach into the small intestine, patients may experience nausea, cramps, and diarrhea. It is also called rapid gastric emptying.
Fenfluramine	Structural analog of amphetamine that was developed in the 1960s to have appetite suppressant effects without stimulant or serotonin transmission in the brain. Withdrawn from the clinical market owing to the side effect of pulmonary hypertension.
Ghrelin	Peptide released from enteroendocrine cells, primarily in the stomach, during fasting. An injection of ghrelin to animals stimulates food intake.
GLP-1RAs or GLP-1 receptor agonists	A class of weight loss drugs which interact with the glucagon-like peptide-1 receptor.

Intermittent fasting	This is a form of fasting where a person restricts their food intake to specific time periods of the day. They are only permitted to eat during those times and refrain from eating outside that window of time. Intermittent fasting may be within a day or across days.
Leptin	Peptide released from adipose (fat) cells in approximate relation to their fat content. Thus, blood concentrations of leptin are a rough measure of the amount of body fat. Several cells in the brain involved in feeding have receptors for and respond to circulating leptin.
Olestra	A fat substitute in which fatty acid chains are bonded to a sucrose molecule, with a resultant molecule that has the "mouth feel" of fat but cannot be broken down and absorbed in the intestine. It was originally developed as a drug to lower cholesterol levels but was instead approved as a food additive.
Orlistat	An inhibitor of intestinal and pancreatic lipase: Blocks or attenuates the absorption of triglycerides from the gastrointestinal tract.
Phentermine	A structural analog of amphetamine that is both a stimulant and an appetite suppressant.
Qsymia	Newly approved combination drug treatment consisting of phentermine and topiramate that acts centrally to reduce appetite and promote weight loss and improvement of type 2 diabetes.
Saccharin	Non-caloric artificial sweetener.
Serotonin	Monoamine neurotransmitter abundant in many regions of the brain; has 14 receptor subtypes, of which the 2c receptor may be the one most prominently involved in appetite.
Sibutramine	Centrally acting appetite suppressant drug, structurally related to amphetamine and having a dual neurochemical action that increases the amounts of norepinephrine and serotonin in active synapses.
Sucralose	The most recently approved (USA, 1998; EU, 2004) artificial sweetener; a structural analog of sucrose, known by the additive code E955 in the European Union; sucralose is sweeter than either aspartame or saccharin and is non-caloric because it is not metabolized.

Supplement	A dietary supplement is an additive to a natural food or foods; because many of these are regulated only loosely (if at all), it is sometimes difficult to assess their safety and efficacy.

REFERENCES

Anderson, G., Foreyt, J., Sigman-Grant, M., & Allison, D. (2012). The use of low-calorie sweeteners by adults: Impact on weight management. *The Journal of Nutrition, 142* (6), 1163S–1169S.

Arble, D., Bass, J., Laposky, A., Vitaterna, M., & Turek, F. (2009). Circadian timing of food intake contributes to weight gain. *Obesity (Silver Spring), 17* (11), 2100–2102.

Azuri, J., Hammerman, A., Aboalhasan, E., Sluckis, B., Arbel, R. (2023). Tirzepatide versus semaglutide for weight loss in patients with type 2 diabetes mellitus: A value for money analysis. *Diabetes Obesity and Metabolism, 25* (4), 961–964.

Buchwald, H., Estok, R., Fahrbach, K., Banel, D., & Sledge, I. (2007). Trends in mortality in bariatric surgery: A systematic review and meta-analysis. *Surgery, 142* (4), 621–635.

Cabou, C., Burcelin, R. (2011). GLP-1, the gut-brain, and brain–periphery axes. *Review of Diabetic Studies, 8* (3), 418–431.

Catenacci, V., Pan, Z., Ostendorf, D., Brannon, S., Gozansky, W., Mattson, M., Bronwent, M., MacLean, P., Melanson, E., & Troy Donahoo, W. (2016). A randomized pilot study comparing zero-calorie alternate-day fasting to daily caloric restriction in adults with obesity. *Obesity (Silver Spring), 24* (9), 1874–1883.

Chaix, A., Zarrinpar, A., Miu, P., & Panda, S. (2014). Time-restricted feeding is a preventative and therapeutic intervention against diverse nutritional challenges. *Cell Metabolism, 20* (6), 991–1005.

Chambers, A. P., Jessen, L., Ryan, K. K., Sisley, S., Wilson-Pérez, H. E., Stefater, M. A., Gaitonde, S. G., Sorrell, J. E., Toure, M., Berger, J., D'Alessio, D. A., Woods, S. C., Seeley, R. J., & Sandoval, D. A. (2011). Weight-independent changes in blood glucose homeostasis after gastric bypass or vertical sleeve gastrectomy in rats. *Gastroenterology, 141* (3), 950–958.

Chellappa, S. L., Qian, J., Vujovic, N., Morris, C. J., Nedeltcheva, A., Nguyen, H., Rahman, N., Heng, S. W., Kelly, L., Kerlin-Monteiro, K., Srivastav, S., Wang, W., Aeschbach, D., Czeisler, C. A., Shea, S. A., Adler, G. K., Garaulet, M., Scheer, F. A. J. L. (2021). Daytime eating prevents internal circadian misalignment and glucose intolerance in night work. *Science Advances, 7* (49), eabg9910. doi:10.1126/sciadv.abg9910

Chin, S., Keum, C., Woo, J., Park, J., Choi, H., Woo, J., & Rhee, S. (2016). Successful weight reduction and maintenance by using a smartphone application in those with overweight and obesity. *Scientific Report, 6*, 34563. doi:10.1038/srep34563

Christou, N. V., Look, D., Maclean, L. D. (2006). Weight gain after short- and long-limb gastric bypass in patients followed for longer than 10 years. *Annals of Surgery, 244* (5), 734–740.

Cremieux, P. Y., Buchwald, H., Shikora, S. A., Ghosh, A., Yang, H. E., & Buessing, M. (2008). A study on the economic impact of bariatric surgery. *American Journal of Managed Care, 14* (9), 589–596.

Cummings, D. E., Overduin, J., & Foster-Schubert, K. E. (2004). Gastric bypass for obesity: Mechanisms of weight loss and diabetes resolution. *The Journal of Clinical Endocrinology & Metabolism, 89* (6), 2608–2615.

Cummings, D. E., & Schwartz, M. W. (2003). Genetics and pathophysiology of human obesity. *Annual Review of Medicine, 54*, 453–471.

Davies, N. K., O'Sullivan, J. M., Plank, L. D., & Murphy, R. (2019). Altered gut microbiome after bariatric surgery and its association with metabolic benefits: A systematic review. *Surgery for Obesity and Related Diseases*. Advanced Online Publication doi:10.1016/j.soard.2019.01.033

DeMaria, E., English, W. J., Mattar, S. G., Brethauer, S., Hutter, M., & Morton, J. M. (2018, November). *State variation in obesity, bariatric surgery, and economic ranks – a tale of two Americas (A198)*. Poster presented at Obesity Week, Nashville, TN. Retrieved from https://asmbs.org/articles/new-study-finds-most-bariatric-surgeries-performed-in-northeast-and-fewest-in-south-where-obesity-rates-are-highest-and-economies-are-weakest on December 8, 2018.

Dobbs, R., Sawers, C., Thompson, F., Manyika, J., Woetzel, J. R., Child, P., McKenna, S., & Spatharou, A. (2014). *Overcoming obesity: An initial economic analysis*. Jakarta, Indonesia: McKinsey Global Institute.

Donnelly, J., & Smith, B. (2005). Is exercise effective for weight loss with ad libitum diet? Energy balance, compensation, and gender differences. *Exercise and Sport Sciences Reviews, 33* (4), 169–174.

Dymek, M. P., le Grange, D., Neven, K., & Alverdy, J. (2002). Quality of life after gastric bypass surgery: A cross-sectional study. *Obesity Research, 10* (11), 1135–1142.

Fothergill, E., Guo, J., Howard, L., Kerns, J. C., Knuth, N. D., Brychta, R., ... Hall, K. D. (2016). Persistent metabolic adaptation 6 years after "The Biggest Loser" competition. *Obesity (Silver Spring), 24* (8), 1612–1619.

Garland, T., Schutz, H., Chappell, M. A., Keeney, B. K., Meek, T. H., Copes, L. E., Acosta, W., Drenowatz, C., Maciel, R. C., van Dijk, G., Kotz, C. M., ... Eisenmann, J. C. (2010). The biological control of voluntary exercise, spontaneous physical activity and daily energy expenditure in relation to obesity: human and rodent perspectives. *The Journal of Experimental Biology, 214* (2), 206–229.

Ghelani, D. P., Moran, L. J., Johnson, C., Mousa, A., & Naderpoor, N. (2020). Mobile apps for weight management: A review of the latest evidence to inform practice. *Frontiers in Endocrinology, 11*, 412.

Hatori, M., Vollmers, C., Zarrinpar, A., DiTacchio, L., Bushong, E., Gill, S., Leblanc, M., Chaix, A., Joens, M. J., Fitzpatrick, A. J., Ellisman, M. H., and Panda, S. (2012). Time-restricted feeding without reducing caloric intake prevents metabolic diseases in mice fed a high-fat diet. *Cell Metabolism, 15* (6), 848–860.

Higa, K. D., Boone, K. B., & Ho, T. (2000). Complications of the laparoscopic Roux-en-Y gastric bypass: 1,040 patients – what have we learned? *Obesity Surgery, 10*, 509–513.

Hutch, C. R., & Sandoval, D. (2017). The role of GLP-1 in the metabolic success of bariatric surgery. *Endocrinology, 158* (12), 4139–4151.

Hutter, M. M., Schirmer, B. D., Jones, D. B., Ko, C. Y., Cohen, M. E., Merkow, R. P., & Nguyen, N. T. (2011). First report from the American College of Surgeons Bariatric Surgery Center Network: Laparoscopic sleeve gastrectomy has morbidity and effectiveness positioned between the band and the bypass. *Annals of Surgery, 254* (3), 410–420; discussion 420–422.

International Federation for the Surgery of Obesity and Metabolic Disorders (IFSO). (2023). International Federation for the Surgery of Obesity and Metabolic Disorders report. Retrieved from www.ifso.com/pdf/8th-ifso-registry-report-2023.pdf on January 18, 2024.

Jakubowicz, D., Barnea, M., Wainstein, J., & Froy, O. (2013). High caloric intake at breakfast vs. dinner differentially influences weight loss of overweight and obese women. *Obesity, 21*, 2504–2512.

Jelalian, E., Mehlenbeck, R., Lloyd-Richardson, E. E., Birmaher, V., & Wing, R. R. (2006). "Adventure therapy" combined with cognitive-behavioral treatment for overweight adolescents. *International Journal of Obesity, 30* (1), 31–39.

Kroke, A., Liese, A., Schulz, M., Bergmann, M., Klipstein-Grobusch, K., Hoffmann, K., & Boeing, H. (2002). Recent weight changes and weight cycling as predictors of subsequent two year weight change in a middle-aged cohort. *International Journal of Obesity, 26* (3), 403–409.

Laferrère, B., Teixeira, J., McGinty, J., Tran, H., Egger, J. R., Colarusso, A., Kovack, B., Bawa, B., Koshy, N., Lee, H., Yapp, K., & Olivan, B. (2008). Effect of weight loss by gastric bypass surgery versus hypocaloric diet on glucose and incretin levels in patients with type 2 diabetes. *Journal of Clinical Endocrinology and Metabolism, 93* (7), 2479–2485.

Laing, B. Y., Mangione, C. M., Tseng, C. H., Leng, M., Vaisberg, E., Mahida, M., Bholat, M., Glazier, E., Morisky, D. E., and Bell, D. S. (2014). Effectiveness of a smartphone application for weight loss compared with usual care in overweight primary care patients: A randomized, controlled trial. *Annals of Internal Medicine, 161* (10 Suppl.), S5–12.

Livingston, E. H., & Ko, C. Y. (2004). Socioeconomic characteristics of the population eligible for obesity surgery. *Surgery, 135*, 288–296.

Magro, D. O., Geloneze, B., Delfini, R., Pareja, B. C., Callejas, F., & Pareja, J. C. (2008). Long-term weight regain after gastric bypass: A 5-year prospective study. *Obesity Surgery, 18* (6), 648–651.

Min, T., Prior, S. L., Churm, R., Dunseath, G., Barry, J. D., & Stephens, J. W. (2020). Effect of laparoscopic sleeve gastrectomy on static and dynamic measures of glucose homeostasis and incretin hormone response 4-years post-operatively. *Obesity Surgery, 30* (1), 46–55.

Mistlberger, R., Lukman, H., & Nadeau, B. (1998). Circadian rhythms in the Zucker obese rat: Assessment and intervention. *Appetite, 30* (3), 255–267.

Moore, S. C., Patel, A. V., Matthews, C. E., Berrington de Gonzalez, A., Park, Y., Katki, H. A., Linet, M. S., Weiderpass, E., Visvanathan, K., Helzlsouer, K. J., Thun, M., Gapstur, S. M., Hartge, P., … Lee, I. M. (2012). Leisure time physical activity of moderate to vigorous intensity and mortality: A large pooled cohort analysis. *PLoS Medicine, 9* (11), e1001335.

National Institutes of Health (NIH). (2016). Potential candidates for bariatric surgery: Who is a good adult candidate for bariatric surgery? Retrieved from www.niddk.nih.gov/health-information/weight-management/bariatric-surgery/potential-candidates on December 7, 2018.

Noria, S. F., Shelby, R. D., Atkins, K. D., Nguyen, N. T., & Gadde, K. M. (2023). Weight regain after bariatric surgery: Scope of the problem, causes, prevention, and treatment. *Current Diabetes Reports, 23* (3), 31–42.

Our World in Data. (2019). Obesity. Retrieved from https://ourworldindata.org/obesity on January 17, 2024.

Patel, R., Sulzberger, L., Li, G., Mair, J., Morley, H., Shing, M., O'Leary, C., Prakash, A., Robilliard, N., Rutherford, M., Sharpe, C., Shie, C., Sritharan, L., Turnbull, J., Whyte, I., Yu, H., Cleghorn, C., Leung, W., & Wilson, N. (2015). Smartphone apps for weight loss and smoking cessation: Quality ranking of 120 apps. *New Zealand Medical Journal, 128* (1421), 73–76.

Perri, M. G., Nezu, A. M., McKelvey, W. F., Shermer, R. L., Renjilian, D. A., & Viegener, B. J. (2001). Relapse prevention training and problem-solving therapy in the long-term management of obesity. *Journal of Consulting and Clinical Psychology, 69* (4), 722–726.

Quinlan, M. E., & Jenner, M. F. (2006). Analysis and stability of the sweetener sucralose in beverages. *Journal of Food Science, 55* (1), 244–246.

Pietiläinen, K., Saarni, S., Kaprio, J., & Rissanen, A. (2012). Does dieting make you fat? A twin study. *International Journal of Obesity, 36* (3), 456–464.

Pratt, J. S. A., Browne, A., Browne, N. T., Bruzoni, M., Cohen, M., Desai, A., Inge, T., Linden, B. C., Mattar, S. G., Michalsky, M., Podkameni, D., Reichard, K. W., Stanford, F. C., Zeller, M. H., & Zitsman, J. (2018). ASMBS pediatric metabolic and bariatric surgery guidelines, 2018. *Surgery for Obesity and Related Diseases, 14* (7), 882–901.

Rangel, A. (2013). Regulation of dietary choice by the decision-making circuitry. *Nature Neuroscience, 16* (12), 1717–1724.

Ríos-Hoyo, A., & Gutiérrez-Salmeán, G. (2016). New dietary supplements for obesity: What we currently know. *Current Obesity Reports, 5* (2), 262–270.

Rolls, B. J., Pirraglia, P. A., Jones, M. B., & Peters, J. C. (1992). Effects of olestra, a noncaloric fat substitute on daily energy and fat intakes in lean men. *American Journal of Clinical Nutrition, 56*, 84–92.

Rubino, D. M., Greenway, F. L., Khalid, U., O'Neil, P. M., Rosenstock, J., Sørrig, R., Wadden, T. A., Wizert, A., Garvey, W. T, & STEP 8 Investigators. (2022). Effect of weekly subcutaneous semaglutide vs daily liraglutide on body weight in adults with overweight or obesity without diabetes: The STEP 8 randomized clinical trial. *JAMA, 327* (2)m 138–150.

Ruiz-Lozano, T., Vidal, J., De Hollanda, A., Scheer, F., Garaulet, M., & Izquierdo-Pulido, M. (2016). Timing of food intake is associated with weight loss evolution in severe obese patients after bariatric surgery. *Clinical Nutrition, 35* (6), 1308–1314.

Salem, L., Devlin, A., Sullivan, S. D., & Flum, D. R. (2008). Cost-effectiveness analysis of laparoscopic gastric bypass, adjustable gastric banding, and nonoperative weight loss interventions. *Surgery for Obesity and Related Diseases, 4* (1), 26–32.

Santo, M. A., Riccioppo, D., Pajecki, D., Kawamoto, F., de Cleva, R., Antonangelo, L., Marçal, L., & Cecconello, I. (2016). Weight regain after gastric bypass: Influence of gut hormones. *Obesity Surgery, 26* (5), 919–925.

Semper, H., Povey, R., & Clark-Carter, D. (2016). A systematic review of the effectiveness of smartphone applications that encourage dietary self-regulatory strategies for weight loss in overweight and obese adults. *Obesity Reviews, 17* (9), 895–906.

Sethi, P., Thillai, M., Nain, P. S., Ahuja, A., Aulakh, N., & Khurana, P. (2018). Role of hunger hormone "ghrelin" in long-term weight loss following laparoscopic sleeve gastrectomy. *Nigerian Journal of Surgery, 24* (2), 121–124.

Seino, Y., Fukushima, M., & Yabe, D. (2010). GIP and GLP-1, the two incretin hormones: Similarities and differences. *Journal of Diabetes Investigation, 1* (1–2), 8–23.

Shah, M., & Vella, A. (2014). Effects of GLP-1 on appetite and weight. *Reviews in Endocrine and Metabolic Disorders, 15* (3), 181–187.

Slentz, C., Duscha, B., Johnson, J., Ketchum, K., Aiken, L., Samsa, G., Houmard, J., Bales, C., & Kraus, W. (2004). Effects of the amount of exercise on body weight, body composition, and measures of central obesity: STRRIDE – a randomized controlled study. *Archives of Internal Medicine, 164* (1), 31–39.

Sogg, S., & Mori, D. L. (2004). The Boston interview for gastric bypass: Determining the psychological suitability of surgical candidates. *Obesity Surgery, 14* (3), 370–380.

Sugerman, H. J., Wolfe, L. G., Sica, D. A., & Clore, J. N. (2003). Diabetes and hypertension in severe obesity and effects of gastric bypass-induced weight loss. *Annals of Surgery, 237* (6), 751–758.

Sundfør, T., Svendsen, M., & Tonstad, S. (2018). Effect of intermittent versus continuous energy restriction on weight loss, maintenance and cardiometabolic risk: A randomized 1-year trial. *Nutrition, Metabolism, and Cardiovascular Diseases, 28* (7), 698–706.

Swinburn, B. B., Gill, T. T., & Kumanyika, S. S. (2005). Obesity prevention: A proposed framework for translating evidence into action. *Obesity Reviews, 6* (1), 23–33.

Sylvetsky, A. C., & Rother, K. I. (2016). Trends in the consumption of low-calorie sweeteners. *Physiology & Behavior, 164* (Pt B), 446–450.

Taylor, R. W., McAuley, K. A., Barbezat, W., Strong, A., Williams, S. M., & Mann, J. I. (2007). APPLE Project: 2-y findings of a community-based obesity prevention program in primary school–age children. *American Journal of Clinical Nutrition, 86*, 735–742.

Thomas, D., Kyle, T., & Stanford, F. (2015). The gap between expectations and reality of exercise-induced weight loss is associated with discouragement. *Preventive Medicine, 81*, 357–360.

Truvia. (2018). Truvia FAQ: Health information and safety. Retrieved from www.truvia.com/faq#faq_8 on December 2,2018.

Tsai, A., & Wadden, T. A. (2005). Systematic review: An evaluation of major commercial weight loss programs in the United States. *Annals of Internal Medicine, 142* (1), 56–66.

Turton, M. D., O'Shea, D., Gunn, I., Beak, S. A., Edwards, C. M., Meeran, K., Choi, S. J., Taylor, G. M., Heath, M. M., Lambert, P. D., Wilding, J. P., Smith, D. M., Ghatei, M. A., Herbert, J., Bloom, S. R. (1996). A role for glucagon-like peptide-1 in the central regulation of feeding. *Nature, 379*(6560), 69–72.

Uchida, A., Zigman, J. M., & Perelló, M. (2013). Ghrelin and eating behavior: Evidence and insights from genetically-modified mouse models. *Frontiers in Neuroscience, 7*, 121.

U.S. Department of Health and Human Services. (2018). Physical activity guidelines for Americans, 2nd edition. Retrieved from https://health.gov/paguidelines/second-edition/pdf/Physical_Activity_Guidelines_2nd_edition.pdf

U.S. Food and Drug Administration. (2018). Additional information about high intensity sweeteners permitted for use in food in the United States. Retrieved from www.fda.gov/food/ingredientspackaginglabeling/foodadditivesingredients/ucm397725.htm

Wang, Y., Cai, L., Wu, Y., Wilson, R. F., Weston, C., Fawole, O., Bleich, S. N., Cheskin, L. J., Showell, N. N., Lau, B. D., Chiu, D. T., Zhang, A., … Segal, J. (2015). What childhood obesity prevention programmes work? A systematic review and meta-analysis. *Obesity Reviews, 16* (7), 547–565.

Wang, X., Zhou, G., Zeng, J., Yang, T., Chen, J., & Li, T. (2018). Effect of educational interventions on health in childhood: A meta-analysis of randomized controlled trials. *Medicine, 97* (36), e11849.

Wankhade, Shraddha. (2023). U.S. weight loss market size, forecast, analysis & share surpass US$ 305.30 billion by 2030, at 9.7% CAGR. Retrieved from www.linkedin.com/pulse/latest-us-weight-loss-market-size-forecast-analysis-share-wankhade/

Westerterp, K., Meijer, G., Janssen, E., Saris, W., & Hoor, F. (1992). Long-term effect of physical activity on energy balance and body composition. *British Journal of Nutrition, 68* (1), 21–30.

Wing, R. R., & Phelan, S. (2005). Long-term weight loss maintenance. *American Journal of Clinical Nutrition, 8,* 2222S–225S.

World Obesity Federation. (2024). Economic impact of overweight and obesity to surpass $4 trillion by 2035. Retrieved from www.worldobesity.org/news/economic-impact-of-overweight-and-obesity-to-surpass-4-trillion-by-2035 on January 19, 2024.

Ye, J., Hao, Z., Mumphrey, M. B., Townsend, R. L., Patterson, L. M., Stylopoulos, N., Münzberg, H., Morrison, C. D., Drucker, D. J., Berthoud, H. R. (2014). GLP-1 receptor signaling is not required for reduced body weight after RYGB in rodents. *American Journal of Physiology – Regulatory, Integrative and Comparative Physiology, 306* (5), R352–362.

CHAPTER 13

Institutional Approaches to Healthful Eating

After reading this chapter, you will

- Have a better idea about the types of interventions that could work to combat obesity.
- Understand the implications of overpopulation for our food and climate systems.
- Understand the importance, challenges, and need for technological innovation to keep food production on a par with population growth.
- Develop an understanding of how much food we waste, and how reducing this can help us meet our food production goals for the future.

Are individuals solely responsible for the global obesity epidemic? This chapter will examine the roles of industry and government in treating obesity as a public health problem. Also addressed are the global environmental impact of feeding 10 billion souls and the ways in which technological solutions such as GMOs and agrochemicals affect the environment. We will conclude with a discussion on the economics of food and food waste.

ROLE OF INDUSTRY AND GOVERNMENT IN ADDRESSING THE OBESITY EPIDEMIC

Historically, being overweight or obese was viewed as a personal matter. Conventional thinking was that a person becomes overweight or obese due to their own choices, and that the adverse consequences of being overweight or obese were borne by the individual alone. Neither of these premises is accurate: Obesity is strongly influenced by factors outside an individual's control, and the costs of obesity are borne widely across society, with significant economic and environmental impacts. Does the recognition that individual choices are not solely responsible for obesity obligate society to bear some of the costs to the individual? Does the recognition that obesity creates costs and harms external to the obese individual give society a right or obligation to intervene and perhaps make choices on behalf of that individual? Should the government be developing policies to curtail individual freedoms when it comes to food selection? Or should the government be developing policies that curtail the sale of foods high in sugar and/or fat, products which, when consumed in moderation, are not detrimental to our health but, when consumed

DOI: 10.4324/9781032621401-13

in excess over the course of many years, can prove to be seriously harmful to us? Is addressing the obesity epidemic a personal/individual responsibility or do we have a collective responsibility to address it? We will now discuss the following topics: Financial incentives, food deserts, taxation, and incremental lifestyle and environmental changes and their effectiveness in promoting weight loss.

Will You Lose Weight if You Get Paid to Do It?

Several modern institutions have financial or other interests in preventing their constituents from becoming overweight or obese and in reversing these conditions when they occur. Governments, health care providers, and employers have experimented with preventing and reversing obesity. Financial incentives to lose weight sound like a great idea – lose weight, make some money – it sounds like a win–win situation. Unfortunately, the research suggests that these short-term financial incentives only work to produce behavioral change for the duration of the incentive. The behavioral change goes away once the incentive ends, and people tend to gain the weight back. If the incentive remains in place, however, then the behavioral change appears to be maintained (Ananthapavan et al., 2018). This suggests that, as a society, we need to do a cost–benefit analysis of whether it is more cost-effective to provide long-term (ideally lifelong) financial incentives to motivate people to engage in healthy behaviors or to pay for long-term health care costs associated with obesity.

Food Deserts and the Built Environment

Much work has been done on the impact of **food deserts** and the **built environment** (human-made environment) on the obesity epidemic (Drewnowski et al., 2019; Epstein et al., 2012; Papas et al., 2007). The term food desert does not have a single, clear definition, which adds to the confusion about how to precisely identify a food desert, and then how to measure its impact on food choice and BMI for those living in its vicinity. The term food desert can be broadly defined as a region where people do not have access to healthy and affordable food. The built or human-made environment can create barriers to a healthy lifestyle and a healthy diet; these include the absence of quality grocery stores, transportation-related limitations, walkability/safety issues in the neighborhood, access to parks for recreation, and so on. While food deserts and limitations of the built environment have been reported to be associated with obesity and obesity-related diseases, the picture is not quite that simple. A study examining the effects of the built environment and neighborhood socioeconomic status on BMI found that neither factor completely explained BMI differences seen across different racial groups (Sharifi et al., 2016). There is also a growing body of research that reveals that increasing access to grocery stores does not produce corresponding positive changes in food selection (Cummins et al., 2014; Handbury et al., 2016).

Food Insecurity and the COVID-19 Pandemic

Food security, as defined by the U.S. Department of Agriculture (USDA), is when people have access to enough food at all times for an active, healthy life. The Food and Agriculture Organization (FAO) of the United Nations defines food insecurity as when a person lacks regular access to enough safe and nutritious food for normal growth and development and an active and healthy life. Globally, population levels of food insecurity vary considerably from continent to continent: In 2021, Africa, ~20%; Asia, 9.1%; Latin America and the Caribbean, 8.6%; Oceania, 5.8%; and less than 2.5% in Northern America and Europe (Carvajal-Aldaz et al., 2022). Food insecurity can range from mild food insecurity (uncertainty in ability to secure food) to severe food insecurity (not having eaten any food for a day or more).

You might be surprised to know that even affluent countries, such as the U.S., have a national average of 10.5% of households that experience some degree of food insecurity (Healthy People 2030, n.d.). This is usually related to low income and is disproportionately represented in racial and ethnic minorities (Odoms-Young, 2018). Households with children also tend to be more vulnerable to food insecurity (Paslakis et al., 2021).

These "normal" statistics are greatly impacted by natural epidemics and disasters, such as the COVID-19 pandemic. For example, in the U.S., the rate of food insecurity more than tripled, from 11% in 2018 to 38% in 2020 (Kakaei et al., 2022). This was owing in part to lost income and in part to rising food prices (United Nations [UN], 2024). There is evidence that food insecurity can trigger eating disorders (Becker et al. 2017), which can last far beyond the precipitating insecurity.

If we are to "solve" the challenge of food insecurity, we must do so with a multi-pronged solution which addresses the socioeconomic factors (poverty, unemployment, racial disparities, etc.), the climate-related factors (which influence food production), as well as sociopolitical factors (e.g., taxation policies on import and export of foods, political instability, etc.).

Carrot or Stick? Taxing "Unhealthy" Foods or Subsidizing "Healthy" Foods

Tax policy is a powerful tool that governments can use to enact policy and effect change. Tax-subsidized retirement accounts encourage us to save for retirement (IRS, 2018), while "sin" taxes discourage us from smoking and drinking (W.Z., 2018). However, tax policy can also be used imprudently; for example, Sweden enacted an "**obesity tax**" levied on obese people in the 1920s (*New York Times*, 1998)! Taxing obese people is imprudent for many reasons; in our society, it would be a regressive tax as it would disproportionately impact low-income people, and holding an individual directly responsible for becoming obese ignores the multifaceted nature of this epidemic. Ideas of taxing foods based on their nutritional status often elicit passionate discourse by folks on either side of this controversial topic.

But which would be more effective when it comes to encouraging healthy food choices – sin taxes or subsidies? A study conducted in a simulated grocery store environment set about trying to answer this question (Epstein et al., 2010). The study participants consisted of 42 lean and overweight mothers (45% were obese as per BMI measures ≥30); approximately half had incomes below $50,000, and half above. They were given $22.50 per family member and were instructed to go on a two-hour grocery trip to purchase food for their household for a week. Each participant went on five separate shopping trips; the first time, the grocery store prices were set to be the same as those found at real grocery stores. The next four times, however, the experimenters manipulated the prices either to decrease the cost of the "healthy foods" by 12.5% or 25% or to increase the cost of the unhealthy foods by the same percentages. As one would expect, decreasing the cost of healthy foods resulted in increased healthy food purchases, but this healthy food subsidy had an unanticipated outcome – the mothers used the money they saved on healthy foods to buy more unhealthy foods so that overall caloric intake increased! However, when the unhealthy options were taxed, the mothers purchased fewer unhealthy foods and used that money to purchase healthier options, resulting in an overall reduction in caloric intake. The results of this study suggest that sin taxes would be more effective than health-food subsidies to reduce overall caloric intake.

In the past decade, several countries have taxed sugary drinks or fatty foods (Wikipedia, 2019). Norway, for example, has had a "sugar tax" since the 1920s and massively increased that tax in 2018, so that sweets and chocolates are now taxed at $2.13 per pound (Harris, 2018). It is of value to note that the average Norwegian consumes approximately 59 lbs (27 kg) of sugar per year, while the average American consumes 75 lbs (35 kg) of sugar annually (Harris, 2018).

In contrast to our Scandinavian neighbors, the U.S. has lagged behind; there are no similar taxes at the federal or state level; however, several city governments have enacted sugary-drink taxes; Berkeley, CA, was the first city in the U.S. to pass a soda tax in 2015 (Barone, 2017). Since then, other cities have followed suit, including Philadelphia, Boulder, Seattle, and San Francisco (Wikipedia, 2019). Unlike sugary drinks, Americans have had trouble swallowing sugary-drink taxes. Resistance is fueled by an American philosophy of personal responsibility and a well-funded sugar lobby which forecasts dire

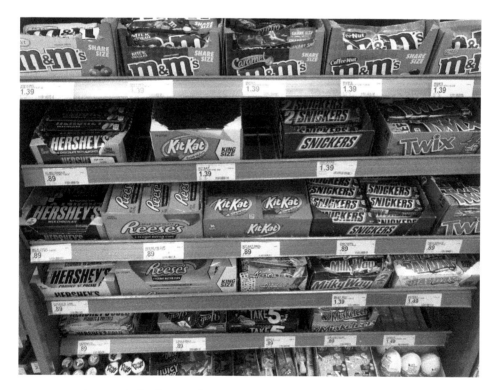

IMAGE 13.1 A typical checkout aisle in the U.S. How might this influence our shopping decisions at the last minute? Consider the soda tax versus an added-sugar tax. How might this influence our shopping decisions?

economic consequences while loudly reminding Americans of their dislike of government intervention in personal matters. At the center of this controversy is the notion of personal choice versus public good. But we must acknowledge that, when it comes to diet, personal choices are not personal. Obesity causes harm past the individual, and society bears those costs – both financial and emotional. Ultimately, we must balance these two opposing viewpoints, ideally preserving a society that values individual choices while minimizing the negative externalities of those choices. Scholars often draw parallels with the decline in tobacco use – a triumph of public health (Wan, 2017). The decline in tobacco use followed slow change in attitudes concerning the magnitude of the harm and damage to others. Over time, we changed our minds about where, when, and who should smoke, despite the objections of the tobacco industry, which regularly tried to manipulate the research and cast doubt on the consequences of smoking and second-hand smoke (Bero, 2005). A 2016 study found that the sugar industry (specifically the Sugar Research Foundation) sponsored research studies in the 1960s and 1970s which would ultimately downplay the significant role of sugar in the development of coronary heart disease and instead shifted the focus to dietary fat (Kearns et al., 2016). The American Beverage Association, which represents the U.S. beverage industry, has spent millions of dollars lobbying against soda taxes (Otterbein, 2016). If our experience with tobacco is a guide, there will be many factors which slowly change our attitudes toward how we nourish our bodies, but increasing the direct financial costs through taxation will be a critical step toward kicking a dangerous habit.

Nudging Our Way Out of the Obesity Epidemic

So, what does this all mean? Are things so bleak that seemingly no interventions will effectively address the obesity epidemic we are facing today? No; it means that we need to think creatively about solutions. A single intervention might not be the answer; perhaps smaller, more subtle interventions will create incremental changes in our behavior and help move the obesity epidemic in the right direction. This theory of small changes has been referred to as **nudge theory**, and it has been gaining a good deal of traction around the world. Starting in 2010, the United Kingdom created what is officially called the Behavioural Insights Team but is unofficially referred to as the "Nudge Unit." A nudge is defined as any modification of the environment that alters people's behavior in a predictable way without forbidding any options or significantly changing their economic incentives. "To count as a nudge, the intervention must be easy and cheap to avoid. Nudges are not mandates. Putting fruit at eye level counts as a nudge. Banning junk food does not" (Thaler & Sunstein, 2008, p. 6).

It is important to note that nudging alters the presentation of options for the consumer but does not create any penalties (beyond those they would have already borne had they not been exposed to the nudge) if the consumer does not engage in the hoped-for behavior. A dramatic example might be stocking checkout aisles with fruits and vegetables rather than candy bars. Perhaps, if we implement enough changes in our lifestyle and our environment, the cumulative effects of these changes/nudges could benefit our health and weight.

When we reexamine the interventions discussed earlier in this chapter with a "nudge theory lens," we might discover partial yet feasible solutions. Consider **incentivized weight loss**: The data indicate that weight loss tends to be sustained if it continues to be incentivized. So, health insurance companies need to experiment with long-term (possibly lifelong) incentives to see if that might result in sustained and improved behavioral choices.

An interesting study examined the impact of changes to the built environment (Bassett et al., 2013). The study found that changes in the built environment that permitted walking/biking to school resulted in increased levels of physical activity in children.

With regard to the role of industry, the news is not all bad. In 2009, 16 major food conglomerates formed the Healthy Weight Commitment Foundation and committed to reduce the number of calories they sell by 1.5 trillion by 2015 (Binks, 2016). Adjusted for population increase and validated by external researchers, this caloric decrease is equivalent to 99 kcal/capita/day (Ng et al., 2014). A study funded by the Healthy Weight Commitment Foundation in 2013 found that, for the companies that are part of this foundation, 82% of sales growth between 2006 and 2011 was driven by low-calorie products (Cardello & Wolfson, 2013); this suggests that industry focus on low-calorie initiatives are beneficial not just from a public health standpoint but also from a business standpoint.

Perhaps the most likely solution to the obesity epidemic is the summative effect of these nudges; by themselves they are inconsequential but, taken together, they might be the silver bullet that we are all searching for.

HUMAN POPULATION, ENVIRONMENTAL IMPACT, AND TECHNOLOGICAL SOLUTIONS

We will now shift gears and discuss changes in human population over the millennia, and the impact human overpopulation is having on our environment. Following this, we will discuss the technological achievements which averted mass famine in the latter part of the 20th century and the new technological solutions we will need to sustain future population growth.

Human Population, Then and Now

Modern humans first appear in the archaeological record around 200 kya (thousand years ago), and, for the first 95% of our time on this planet, we clung to existence in small nomadic groups, often following herds of prey animals while gathering wild plant material for food. The human population was relatively small for the vast majority of human history; population estimates for humans living 10 kya suggest a number somewhere at or below 1 million humans worldwide (Baird, 2011, p. 24). Then, somewhere between 12 and 4 kya, communities in different parts of the world began to make the switch to an agrarian lifestyle (Bellwood, 2005, p. 2). Rather than merely gathering wild plants, we domesticated them. We deliberately planted and harvested, and in doing so we changed the fundamental nature of the plants. Through selective breeding, a form of **genetic engineering**, we transformed wild grains into crops that provided more harvestable material for our consumption. We began to engage in **animal husbandry**, domesticating wild animals to provide us with food, clothing, and a source of assistance for labor-intensive farming practices. That this shift from a hunter-gatherer lifestyle to a settled agrarian lifestyle resulted in an explosion in our numbers is evidenced by the larger archaeological sites unearthed in the Fertile Crescent (often referred to as the cradle of civilization), sites that show a tenfold increase in size, moving from 0.2 hectares to 2–3 hectares (Pringle, 1998). The invention of agriculture and a move to a non-nomadic life-style had such a profound and rapid effect that it is called the Neolithic Revolution and it occurred sometime between 10 and 12 kya.

The domestication of plants and animals brought efficiencies to the food production process, allowing humans to delegate the production of food to only some people. Humans, now freed from the perpetual chore of feeding themselves, were free to settle down in one place and specialize their labor, and so we built cities, exchanged ideas, and invented new tools. The way we produced food changed the way most humans lived, and our population exploded from a few million to hundreds of millions. As we changed ourselves and species of plants and animals, we also changed our environment. We cleared land for fields and redirected rivers to irrigate our crops. As we became more technologically sophisticated, the speed and efficiency with which we could (can) modify our environment increased.

The human population continued to grow until the next seismic technological leap that accelerated our transformation of the planet and caused an explosive growth in the human population – the Industrial Revolution. The Industrial Revolution began in Great Britain, sometime in the mid-1700s. It was a turning point for humans in terms of changes in production (machines began to replace manual labor) and farming techniques, and medical and scientific advancements. By the 1800s, the world population had reached 1 billion, and, by the 1950s, we were at 2.5 billion people (Bongaarts, 2009). Population growth continued at unprecedented levels through most of the 20th century, bringing us to 7.6 billion as of 2017 (United Nations [UN], 2017). Population projections based on current growth rates (which are declining, but not fast enough) suggest that the global population will reach 9.7 billion in 2050, and 10.9 billion in 2100 (UN, 2019). These are sobering numbers.

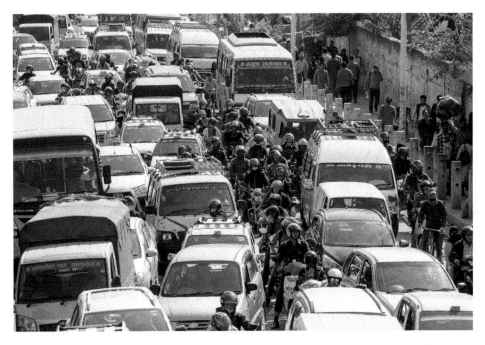

IMAGE 13.2 Traffic jams in urban areas are a familiar sight and contribute to air pollution and increased emissions

Environmental Impact of Human Overpopulation

This exponential growth in the human population has placed an enormous strain on the environment and our planet's limited resources; indeed, human overpopulation is at the center of all our environmental and sociocultural issues: Climate change, air pollution, ozone depletion, depletion of fresh water sources, **eutrophication**, habitat encroachment, **deforestation**, **desertification**, species extinction, overfishing, declines in biodiversity, poverty, sanitation, unemployment, and more.

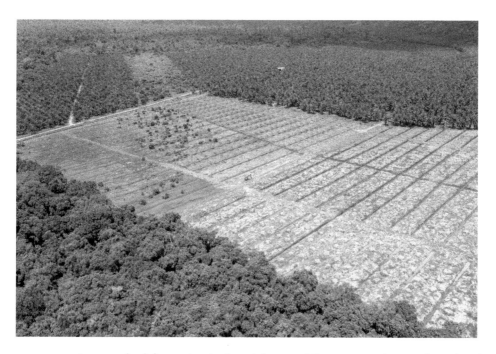

IMAGE 13.3 Large-scale deforestation in the rainforests of Borneo to make way for palm-oil plantations

It is easy to look at developing regions of the world with booming populations (e.g., China and India) and erroneously conclude that these countries are primarily "responsible" for much of the environmental degradation that we are witnessing today. However, it is equally important to consider the disproportionate resource consumption seen in developed countries (perhaps in particular the U.S.) and recognize that lifestyles and diets in these parts of the world are also major offenders when it comes to harming the environment on a global scale. Figure 13.1 compares energy consumption and CO_2 emissions by a few developed and developing world countries relative to their populations. The U.S., which accounts for 4% of the world's population (UN, 2017), consumes 17% of the world's primary energy resources (BP, 2018), while India, which accounts for 19% of the world's population, consumes a mere 6% of the world's primary energy resources.

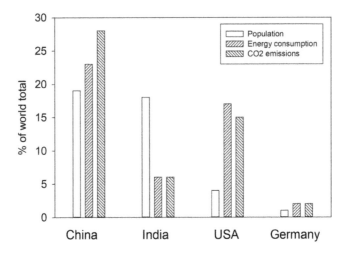

FIGURE 13.1 Comparing energy consumption, population, and CO_2 emissions across two developing and two developed countries. Energy consumption is presented in tonnes of oil equivalent, or "toe." This is a unit of energy and is defined as the amount of energy released by the burning of 1 tonne of crude oil (~ 42 gigajoules of energy). CO_2 emissions are based on fuel combustion and are presented in million metric tonnes

Source: BP (2018) and UN (2017). Source: CO2 emissions: Union of Concerned Scientists (2018; based on data compiled in 2015 by the International Energy Agency).

Environmental Impact of Agriculture (Crops and Livestock)

Agriculture is estimated to account for nearly 80% of the world's deforestation (Kissinger et al., 2012). Food production and distribution (including growing crops and livestock, fertilizer production, storage and transportation of food, etc.) account for somewhere between 19% and 29% of **greenhouse gas (GHG)** emissions; direct agricultural practices (crops and livestock) account for 80% of this figure (Vermeulen et al., 2012). Agricultural practices also account for 70% of freshwater use (Aleksandrowicz et al., 2016). Livestock production is a major emitter of GHGs. On a global scale, the livestock sector is estimated to be responsible for 14.5% of all anthropogenic GHG emissions (Food and Agriculture Organization of the United Nations [FAO-UN], 2013). Cattle production (including beef and dairy cattle, and cattle used for draft/pulling power) is by far the most significant contributor to GHG emissions, accounting for approximately 65% of the livestock sector's emissions (FAO-UN, 2013). In comparison, pork, buffalo milk and meat, chicken meat and eggs, and small ruminant milk and meat together account for 31% of the livestock sector's emissions; the remaining 4% is accounted for by other poultry species and non-edible products (FAO-UN, 2013). GHG emissions from livestock are predominantly the result of feed production and processing (this includes the decrease in forests as pasture and feed crop land use increases), the natural digestive process of ruminants (**methane** is a natural byproduct of their digestive process), and decomposition of manure (FAO-UN, 2014). These data reflect the greater environmental toll that results from cattle farming. To put this in starker contrast, one study reports that an energy equivalent quantity of beef requires 28 times more land and 11 times more water than dairy, poultry, pork, and eggs and produces 5 times more GHGs (Eshel et al., 2014).

The impacts of increased GHG emissions are too varied to detail here, but, on a basic level, they include higher global temperatures and reduced rainfall; these factors will undoubtedly impact the landscape of agriculture and food as we know it today. As our population continues to grow, global agricultural systems will struggle to meet the nutritional needs of all the humans on the planet. Food production demands are going to continue to increase and, unless they can at the minimum meet (if not exceed) population growth, the consequences of overpopulation are clear: Famine and starvation. This is referred to as a Malthusian catastrophe, named after the English cleric and scholar Thomas Robert Malthus who wrote on the dangers of overpopulation in the late 1700s (Malthus, 1798). Technological solutions (in the form of genetically modified organisms, improved **agrochemicals**, and sustainable farming practices) and social change (sustainable diets which are less reliant on meat, reduction in food waste, and reduction in energy consumption) are critical to our future survival.

TECHNOLOGICAL SOLUTIONS

The explosion in our population during the latter half of the 20th century is attributed to a combination of people living longer and lower infant mortality. However, it would not have been possible without food production keeping pace with population growth rates.

The end of the 1960s is now referred to as the beginning of the "Green Revolution." The Green Revolution resulted in global increases in crop production and was the result of significant advances in agricultural production techniques, including the development of high-yield varieties of crops which had a shorter time to maturity (Pingali, 2012). These high-yielding varieties were developed by **cross-breeding** different strains of the same crop so that the next generation of the crop had specific desirable traits (e.g., rust resistance and dwarfism in wheat crops). These cross-bred strains were used in conjunction with higher-quality fertilizers and pesticides, better irrigation methods, and increased mechanization of the harvesting process (Borlaug, 1970). Had it not been for these agricultural innovations, the 1960s and 1970s would have been characterized by mass famines in many parts of the developing world. Dr. Norman Borlaug (1914–2009) is credited as being the Father of the Green Revolution; estimates say that the high-yield, disease-resistant varieties of wheat and rice he was involved in creating may have saved more than 1 billion human lives from hunger (James, 2014). For this work, he was awarded the Nobel Peace Prize in 1970. Despite his scientific and humanitarian contributions to the world, his work was considered controversial by some as it involved cross-breeding to produce desirable traits in the offspring. This may be considered a precursor to the more modern (and targeted) technology of genetic modification of plants and animals.

Genetically Modified Organisms (GMOs)

A GMO may be a plant, an animal, or even a bacterium or a fungus. The organism in question is "genetically modified" by the insertion of one or more genes from a different organism, and the now-modified organism exhibits the desired trait. Some examples of desirable traits include nutrition enhancement, pest resistance, herbicide tolerance, decreased time to maturity, and **drought resistance**. See Table 13.1 for some of the most common GMO modifications in certain crops.

TABLE 13.1 Examples of the Most Common Genetic Modifications

Most common modifications	Reason for modification	Benefits	Crops
Herbicide tolerance	GM crops can be sprayed with herbicides and not be harmed (while weeds in the same region are killed)	Improved weed management; less herbicide used; fuel savings due to fewer applications of herbicides	Corn, cotton, canola, soybeans, sugar beets, alfalfa
Insect resistance	GM crops produce a protein which is poisonous to insects	Improved pest management; less pesticide use; fuel savings due to fewer applications of pesticide	Corn, cotton, brinjal
Resistance to environmental stress	GM crops can grow in harsh environments (regions with low rainfall, or regions prone to flooding)	Given global climate change predictions of reduced rains and rising water levels, these traits will be critical for crop production	Flood-tolerant rice, drought-resistant maize[*]
Disease resistance	These crops can fight off specific diseases	Increase in crop yields; fewer applications of chemicals to protect the plant; fuel savings due to fewer applications of agrochemicals	Rainbow papaya,[*] innate potato,[*] soybeans[*]
Nutrition enhancement	These crops have either additional nutrients (e.g., vitamins) or higher caloric yields	Improved nutrition for people; this is especially important in regions dealing with food insecurity; also important to feed our growing population	Golden rice,[**] sweet potatoes

Source: Genetic Literacy Project (2 016); * James (2014); ** Golden Rice Project (n.d.).

GM plants have been approved for use in the U.S. since the 1990s; today, more than 90% of corn, soybean, cotton, canola, and sugar beet grown in the U.S. is GM (Genetic Literacy Project, 2016). But this acceptance of GM technology is not limited to the U.S. Between 1996 and 2013, we have seen a 100-fold increase in the global area on which GM crops are grown; the top five countries that plant GM crops are the U.S., Brazil, Argentina, India, and Canada (James, 2014). This increase in adoption of GM crop technology is indicative of the enormous economic and environmental benefits producers and consumers gain from GMOs.

While GM plants have been part of our food supply for nearly two decades now, this has not been the case for GM animals. However, in order to meet food demand, GM animals will likely enter our food supply in the coming years; there is already significant research that is being done to produce virus-resistant animals (McColl et al., 2013). In 2015, Atlantic salmon became the first genetically modified animal to have been approved for consumption by the U.S. Food and Drug Administration (Ledford, 2015). This salmon (known as AquaAdvantage® salmon) has been genetically modified so that it matures faster, reaching market size in half the time taken by conventional Atlantic salmon (Clifford, 2014).

Despite their broad use and acceptance, GMOs remain the subject of social, political, and scientific debate. The increase in the adoption of GM technology has increased the public's concern regarding the safety of GMOs, both with regard to their impact on the environment and how they may affect the health of the consumer. Some of the major concerns and/or controversies surrounding the use of GMOs are outlined in Table 13.2. It is of interest to point out that, despite all the controversy swirling around the "dangers" of GMO products in the **food supply chain**, diabetics around the world have been using insulin produced by GM bacteria since the 1980s (Walsh, 2005).

TABLE 13.2 Concerns and controversies surrounding GMOs

Concerns	Evaluation of the concerns	Interpretation
GM corn's carcinogenic effects in rats (2012): Toxicity concerns were raised in a 2012 publication which asserted that GM corn caused cancer in the rats (Séralini et al., 2012)	The 2012 article was retracted owing to poor study design (e.g., rats were given Roundup to drink). The authors republished their results in a different journal (Séralini et al., 2014) Studies in GM potatoes, sweet peppers, and tomatoes have found no differences in the health of animals fed the GM products versus the non-GM products (Norris, 2015)	Given the problems with the design of the study, it is reasonable to say that the results are inconclusive. However, this does not preclude the need for better-designed studies to help shed light on this important issue Of interest: The International Agency for Research on Cancer (IARC; affiliated with the World Health Organization) announced that glyphosate might be carcinogenic (IARC, 2016)
GMO effects on our children (i.e., intergenerational effects)	Multigenerational studies in rats fed GM corn and GM potatoes: The researchers studied health of the embryos and tracked the health of each generation. They could find no differences between the rats fed the GM products versus the rats fed non-GM products (Norris, 2015)	The concern is low
Are the "modified" genes unstable and, after we consume them, can they change our DNA?	Research shows that DNA from GMOs is not different in its stability than DNA from non-GMO plants (Norris, 2015)	The concern is low

TABLE 13.2 (Continued)

Concerns	Evaluation of the concerns	Interpretation
Impact of GM corn pollen on the health of monarch butterfly larvae (1999): A study compared growth and mortality in monarch butterfly larvae which were fed either milkweed (the larvae's natural food) dusted with non-GMO corn pollen (Control Group 1), or GMO corn pollen (Experimental Group 2). They reported that growth rates were lower and mortality was higher in Group 2 (Losey et al., 1999)	Lab-based study; concerns about the ecological validity of this study. Factors which would reduce larval exposure to GM corn pollen include: • Bt toxin* levels in pollen is very low. • Rain would reduce pollen levels on leaves. • Pollen shedding times and the larval stage of the monarch do not overlap perfectly. (Raman, 2017; Sears et al., 2001)	Additional research is needed to examine the effects of GM crops on non-target insect species Concerns about impact of GM corn pollen on monarch larvae are negligible When considered in the context of reduced pesticide use, the GM corn is the environmentally superior choice
Concern: Herbicide drift: Application of herbicides such as Roundup (glyphosate) and Dicamba to herbicide-resistant crops has resulted in neighboring non-herbicide-resistant fields of crops being exposed and harmed (Charles, 2016; Dewey, 2017)	This is an ongoing problem with the development of herbicide-resistant GM plants. Weeds that these herbicides are designed to kill evolve their own genetic resistance, resulting in the need for more applications of the herbicides or the development of new chemical formulations (Charles, 2016; Dewey, 2017)	The concern is real. The problem arises when these farmers either accidentally or negligently apply the herbicides and contaminate their neighbors' non-GM crops (Charles, 2016; Dewey, 2017)
Concern: Big Ag (e.g., Monsanto, Dow Chemical, Syngenta, etc.) is a bully 1 Big Ag sues farmers for contract violations pertaining to GM seed use. 2 Big Ag sues farmers whose fields "accidentally" get contaminated by GM pollen.	1 The companies which produce GM seeds require that farmers using their GM products agree to not save and replant seeds they obtained from plants grown from purchased GM seeds. 2 There are no cases of the Big Ag companies suing farmers whose crops had been accidentally contaminated	Big Ag has gone after farmers for using GM seeds saved from a previous harvest. Their argument is that, if the companies developing this technology are not paid for their product, they cannot stay in business, and that it is unfair to farmers who repurchase seeds every year

* See the Agrochemicals section ahead for an explanation of what Bt toxin is.

BOX 13.1 A SPECIAL GMO: THE GOLDEN RICE PROJECT. A HUMANITARIAN EFFORT TO ADDRESS GLOBAL VITAMIN A DEFICIENCY AND BLINDNESS

The development of Golden Rice has been a decades-long humanitarian project to address the global public health problem of vitamin A deficiency (VAD).

VAD is a leading cause of reduced immunity, blindness, and death in children under five and pregnant women in many parts of the world; it is estimated that between 250,000 and 500,000 children under five become blind each year as a result of vitamin A deficiency, and half of them die within a year of becoming blind (WHO, n.d.).

Rice, which is a staple food for nearly half the world's population (Mohanty, 2013), is naturally low in micronutrients, including **β-carotene**, which is the precursor to vitamin A. Foods naturally high in β-carotene include leafy green vegetables and eggs, which are too expensive for people living in many of the low-income countries suffering from VAD.

Traditional rice was genetically modified so that it would produce and store β-carotene. This storage of β-carotene is what gives Golden Rice its yellow color (as opposed to the white/brown color of traditional rice). Upon consumption, the β-carotene is then either stored or converted to vitamin A (Golden Rice Project, n.d.). The application and spread of Golden Rice have been hampered by anti-GMO activists and GMO-related fearmongering.

As of this writing, 141 Nobel laureates have signed a petition supporting GMOs. The petition specifically asks Greenpeace to abandon its campaign against Golden Rice (Nobel Laureates, 2016). For more information on Golden Rice, visit the Golden Rice Project: www.goldenrice.org/Content3-Why/why3_FAQ.php#Everything_about

Agrochemicals

The advent of the Green Revolution saw a dramatic increase in the use of agrochemicals such as fertilizers, pesticides, herbicides, and so on (Nair, 2014). However, the use of these chemicals was not (and is not) without consequences. Excessive use of fertilizers in some regions has contaminated surface water and groundwater and, ultimately, devastated marine ecosystems, resulting in dead zones (Diaz & Rosenberg, 2008). This process is referred to as **eutrophication** and involves the creation of a dead zone, which is a hypoxic (or low-oxygen) zone in the ocean which tends to result in the death of marine animal life. The low oxygen levels are the result of the action of the fertilizers which cause an overgrowth of marine plant life; this abundant plant life subsequently decomposes, and this decomposition process consumes the oxygen in the water, resulting in a hypoxic zone which is incompatible with marine animal life (NOAA, 2018). Pesticides are chemicals designed to kill pests (i.e., insects or worms which eat or in some way damage crops). Herbicides are chemicals designed to kill weeds which compete with agricultural crops for resources. Other agrochemicals include growth-promoting fertilizers, chemicals which alter the pH of the soil (i.e., how acidic or alkaline soil is) according to the needs of the plant, and antibiotics and chemicals applied to livestock to reduce disease and promote growth.

Exposure to these agrochemicals, be it acute or chronic, has sometimes resulted in serious adverse outcomes for humans and animals. GM technology, for the most part, has resulted in reductions in the need for these agrochemicals, which is seen as an advantage of GM technology. An example of this is a reduction in the wide-spectrum application of insecticides in plants such as potatoes, corn, and cotton after they were genetically modified to carry a gene from the bacterium *Bacillus thuringiensis*. This bacterium produces a natural insecticide called Bt toxin which is toxic to many insects (Niederhuber, 2015). The GM crops (called BT crops) now produce this toxin, making them toxic to insects. However, in the case of the herbicide glyphosate, the reverse situation has occurred in some instances. **Glyphosate** is a herbicide, and crops which are resistant to glyphosate will not die when sprayed with this chemical. However, neighboring weeds will die, which is why glyphosate resistance was developed in crops. Some farmers growing glyphosate-resistant crops began to overtreat their crops with glyphosate, resulting in the development of weeds that are resistant to the effects of glyphosate (Brookes & Barfoot, 2013).

The need for agrochemicals is clear given our population explosion. But their toxicity, frequency of application, and specificity need both oversight and improvements, with further advances in agricultural and chemical technology.

CRISPR – The Future of Gene-Edited Food?

For those who continue to be uneasy about the risks associated with GMOs, and specifically the risks of mingling DNA from different organisms, CRISPR/Cas9 (clustered regularly interspaced short palindromic repeats/CRISPR-associated 9) is a relatively new technology which might put your mind at ease. This technology is derived from the defense system of bacteria (Li, 2018). In 2020, Emmanuelle Charpentier and Jennifer A. Doudna received the Nobel Prize in Chemistry for their contributions and work on the CRISPR/Cas9 system. Interestingly, the CRISPR modification of a plant does not make the resulting plant a GMO (as per the current regulatory guidelines). This is because there is no addition of foreign genetic material to the target plant. Instead, CRISPR allows us to introduce a new trait by rewriting the plant's genetic code (Li, 2018). This is a critical characteristic distinguishing such plants from GMOs, given that, in 2018, the U.S. Secretary of Agriculture announced that the USDA would not regulate plants produced using technologies which create plants that could have been developed using traditional breeding techniques (USDA, 2018). Despite the infancy of the CRISPR technology, there are already several plant products that have been modified using CRISPR, ranging from mushrooms that resist browning to soybeans that exhibit drought-resistant and salt-resistant traits (Waltz, 2018). Scientists around the world are exploring the many applications this disruptive new technology promises, ranging from crops and livestock with advantageous traits to curing cancer in humans.

Balancing Issues of Population Growth with the Need to Produce More Food

Given the population estimates for the year 2050, reports from the United Nations suggest that food production will have to increase by 70% above today's levels to keep pace (FAO-UN, 2009). This increase in food production will need to be done efficiently, sustainably, and cost-effectively. With regard to the issue of crop efficiencies (yields per area of crops planted), it is estimated that global crop yields increased by more than 370 million **tonnes** during 1996–2013 as a result of the adoption of GMO crops (Zhang et al., 2016). With regard to the issue of **sustainability**, it is estimated that global adoption of GM technologies in agriculture between 2006 and 2011 has reduced GHG emissions to the equivalent of removing 10.22 million cars from the roads (Brookes & Barfoot, 2013).

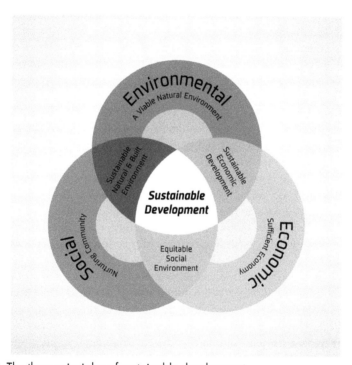

FIGURE 13.2 The three principles of sustainable development

Ultimately, our wariness toward technological innovations in our food supply needs to be balanced with the reality of our planet's human population problem. We need to grow food that is environmentally sustainable and nutrient dense. Technologically modified food is the only solution, in the absence of effective population control measures. However, despite a scientist's best intentions, a technological innovation can have unintended and sometimes harmful consequences. Therefore, critical evaluation of unbiased research combined with fair and appropriate regulatory oversight is vital to ensure that the future of food is a safe one.

ECONOMICS OF FOOD AND FOOD WASTE

The FAO-UN reports that nearly a third of global food produced is either lost or wasted (FAO-UN, n.d.). The industrialized world wastes considerably more food than that wasted in developing countries. The FAO-UN estimates that consumers in Europe and North America waste approximately 230 lbs of food per year (~100 kg/year), compared with approximately 20 lbs of food per year (~10 kg/year) in Sub-Saharan Africa and South and Southeast Asia (Gustavsson et al., 2011). According to the National Resources Defense Council, the U.S. wastes closer to 40% of all the food it produces (Gunders, 2012). In the U.S., it is estimated that the standard family of four will throw out wasted food worth between $1,350 and $2,275 per year (Bloom, 2011, p. 187).

Food loss is broadly defined as the loss of edible food from parts of the supply chain system prior to food retailers and end consumers, while food waste refers to food discarded or in some way mismanaged by the retailers and end consumers (Parfitt et al., 2010, as cited by Gustavsson et al., 2011). If these definitions seem somewhat esoteric, the U.S. Environmental Protection Agency's (EPA) definition of food waste is perhaps more concrete: "Uneaten food and food preparation wastes from residences and commercial establishments such as grocery stores, restaurants, and produce stands, institutional cafeterias and kitchens, and industrial sources like employee lunchrooms" (EPA, n.d.).

We see different reasons for food loss and waste (FLW) in developed countries than in developing countries. In developing countries, food loss is related to pest infestations (prior to harvest or during storage) and, more broadly, to supply chain issues including inadequate infrastructure for properly storing and packing food for transportation, inadequate transportation options, political and social problems with delivering the food to markets, and so on. Food waste, which is substantially lower in the developed world, occurs on the supply chain side (e.g., fruits or vegetables discarded because they are not ideal in shape, size, or color) and is done by food retailers (e.g., discarding food close to or beyond the best-by date), as well as households over-purchasing and then discarding excess food (FAO-UN, n.d.).

FLW has obvious economic implications for producers of food, distributors of food, and, finally, the households which ultimately consume the food. The social dilemma of FLW is starkly evident when viewed through the lens of the millions of people in the developed and developing worlds who are experiencing food insecurity, hunger, malnutrition, and/or undernutrition. And, finally, the environmental implications of FLW are staggering: Global FLW is said to account for 4.4 gigatonnes of greenhouse gas emissions (FAO-UN, as cited by Hanson et al., 2015). To put this in more relatable terms, if FLW were its own country, it would be the third largest emitter of greenhouse gases in the world, surpassed only by China and the U.S. (Hanson et al., 2015).

Awareness regarding food waste is growing, as is evidenced by the increase in marketing campaigns run by the Ad Council and the NRDC for organizations such as Savethefood.com. Grocery stores such as Daily Table provide low-cost food options to their consumers by either accepting donations from other food producers and retailers and/or purchasing excess food from food distributors and selling food close to or past its "best-by" and "use-by" dates. In order to combat food waste due to imperfections in appearance, organizations such as Imperfect Produce purchase this "ugly" produce from farmers and then sell it at a discount to consumers willing to eat an imperfectly shaped vegetable (Imperfect Produce, 2019). Finally, in line with the United Nations'

Sustainable Development Goals (adopted in 2015), the USDA and EPA have announced a domestic goal of reducing U.S. food waste by half by 2030 (EPA, 2015).

CONCLUDING REMARKS

When we view the issues of obesity, food insecurity, overpopulation, GMOs, climate change, and food waste, it becomes clear that these issues, which at first glance may seem quite disparate, are intractably linked to one another, and improvements in one area could well have tremendous impacts on another one of these areas. If we are to combat the obesity epidemic, feed our growing population, combat climate change, and reduce food insecurity, not only will we need to amplify our food production, but it is equally critical that we reduce our overconsumption, reduce our food waste, and reduce our fuel use, as we progress into the 22nd century.

GLOSSARY

Agrochemicals	Chemicals used in agriculture; these include chemicals to resist pests (pesticides), kill weeds (herbicides), kill worms (nematicides), and kill fungi (fungicides). They also protect crops from disease. Also included are fertilizers, which promote growth in plants, chemicals that alter soil pH to support plant growth, and antibiotics and hormones used for plants and animals.
Animal husbandry	The agricultural practice of rearing, caring for, and selectively breeding animals for the purpose of harvesting their fur, eggs, milk, or meat. This is an ancient practice which dates from the dawn of the Neolithic era approximately 13,000 years ago.
β-carotene	A precursor to vitamin A, which is essential for vision, normal development, and immune functioning. We cannot synthesize β-carotene and must derive it from our diet. It is found in red-orange-colored fruits and vegetables, such as mangoes and sweet potatoes, and in green, leafy vegetables, such as spinach. It is also found in Golden Rice.
Built environment	Refers to the human-made environment in which we live.
CRISPR gene editing	(clustered regularly interspaced short palindromic repeats) A new method of precision genomic editing.

Cross-breeding	The process of breeding two animals from different populations with the intention of creating a new organism that has traits of both parents.
Deforestation	The removal of forests and trees and conversion of that land to non-forest use.
Desertification	The conversion of an area into a desert, usually preceded by the death of local vegetation and wildlife. This may occur through natural means or as a result of human actions such as climate change or overgrazing.
Drought resistance	The ability of plants to survive for extended periods of time without enough water. While some plants have naturally occurring drought resistance, scientists have genetically modified certain crops to endow them with drought resistance, allowing them to grow under low-water conditions.
Eutrophication	Occurs when a body of water becomes overly nourished by pollutants that contain nitrates and phosphates, often from detergents and fertilizers. The excess nutrition causes plant and algae blooms, which may block enough light to cause the plant life on the bottom to die. When the algae die, they, along with the dead plant life, decompose in a process which consumes much of the oxygen in the body of water, which renders the body of water uninhabitable for many organisms.
Food deserts	Areas or neighborhoods that lack easy access to healthy foods such as fresh fruit and vegetables. Food deserts are often found in low-SES neighborhoods.
Food supply chain	The process by which food from a farm eventually reaches our tables. This process begins with the production of food, followed by its processing, transportation, and distribution. It ends with the consumption and disposal of food.
Genetic engineering	The process of adding or removing genetic material from an organism. Since the early 1970s, genetic engineering has been the domain of biotechnology; however, humans have engaged in selective breeding of crops and domestication for thousands of years,

	which may sometimes be considered genetic engineering.
Glyphosate	A herbicide that is used by farmers to kill weeds. It became an especially popular herbicide following the creation of glyphosate-resistant crops, which allowed farmers to spray their crops with this herbicide without harming them. Overuse of this herbicide has resulted in the development of glyphosate-resistant weeds.
Greenhouse gases (GHGs)	Greenhouse gases are gases in our atmosphere that absorb thermal solar radiation. Carbon dioxide is the most commonly discussed greenhouse gas, but there are many other GHGs such as methane, ozone, and even water in vapor form. GHGs are byproducts of many modern manufacturing and power-generation processes. Excess GHG production by humans is causing global climate change, which includes higher temperatures and extreme weather events.
Incentivized weight loss	Weight loss due to the offering of an incentive, often financial. Researchers and governments have experimented with incentivized weight loss with varying degrees of success.
Methane	Methane, or CH_4, is a colorless, odorless gas and is an important contributor to global warming as it absorbs much more heat from the sun than carbon dioxide (CO_2). Microorganisms inhabiting the digestive tracts of ruminants (e.g., cattle, sheep, etc.) also produce significant amounts of methane and thus contribute to global warming.
Nudge theory	Attempts to influence behavior through indirect environmental stimulus. Many nudges involve making the desired behavior the default choice or the easier choice. For example, a school cafeteria seeking to improve nutrition might place fruit in a convenient display while relocating candy to a more obscure area.
Obesity tax	Also known as "fat tax"; a tax on overweight individuals or on foods and beverages that cause obesity. The goal may be to reduce obesity and/or to reimburse society for the negative externalities due to obesity.
Sustainability	A philosophy where development and progress are managed so that we can meet both the needs of the present and the needs of the future.

	Three key overlapping principles of sustainable development include social factors, economic factors, and environmental factors.
Tonne (aka metric ton)	A non-SI unit of mass with slightly different meanings around the world. In the U.S., a ton is equal to 2000 lbs. Outside the U.S. a tonne or metric ton is equal to 2,204.6 lbs (1,000 kg).

REFERENCES

Aleksandrowicz, L., Green, R., Joy, E. J. M., Smith, P., & Haines, A. (2016). The impacts of dietary change on greenhouse gas emissions, land use, water use, and health: A systematic review. *PLoS One, 11*, e0165797.

Ananthapavan, J., Peterson, A., & Sacks, G. (2018). Paying people to lose weight: The effectiveness of financial incentives provided by health insurers for the prevention and management of overweight and obesity: A systematic review. *Obesity Reviews, 19* (5), 605–613.

Baird, V. (2011). *The no-nonsense guide to world population.* Oxford: New Internationalist.

Barone, J. (2017, October 12). Why soda taxes work. Retrieved from www.berkeleywellness.com/heal thy-community/health-care-policy/article/why-soda-taxes-work

Bassett, D. R., Fitzhugh, E. C., Heath, G. W., Erwin, P. C., Frederick, G. M., Wolff, D. L., Welch, W. A., & Stout, A. B. (2013). Estimated energy expenditures for school-based policies and active living. *American Journal of Preventive Medicine, 44* (2), 108–113.

Becker, C. B., Middlemass, K., Taylor, B., Johnson, C., & Gomez, F. (2017). Food insecurity and eating disorder pathology. *International Journal of Eating Disorders, 50* (9), 1031–1040.

Bellwood, P. (2005). *First farmers: The origins of agricultural societies.* Oxford: Blackwell.

Bero, L. A. (2005). Tobacco industry manipulation of research. *Public Health Reports (Washington, D.C.: 1974), 120* (2), 200–208.

Binks, M. (2016). The role of the food industry in obesity prevention. *Current Obesity Reports, 5* (2), 201–207.

Bloom, J. (2011). *American wasteland: How America throws away nearly half of its food (and what we can do about it).* Cambridge, MA: Da Capo Lifelong Books.

Bongaarts, J. (2009). Human population growth and the demographic transition. *Philosophical Transactions of the Royal Society of London. Series B, Biological Sciences, 364* (1532), 2985–2990.

Borlaug, N. (1970, December 11). Norman Borlaug Nobel lecture: The green revolution, peace and humanity. Retrieved from www.nobelprize.org/prizes/peace/1970/borlaug/lecture/

BP. (2018). Statistical review of world energy. 67th edition. Retrieved from www.bp.com/content/dam/ bp/en/corporate/pdf/energy-economics/statistical-review/bp-stats-review-2018-full-report.pdf

Brookes, G., & Barfoot, P. (2013). Key environmental impacts of global genetically modified (GM) crop use 1996–2011. *GM Crops & Food, 4* (2), 109–119.

Cardello, H., & Wolfson, J. (2013, May). Lower-calorie foods and beverages drive Healthy Weight Commitment Foundation Companies' sales growth interim report. Retrieved from www.hudson.org/ content/researchattachments/attachment/1107/lowercalhealthyweightcommitment–may2013.pdf

Carvajal-Aldaz, D., Cucalon, G., & Ordonez, C. (2022). Food insecurity as a risk factor for obesity: A review. Frontiers in Nutrition, 9, 1012734.

Charles, D. (2016, August 1). How Monsanto and Scofflaw farmers hurt soybeans in Arkansas. Retrieved from www.npr.org/sections/thesalt/2016/08/01/487809643/crime-in-the-fields-how-monsanto-and-scofflaw-farmers-hurt-soybeans-in-arkansas

Clifford, H. (2014). AquaAdvantage Salmon: A pioneering application of biotechnology in aquaculture. *BMC Proceedings, 8* (Suppl. 4), O31. doi: 10.1186/1753-6561-8-S4-O31

Cummins, S., Flint, E., & Matthews, S. (2014). New neighborhood grocery store increased awareness of food access but did not alter dietary habits or obesity. *Health Affairs, 33* (2), 283–291.

Dewey, C. (2017, August 29). This miracle weed killer was supposed to save farms. Instead, it's devastating them. Retrieved from www.washingtonpost.com/business/economy/this-miracle-weed-killer-was-supposed-to-save-farms-instead-its-devastating-them/2017/08/29/33a21a56-88e3-11e7-961d-2f373b3977ee_story.html?noredirect=on&utm_term=.c3c040758325

Diaz, R. J., & Rosenberg, R. (2008). Spreading dead zones and consequences for marine ecosystems. *Science, 321*, 926–929.

Drewnowski, A., Arterburn, D., Zane, J., et al. (2019). The Moving to Health (M2H) approach to natural experiment research: A paradigm shift for studies on built environment and health. *SSM - Population Health, 7*, 100345.

Epstein, L. H., Dearing, K. K., Roba, L. G., & Finkelstein, E. (2010). The influence of taxes and subsidies on energy purchased in an experimental purchasing study. *Psychological Science, 21* (3), 406–414.

Epstein, L. H., Raja, S., Daniel, T. O., et al. (2012). The built environment moderates effects of family-based childhood obesity treatment over 2 years. *Annals of Behavioral Medicine, 44*, 248–258.

Eshel, G., Shepon, A., Makov, T., & Milo, R. (2014). Land, irrigation water, greenhouse gas, and reactive nitrogen burdens of meat, eggs, and dairy production in the United States. *Proceedings of the National Academy of Sciences of the United States, 111* (33), 11996.

Food and Agriculture Organization of the United Nations (FAO-UN). (n.d.). Food loss and waste. Retrieved from www.fao.org/food-loss-and-food-waste/en/

Food and Agriculture Organization of the United Nations (FAO-UN). (2009, September 23). 2050: A third more mouths to feed. Retrieved from www.fao.org/news/story/en/item/35571/icode/

Food and Agriculture Organization of the United Nations (FAO-UN). (2013, September 26). Major cuts of greenhouse gas emissions from livestock within reach; key facts and findings. Retrieved from www.fao.org/news/story/en/item/197623/icode/

Food and Agriculture Organization of the United Nations (FAO-UN). (2014, October 21). Tackling climate change through livestock. Retrieved January 31, 2019 from www.fao.org/ag/againfo/resources/en/publications/tackling_climate_change/index.htm

Genetic Literacy Project. (2016). GMO FAQ: Which genetically engineered crops are approved in the U.S.? Retrieved from https://gmo.geneticliteracyproject.org/FAQ/which-genetically-engineered-crops-are-approved-in-the-us/

Golden Rice Project. (n.d.). FAQ. Retrieved from www.goldenrice.org/Content3-Why/why3_FAQ.php#Everything_about

Gunders, D. (2012). Wasted: How America is losing up to 40 percent of its food from farm to fork to landfill. National Resources Defense Council. Retrieved from www.nrdc.org/sites/default/files/wasted-food-IP.pdf

Gustavsson, J., Cederberg, C., Sonnesson, U., van Otterdijk, R., & Meybeck, A. (2011). Global food losses and food waste: Extent, causes and prevention. FAO-UN. Retrieved from www.fao.org/3/a-i2697e.pdf

Handbury, J., Rahkovsky, I., & Schnell, M. (2016). Is the focus on food deserts fruitless? Retail access and food purchases across the socioeconomic spectrum (NBER Working Paper No. 21126). Retrieved January 27, 2019 at 11:00 pm from National Bureau of Economic Research website www.nber.org/papers/w21126

Hanson, C., Lipinski, B., Friedrich, J., O'Connor, C., & James, K. (2015). What's food loss and waste got to do with climate change? A lot, actually. Retrieved from www.wri.org/blog/2015/12/whats-food-loss-and-waste-got-do-climate-change-lot-actually

Harris, B. (2018, March 14). Will a sugar tax help reduce obesity? Retrieved from www.weforum.org/agenda/2018/03/will-a-sugar-tax-help-reduce-obesity/

Healthy People 2030. (n.d.). Retrieved from https://health.gov/healthypeople/priority-areas/social-determinants-health/literature-summaries/food-insecurity on January 11, 2024.

Imperfect Produce. (2019). FAQ. What is imperfect, and how does it work?? Retrieved from https://help.imperfectproduce.com/hc/en-us/articles/115004535013-What-is-Imperfect-and-how-does-it-work-

International Agency for Research on Cancer (IARC). (2016, January 3). Monograph on glyphosate. Retrieved from www.iarc.fr/featured-news/media-centre-iarc-news-glyphosate/

IRS. (2018, August 2). Retirement topics – benefits of saving now. Retrieved from www.irs.gov/retirement-plans/plan-participant-employee/retirement-topics-benefits-of-saving-now

James, C. (2014). Global status of commercialized biotech/GM crops. ISAAA Brief No. 49.

Kakaei, H., Nourmoradi, H., Bakhtiyari, S., Jalilian, M., Mirzaei, A. (2022). Effect of COVID-19 on food security, hunger, and food crisis. *COVID-19 and the Sustainable Development Goals. 2022*, 3–29.

Kearns, C. E., Schmidt, L. A., & Glantz, S. A. (2016). Sugar industry and coronary heart disease research: A historical analysis of internal industry documents. *JAMA Internal Medicine, 176* (11), 1680–1685.

Kissinger, G., Herold, M., & de Sy, V. (2012). Drivers of deforestation and forest degradation: A synthesis report for REDD+ policymakers. Published by the governments of UK and Norway.

Nobel Laureates. (2016, June 29). Letter supporting precision agriculture (GMOs). Retrieved from http://supportprecisionagriculture.org/nobel-laureate-gmo-letter_rjr.html

Ledford, H. (2015, November 23). News: Salmon approval heralds rethink of transgenic animals. *Nature*. Retrieved from www.nature.com/news/salmon-approval-heralds-rethink-of-transgenic-animals-1.18867

Li, Y. (2018, November 15). How scientists are using CRISPR to create non-GMO crops. Retrieved from https://geneticliteracyproject.org/2018/11/15/how-scientists-are-using-crispr-to-create-non-gmo-crops/

Losey, J., Rayor, L., & Carter, M. (1999). Transgenic pollen harms monarch larvae. *Nature, 399* (6733), 214.

Malthus, T. R. (1798). *An essay on the principle of population: Or, a view of its past and present effects on human happiness; with an inquiry into our prospects respecting the future removal or mitigation of the evils which it occasions*, 7th ed. London: J. Johnson. Retrieved from https://books.google.co.uk/books/about/An_Essay_on_the_Principle_of_Population.html?id=kY0VAAAAYAAJ&printsec=frontcover&source=kp_read_button&redir_esc=y#v=onepage&q&f=false.

McColl, K., Clarke, B., & Doran, T. (2013). Role of genetically engineered animals in future food production. *Australian Veterinary Journal, 91*, 113–117.

Mohanty, S. (2013). Trends in global rice consumption. *Rice Today, 12*, 44–45.

Nair, P. K. R. (2014). Grand challenges in agroecology and land use systems. *Frontiers in Environmental Science, 2*, 1.

National Oceanic and Atmospheric Administration, Department of Commerce (NOAA). (2018, June 25). What is a dead zone? Retrieved January 30, 2019 from https://oceanservice.noaa.gov/facts/deadzone.html

New York Times. (1998, February 9). 1923: Obesity tax: In our pages: 100, 75 and 50 years ago. Retrieved from www.nytimes.com/1998/02/09/opinion/IHT-1923-obesity-tax-in-our-pages100-75-and-50-years-ago.html

Ng, S., Slining, M., & Popkin, B. (2014). The healthy weight commitment foundation pledge: Calories sold from U. S. consumer packaged goods, 2007–2012. *American Journal of Preventive Medicine, 47* (4), 508–519.

Niederhuber, M. (2015, August). Insecticidal plants: The tech and safety of GM Bt crops. Retrieved from http://sitn.hms.harvard.edu/flash/2015/insecticidal-plants/

Norris, M. L. (2015, August 10). Will GMOs hurt my body? The public's concerns and how scientists have addressed them. Retrieved from http://sitn.hms.harvard.edu/flash/2015/will-gmos-hurt-my-body/

Odoms-Young, A., & Bruce, M. A. (2018). Examining the impact of structural racism on food insecurity: Implications for addressing racial/ethnic disparities. *Family and Community Health, 41* (Suppl. 2 Food Insecurity and Obesity), S3–S6.

Otterbein, H. (2016, August 2). The beverage lobby spent $10.6 million to kill the soda tax — and failed. Retrieved from www.phillymag.com/citified/2016/08/02/soda-tax-spending-lobbying/

Papas, M., Alberg, A., Ewing, R., Helzlsouer, K., Gary, T., & Klassen, A. (2007). The built environment and obesity. *Epidemiologic Reviews, 29*, 129–143.

Paslakis, G., Dimitropoulos, G., and Katzman, D. K. (2021). A call to action to address COVID-19-induced global food insecurity to prevent hunger, malnutrition, and eating pathology. *Nutrition Reviews, 79* (1), 114–116.

Pingali, P. L. (2012). Green revolution: Impacts, limits, and the path ahead. *Proceedings of the National Academy of Sciences of the United States of America, 109* (31), 12302–12308.

Pringle, H. (1998). The slow birth of agriculture. *Science, 282* (5393), 1446.

Raman, R. (2017). The impact of genetically modified (GM) crops in modern agriculture: A review. *GM Crops & Food, 8* (4), 195–208.

Sears, M. K., Hellmich, R. L., Stanley-Horn, D. E., et al. (2001). Impact of Bt corn pollen on monarch butterfly populations: A risk assessment. *Proceedings of the National Academy of Sciences of the United States of America, 98* (21), 11937–11942.

Séralini, G. E., Clair, E., Mesnage, R., et al. (2012). Long-term toxicity of a Roundup herbicide and a Roundup-tolerant genetically modified maize. *Food and Chemical Toxicology, 50,* 4221–4231. Retraction published in *Food and Chemical Toxicology,* www.sciencedirect.com/science/article/pii/S0278691512005637?via%3Dihub

Séralini, G. E., Clair, E., Mesnage, R., et al. (2014). Republished study: Long-term toxicity of a Roundup herbicide and a Roundup-tolerant genetically modified maize. *Environmental Sciences Europe, 26,* 14.

Sharifi, M., Sequist, T., Rifas-Shiman, S., et al. (2016). The role of neighborhood characteristics and the built environment in understanding racial/ethnic disparities in childhood obesity. *Preventive Medicine, 91,* 103–109.

Thaler, R. H., & Sunstein, C. R. (2008). *Nudge: Improving decisions about health, weight and happiness.* New York: Penguin Books.

Union of Concerned Scientists. (2018, October 11). Each country's share of CO_2 emissions. Retrieved on January 31 at 11:50 pm from www.ucsusa.org/global-warming/science-and-impacts/science/each-countrys-share-of-co2.html#.XFPXTFxKguU

United Nations (UN). (2017). UN World population prospects: The 2017 revision. New York: United Nations Department of Economic and Social Affairs; Population Division.

United Nations (UN). (2019). UN World population prospects: The 2019 revision. New York: United Nations Department of Economic and Social Affairs; Population Division.

United Nations (UN). (2024). United Nations' Sustainable Development Goals – zero hunger. Retrieved from www.un.org/sustainabledevelopment/hunger/ on January 11, 2024.

U.S. Department of Agriculture (USDA). (2018, March 28). Secretary Perdue issues USDA statement on plant breeding innovation. Retrieved from www.usda.gov/media/press-releases/2018/03/28/secretary-perdue-issues-usda-statement-plant-breeding-innovation

U.S. Environmental Protection Agency (EPA). (n.d.). Terminology services. Retrieved from https://iaspub.epa.gov/sor_internet/registry/termreg/searchandretrieve/termsandacronyms/search.do?search=&term=food%20waste&matchCriteria=Contains&checkedAcronym=true&checkedTerm=true&hasDefinitions=false

U.S. Environmental Protection Agency (EPA). (2015). United States 2030 food loss and reduction goal. Retrieved from www.epa.gov/sustainable-management-food/united-states-2030-food-loss-and-waste-reduction-goal

Vermeulen, S. J., Campbell, B. M., & Ingram, J. S. I. (2012). Climate change and food systems. *Annual Review of Environment and Resources, 37* (1), 195–222.

Walsh, G. (2005). Therapeutic insulins and their large-scale manufacture. *Applied Microbiology and Biotechnology, 67* (2), 151–159.

Waltz, E. (2018). With a free pass, CRISPR-edited plants reach market in record time. *Nature Biotechnology, 36* (1), 6–7.

Wan, W. (2017, October 21). Cigarette taxes are the best way to cut smoking, scaring Big Tobacco. Retrieved from www.washingtonpost.com/national/health-science/cigarette-taxes-are-the-best-way-to-cut-smoking-scaring-big-tobacco/2017/10/21/fbf51d04-9f05-11e7-8ea1-ed975285475e_story.html?noredirect=on&utm_term=.5ea6bdc69bbe

Wikipedia. (2019, February 1). Sugary drink tax. Retrieved from https://en.wikipedia.org/wiki/Sugary_drink_tax

World Health Organization (WHO). (n.d.). Micronutrient deficiencies – vitamin A deficiency. Retrieved from www.who.int/nutrition/topics/vad/en/

W.Z. (2018, August 10). Do "sin taxes" work? Retrieved from www. economist. com/the-economist-explains/2018/08/10/do-sin-taxes-work

Zhang, C., Wohlhueter, R., & Zhang, H. (2016). Genetically modified foods: A critical review of their promise and problems. *Food Science and Human Wellness, 5* (3), 116–123.

Index